Cyanide and the Environment

Proceedings of a Conference
Tucson, Arizona
December 11-14, 1984

Volume 1

Conference Organized by:
Department of Civil Engineering
and Engineering Mechanics
The University of Arizona
Tucson, Arizona

Proceedings Edited by
DIRK VAN ZYL

Published by
Geotechnical Engineering Program
Department of Civil Engineering
Colorado State University
Fort Collins, Colorado 80523

1985

ISBN 0-910069-12-3 (Volume 1)
ISBN 0-910069-14-X (Two-volume set)

Second Printing 1988

PREFACE

Cyanides appear in a great variety of forms and in a great number of organic and inorganic compounds in nature. It is widely used in the mining, electroplating and microcomputer industries. There is currently much interest in the mining of precious metals where cyanide is almost exclusively used as a lixiviant. The safe handling of cyanide and the environmentally acceptable disposal of cyanided mine wastes are of interest to a large group of engineers, scientists, regulators and society as a whole.

The Conference on Cyanide and the Environment brought together a diverse group of engineers and scientists representing a wide range of interests in the topic. These proceedings represent a major contribution to the literature in this area. Not only is a broad range of topics covered, but the papers also present data and experiences from a wide range of climatic and environmental conditions. The principal purpose of the conference — to provide an open forum for the presentation of new developments in cyanide chemistry/toxicity and environmental aspects of cyanide use and disposal — has been successfully accomplished.

The conference was organized by the Department of Civil Engineering and Engineering Mechanics, the University of Arizona, Tucson, Arizona. Support was also given by the Department of Soils, Water and Engineering and the College of Mines at the University of Arizona, as well as the Tucson Section of AIME.

I would like to express my appreciation to everyone who supported this effort, especially the authors who contributed their time in preparing the papers. The help and advice received from the organizing committee and the advisory panel members are greatly appreciated. A special word of thanks goes to Kim Clarkin who spent many hours unraveling and editing the discussions taped at the conference. Her help in compiling this final product was invaluable.

Dirk van Zyl
Fort Collins, May 1985

ORGANIZING COMMITTEE

Gary L. Amy, University of Arizona, Tucson, Arizona

Donald R. Baker, Environmental Counselor, Bethlehem, Pennsylvania

Jack B. Bale, Arizona Department of Health Services, Phoenix, Arizona

Wallace H. Fuller, University of Arizona, Tucson, Arizona

Paul H. King, University of Arizona, Tucson, Arizona

Ronald L. Miller, Arizona Department of Health Service, Phoenix, Arizona

David D. Rabb, Consultant, Tucson, Arizona

Srini Raghavan, University of Arizona, Tucson, Arizona

Raymond A. Sierka, University of Arizona, Tucson, Arizona

Dirk van Zyl, Colorado State University, Fort Collins, Colorado (Coordinator)

ADVISORY PANEL

David Crouch, Homestake Mining Company, San Francisco, California

Frederick W. DeVries, E.I. DuPont de Nemours & Company, Wilmington, Delaware

Anton R. Hendriksz, Bechtel Civil & Minerals, Inc., San Francisco, California

Jerry L. Huiatt, U.S. Bureau of Mines, Salt Lake City, Utah

James E. Kerrigan, Amax Environmental Service, Golden, Colorado

Walter Kuit, Cominco Limited, Trail, British Columbia

Gérard Leduc, Concordia University, Montreal, Canada

Kent McGrew, Wharf Resources, Lead, South Dakota

David A. Milligan, Anaconda Minerals Company, Tucson, Arizona

George M. Potter, Consultant, Tucson, Arizona

James S. Scott, Environmental Protection Service, Quebec, Canada

Rodney K. Skogerboe, Colorado State University, Fort Collins, Colorado

Richard E. Speece, Drexel University, Philadelphia, Pennsylvania

Robert V. Thurston, Montana State University, Bozeman, Montana

John D. Welsh, President, J.D. Welsh and Associates, Reno, Nevada

TABLE OF CONTENTS

Volume 1

TABLE OF CONTENTS

Volume 2

RESEARCH UPDATE

Conference Summary

CONFERENCE ON CYANIDE AND THE ENVIRONMENT
Tucson, Arizona . December 1984
Published by Geotechnical Engineering Program • Colorado State University • Fort Collins, Colorado 80523

CONFERENCE SUMMARY

by

Terry Mudder, Ph.D.*

INTRODUCTION

Although cyanidation has been employed commercially in the recovery of gold and silver for more than half a century, only in recent years has attention been focused on the fate and impact of cyanide and cyanidation byproducts in and upon the environment. Research conducted to elucidate, monitor, and control the impact of cyanide-containing wastewaters and solid wastes has been undertaken by a variety of companies, educational institutions, and government agencies located throughout the world. The majority of the individuals involved in the research have been largely unaware of each others' progress and findings. As a result, the National Science Foundation provided a grant to fund a workshop sponsored by the U.S. Bureau of Mines, the Mineral Industries Institute located at the University of Utah, and several minerals industries. The workshop was held at the U.S. Bureau of Mines complex in Salt Lake City, Utah, February 2-3, 1982. Prior to the workshop a working paper was prepared and delivered to the invited participants who were the authors of the final white paper. The paper was used as a guide during panel discussions and formed the basis for the final proceedings document.

The workshop focused on the use of cyanide as it relates to the gold and silver mining industry. Its intent was to discuss πstate of the artπ technology and provide an avenue for exchange of information pertinent to the use, handling, monitoring, treatment, and disposal of cyanide-bearing wastes. No attempt was made to advocate regulatory limits or set policy governing the use of cyanide. The principal topics of discussion included: (1) the chemistry, use and handling of cyanide, (2) the analytical methodology associated with cyanide analyses, (3) the fate of cyanide and cyanidation byproducts in the environment, (4) the control and treatment of liquid and solid cyanidation processing wastes and (5) the toxicity of mining wastes.

During the workshop discussions, the problems associated with cyanide use in the mining industry and areas of insufficient technical information were identified. The areas and direction of research

---

* Terry Mudder, Phd., Chief Environmental Engineer, Homestake Mine, Lead, S.D.

required to understand and resolve potential adverse environmental problems were also identified. It is this research, conducted in the last two years and directed toward answering these questions, that formed the basis for the recent conference held in Tucson, Arizona, December 11-14, 1984. The conference entitled 'Cyanide and the Environment' was hosted by the Department of Civil Engineering and Engineering Mechanics of the University of Arizona and coordinated by Dr. Dirk van Zyl, currently Associate Professor of Civil Engineering at Colorado State University.

There were approximately 200 attendees including individuals from more than 15 states and 5 countries (France, West Germany, Canada, South Africa, and the United States). They included persons from various industries, academic institutions, consulting firms, and state and federal regulatory agencies (U.S. Bureau of Mines, U.S.E.P.A., and Environment Canada). The industries included not only mining industries, but also chemical and oil industries (DuPont, Standard Oil, and Shell Oil), other metals industries (Alcoa, Kaiser, and Eastalco) and a representative from the Chicago Sanitation District. The diversity of the group resulted in an excellent exchange of ideas and recent research developments, leading to the conclusion that considerable progress had been made since the original workshop. The purpose of this review is to summarize the findings and conclusions of the conference with emphasis placed on the progress made in addressing the particular problems and research needs identified in the previous workshop.

THE CHEMISTRY OF CYANIDE, ITS COMPLEXES, AND CYANIDATION BYPRODUCTS

Several papers dealt with the chemistry of the various metal-cyanide complexes and cyanidation byproducts (i.e. thiocyanate). Emphasis was placed upon their stabilities and solubilities, an area of considerable interest at the original workshop. Since the chemical behavior of these compounds in solution is fairly well understood, greater emphasis was placed on the question of stability and mobility of these compunds within and from the solid phase, as in tailings impoundments and abandoned heap leach piles. With respect to tailings impoundments, concerns were primarily with the dissolution and dissociation of these complexes and possible contamination of ground water and surface waters, while with the heap leaches the concern was mainly with the stability of these compounds and their rates of degradation.

One paper by Howe discussed the chemistry of cyanide degradation, while three additional papers—two by Hendrix and coworkers from the University of Nevada, Reno, and one by Engelhardt of Anaconda Minerals Company—contained information concerning the fate and degradation of cyanide and its complexes and the formation of cyanidation byproducts within tailings (thiocyanate). The chemistry of cyanide and its complexes in the solid phase was identified as an area requiring additional research, as the number of heap leach operations increases and greater emphasis is placed on solid waste disposal.

HANDLING AND SAFETY OF CYANIDE AND ITS SOLUTIONS

Although there was limited new information concerning the safety, storage, and handling of cyanide and its solutions, several papers directed toward this topic comprised an entire session at the conference. Many informative discussions evolved as a result of various industries relating their respective experiences with cyanide. Topics included human and aquatic toxicity, in-plant monitoring for safety, the handling and storage of cyanide and its solutions, and personnel training associated with cyanide usage. Although nearly 75,000 tons of cyanide are consumed annually around the world, there is no history of serious accidents recorded in its daily use, a safety record of which the mining industry as a whole can be quite proud. Discussions presented by DeVries of DuPont, Fellows of the Arizona Mine Inspector's Office, Pickett of the Nevada State Division of Mine Inspection, and Stotts of the Superior Mining Company, Stibnite, Idaho, discussed in detail the various aspects of transportation, storage, handling, and training involved with cyanide usage. In addition, Tong of the Poison Control Center at the University of Arizona discussed certain aspects of cyanide toxicity in relation to poison control.

METHODOLOGY FOR ANALYTICAL DETERMINATIONS OF CYANIDES

In order to obtain and interpret data used in elucidating the fate, treatment, and the toxicity of cyanides, samples must be collected and analyzed. The sampling procedure must insure representative sampling of the solution or solid to be analyzed, while the analytical procedure must be sensitive for the particular purpose, accurate at the concentration levels desired, and reliable from analysis to analysis. Significant advances have occurred in the determination of cyanides since the original workshop. There has been a significant increase in our knowledge of specific interferences associated with cyanide analyses and their quantitative effects upon those analyses. An excellent review of these interferences and their effects upon the automated analysis of cyanides was presented by Kelada of the Chicago Sanitary District. It appeared that greater reliance is being placed upon the use of ASTM methods for total and weak-acid-dissociable cyanides to characterize and quantify the various metal-cyanide complexes. Two research areas which were identified in the previous workshop concerned accurate methods of free cyanide analysis, and development of rapid and simple analytical methods for the field measurement of cyanides. Pohlandt, from the Council for Mineral Technology (MINTEK), South Africa, described a new method for the analysis of free cyanide as well as the analysis of individual metal-cyanide complexes using ion chromatography. Also Mathre and DeVries of DuPont presented a modified method for the field evaluation of free cyanide concentrations.

A relatively new area that received considerable attention was the sampling and analysis of solid phase cyanide concentrations. These types of analyses are particularly important in monitoring tailings impoundments and heap leach piles. An approach to sampling and analysis of solids was presented by Ray of the California Regional

Water Quality Control Board. A suggestion was advanced that until reliable methods for solids analyses are developed, attention be focused on the analyses of the liquid phase within these solids. There are many reliable methods for the aqueous phase determination of cyanides, as well as the sampling of the liquid phase through the use of depth-specific lysimeters and piezometers.

Although questions pertaining to the determination of cyanides still remain and require additional investigation, there are at present a sufficient number of sensitive, reliable, and accurate methods of cyanide analysis to collect data for any specific purpose, such as wastewater treatment, ground water monitoring, toxicological investigations, and in-plant monitoring.

FATE OF CYANIDES IN THE ENVIRONMENT

Traditionally, natural degradation of cyanides and cyanidation by-products has been the primary mode of treatment of mine milling wastes. Qualititative aspects of the natural degradation of cyanides, illustrated in Figure 1, are well understood, but interest in its quantitative aspects and possible enhancement is underscored by the number of discussions and papers centering around the topic. An attempt to describe the natural degradation of cyanides in a quantitative manner was presented by Simovic of Environment Canada. Her paper dealt with the development of a mathmatical model to describe the natural degradation occurring in a tailings impoundment. The model was developed through laboratory experiments and calibrated with actual field data. In addition, Fuller from the University of Arizona, in a keynote address, discussed the various chemical, physical, and biological reactions of cyanides occurring naturally in the soil. Howe also treated this topic in a subsequent paper on the chemistry of cyanides degradation and their presence in the natural environment. Reed, from the University of Arizona, discussed the occurrence of cyanide compounds in plants and their effects on animals eating these plants.

THE TREATMENT OF CYANIDATION WASTEWATERS

As expected, there was considerable interest in the various alternatives available for the treatment and disposal of liquid and solid wastes. Two entire sessions at the conference were devoted to this topic. The sessions began with an overview by Scott of Environment Canada of the various wastewater treatment processes currently being employed throughout the world. Again, considerable progress has been made since the workshop held two years ago. The major processes currently in use include natural degradation, acidification/volatilization, hydrogen peroxide, alkaline chlorination, ferrous sulfide precipitation, the Inco SO_2-air process, evaporation, and the biological treatment process employed at the Homestake Gold Mine. The papers were divided into two categories. One category dealt with basic research into various treatment processes and degradation mechanisms, while the other category dealt with actual field experience obtained from pilot and full-scale operations. Gurol from Drexel

University presented a paper on the ozonation of cyanides in industrial wastewaters. Zaidi and Carey of Environment Canada discussed the use of ultraviolet irradiation for the destruction of iron-complexed cyanides. A third paper presented by Layne, based on work performed at the University of North Carolina, described the oxidation of thiocyanate, a cyanidation byproduct, through ozonation. Stevens of Lancy International presented research on the oxidation of cyanides from metal finishing wastewaters through alkaline chlorination. The detection and treatment of ferrocyanides was further discussed with respect to the photographic and electroplating industries in a paper by McGivney and Shelton from the University of Texas, El Paso.

Several additional papers dealt with actual field experience in the treatment of cyanide-containing wastewaters. An excellent paper by Conard of Inco described the successful piloting and full scale commercial application of the Inco SO_2-air process at three mining facilities in Canada. Another paper presented by Baker from Shell Oil Company discussed in detail their experiences in treating cyanide-containing wastewaters with hydrogen peroxide. Although a formal paper was not presented, it was noted by Scott that the full-scale biological treatment facility (Figure 2) at Homestake has been in operation for six months, producing an effluent compatible with the beneficial use (trout fishery) classification of the receiving stream. Von Michaelis of Randol International suggested that further research should be conducted into the enhancement of natural degradation of cyanides. Finally, Kerrigan of AMAX presented an excellent philosophical perspective on our duties and goals when considering alternative solutions to any environmental issue.

As these various papers indicate, there are several viable wastewater treatment alternatives currently available which, employed alone or in combination, can aid in treatment of wastewaters containing various forms of free and complexed cyanides. Indispensable to selection of a viable treatment alternative is an intensive and well-planned pilot testing program supported by sound analytical determinations and in certain instances toxicological evaluations.

THE TOXICITY OF CYANIDES

Another area not fully addressed previously which requires further research pertains to the toxicity of the various forms of cyanide as they occur in 'real' situations. There is a need for additional toxicological testing to aid in selection of viable treatment alternatives and to gather additional quantitative information on the toxicity of cyanide-containing wastewaters. As pointed out in a keynote address by Walline from the U.S. E.P.A., there is a need for industries and regulatory agencies to cooperate in asking the appropriate questions and addressing those questions through a sound scientific approach. Discussions between industries and regulatory agencies concerning permit levels have left many environmental issues unresolved and have led to needless legal confrontations. We must recognize that there are uncertainties in solving environmental issues and we must use all the available scientific tools in solving those issues. One such approach presented by Mudder described the use of toxicological testing to develop discharge criteria at the Homestake Mine in South Dakota. The toxicity data aided the company in the selection of a viable treatment process and the subsequent development of permit discharge criteria. The use of such testing creates a bridge between regulatory agencies and industries and produces quantitative answers to otherwise emotionally debated issues.

A paper by Heming and Thurston, based on work at the Fisheries Bioassay Laboratory at Montana State University, discussed the effects of thiocyanate toxicity on trout under stress conditions. Feigley of Bozeman, Montana described the use of small mammals in identifying and monitoring the impacts of cyanide at a heap leach operation in South Dakota. The area of toxicity testing and biological monitoring is a new area, in which there was considerable interest and an identified need for further research.

CONCLUSIONS

After attending the conference one is left with the impression that there is a great deal of interest in the effects of cyanides on the environment and that a concerted effort is underway to address the difficult environmental issues and formulate long term solutions to them. The association of cyanide with the environment does not involve only a single industry, regulatory agency, or country. The excellent attendance at the conference underscores the dedicated individual and cooperative effort being put forth to deal with the impact of cyanide on the environment. Many advances have been made since the original workshop in Salt Lake City, but many additional questions are being asked and investigated. Efforts are being directed toward cooperation and exchange of ideas and information between industry and the regulatory agencies to find practical and acceptable solutions to long-standing environmental issues and problems. Industries are indicating their concern by increased funding of environmental programs and personnel.

FIGURE 1

THE CYANIDE CYCLE

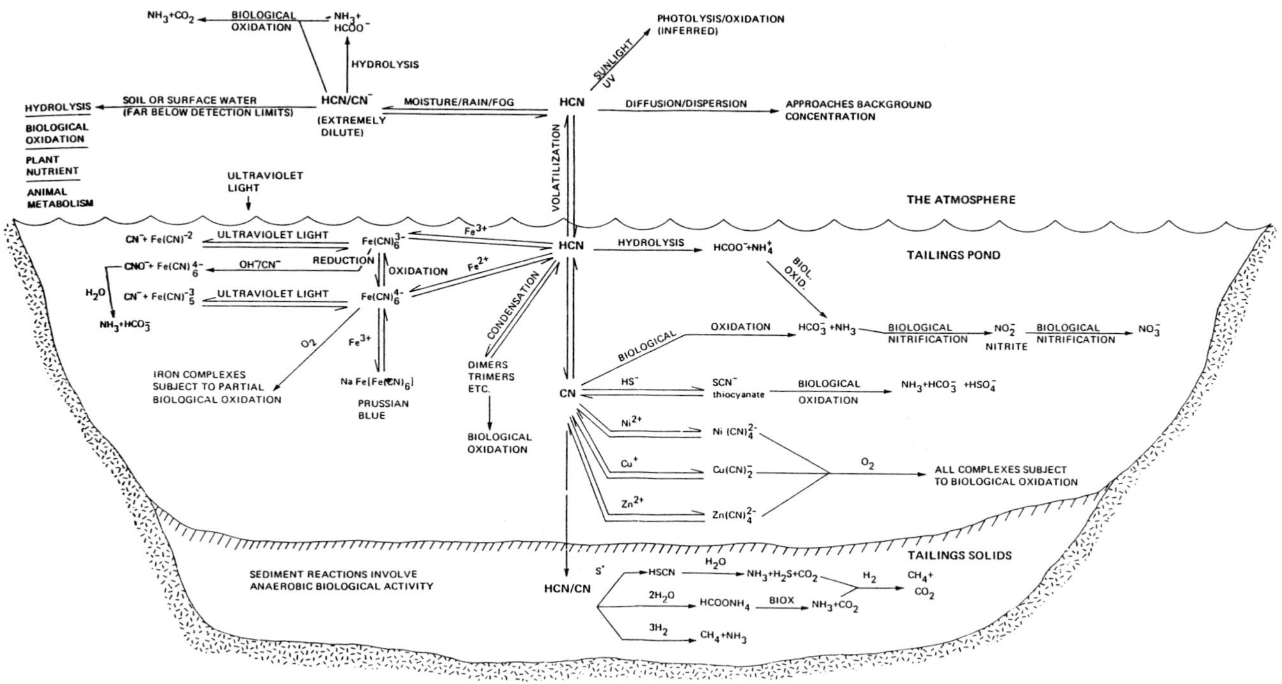

Adapted by CH_2M Hill from a drawing by T. Mudder

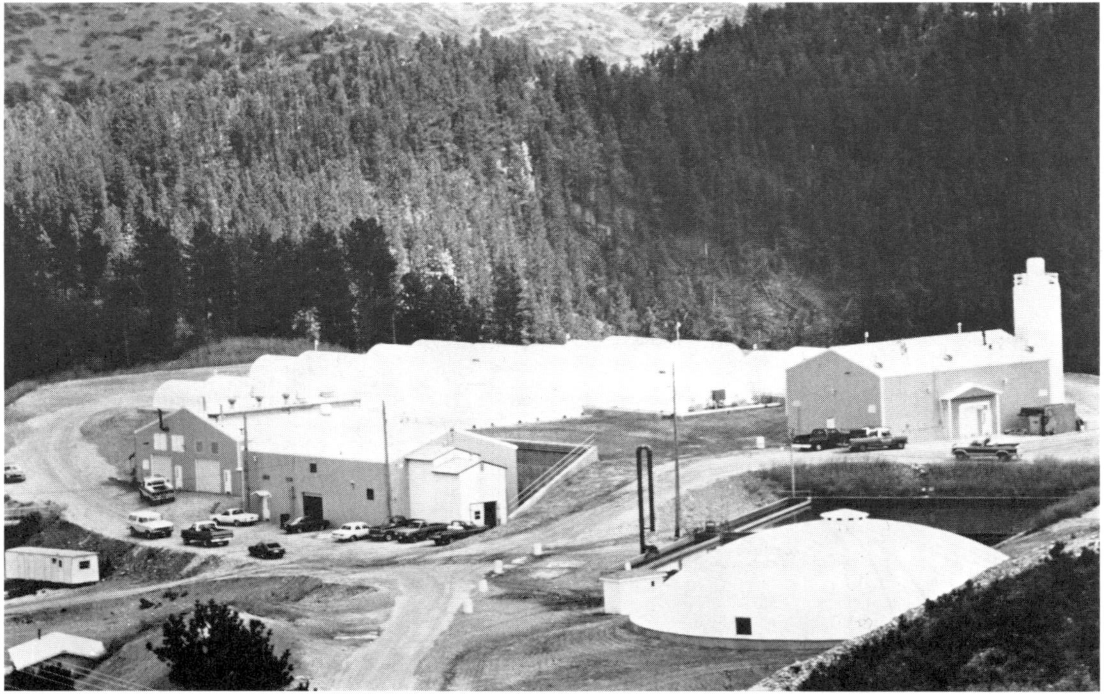

Fig. 2 Homestake Biological Wastewater Treatment Facility

Keynote and Overview

CONFERENCE ON CYANIDE AND THE ENVIRONMENT
Tucson, Arizona • December 1984
Published by Geotechnical Engineering Program • Colorado State University • Fort Collins, Colorado 80523

A PERSPECTIVE ON THE ENVIRONMENTAL REGULATION OF CYANIDE

by

Robert E. Walline

The focus for this discussion of the environmental regulation of cyanide is the mineral process industry. The perspective that will be utilized is a result of experience in the Region VIII Office of EPA in the areas of surface water, ground water and solid waste and includes involvement from site specific permitting to national regulatory development. I think it is fair to say that currently a lot of the issues surrounding the environmental regulation of cyanide bearing wastes from the mineral processing industry have not been resolved. This can be illustrated by the current status of cyanide regulations in the areas of surface water (NPDES), solid waste (RCRA), and environmental assessment (NEPA).

Starting with the NPDES surface water discharge programs, let's look at where the national effluent standards are now. On December 3, 1982, Final Effluent Guidelines were promulgated for the Ore Mining and Dressing Point Source Category. These national technology based effluent standards for the mining industry, which set the minimum effluent standards utilized nationally in NPDES permits, did not set limitations for cyanide. The principal reason for this was the problems with the precision and accuracy of the EPA approved method for analysis of total cyanide. This decision not to promulgate a national effluent standard for cyanide for mining effluents means that under NPDES, discharges of wastewater containing cyanide must be addressed on a case-by-case utilizing Best Professional Judgement authority.

Under the Resource Conservation and Recovery Act, the solid and hazardous waste control statute, the regulation of solid waste from the extracting, benefication and processing of ores and minerals has been excluded until a report on mining wastes has been submitted to Congress and regulations have been promulgated. Thus, the soli wastes from the mineral processing industry which contain cyanide are not currently regulated, but there are still cyanide related issues under RCRA. In order to prepare the report to Congress on mining

---

Environmental Engineer, Chairman of Mining Waste Advisory Group, U.S. Environmental Protection Agency, Region VIII, Denver.

wastes, EPA has conducted studies of mining waste disposal practice and problems. The evaluation of these studies will include wastes containing cyanide. Currently under RCRA, other than the reactivity characteristic, there is no criteria for determining if a waste containing cyanide is hazardous or not. In the report to Congress, EPA will have to evaluate the potential threats to human health and the environment posed by mining wastes containing cyanide without the benefit of an established criterion for comparison. In the future, if some mining wastes containing cyanide are regulated under RCRA, criteria will have to be developed which distinguishes for regulatory purposes those wastes which are of relatively little concern from those that are truly hazardous.

In the area of environmental assessments for new operations, evaluations have to be made now concerning future impacts. Given the current development activity, precious metal operations will make up a large percentage of the new mining facilities in the near term. Since the majority of these facilities will utilize some form of cyanidization, the issues surrounding cyanide will be an important part of the environmental evaluations. Further, since waste disposal in many cases is not currently regulated directly, environmental assessments are particularly important because they may be the primary preoperational evaluation of disposal practices. In many cases, the information that is available in environment assessments is not focused enough to answer the question of what are the potential environmental impacts. Given that for large volume waste disposal, total containment is not feasible and that even closed systems are prone to upset and spills, detailed information on waste characterization, migration potential, natural attenuation, and facility closure are important. Only with this type of specific information can the environmental threats, or lack thereof, of cyanide waste be placed in their proper perspective.

As shown by the examples of the three programs previously discussed, EPA to date has not addressed some of the issues related to the environmental regulation of cyanide in the mineral processing industry. As we move forward from here, more specific questions will have to be answered. The answers will be needed for site specific NPDES permitting and environmental assessments as well as for developing an appropriate regulatory framework for implementing statutes such as RCRA. Examples of what will be necessary include criteria for determining what cyanide wastes are hazardous, improved standard analytical methodology for complex effluents, and field bioassay protocol for aquatic toxicity evaluations of complex wastes. Some of these answers have been developed for specific sides, but there is need for standardization and a more universally recognized set of acceptable procedures. This type of specific information is particularly important for cyanide bearing wastes because in order to evaluate the environmental hazards, waste management options and treatment technologies for a given facility, the nature of cyanide chemistry must be put in the proper perspective.

At this point, you may be wondering what EPA is going to do with all these questions. I cannot speak for the agency as a whole, but I can discuss an approach that is being utilized by Region VIII. The region has established the Mining Wastes Technical Advisory Group made up of regional staff with expertise in the areas of liquid, solid, and hazardous waste management, wastewater treatment, and groundwater protection. The group serves as a regional focal point on issues related to the extractive industries and was designed to be flexible enough to include additional expertise with specific skills and knowledge useful on a given issue. The group has a number of objectives, but one particularly revelant to the environmental regulation of cyanide is the objective to facilitate a better understanding within EPA of issues related to the mineral process industry.

In areas which involve cyanide, the Mine Wastes Group is currently working with the State of South Dakota and EPA water quality standards staff on evaluation of the Homestake Mining Company toxicological testing which Terry Mudder will be discussing this afternoon. In addition, on a national level the group is providing input into the EPA Headquarters Office of Solid Waste on the RCRA Mining Waste Report to Congress and the implementation of the Groundwater Strategy. Hopefully, this approach provides a mechanism by which knowledge that has been generated by site specific work at facilities such as Homestake Mining Company can be utilized and expanded upon for agency actions like any future regulatory development for mining wastes under RCRA.

The region, by utilizing the Mine Wastes Group, has tried to create a forum to facilitate a good understanding of a given situation. Particularly in the case of wastes containing cyanide from the mining industry, it is necessary to ask the hard questions and to be cautious of the simple assumptions. Examples of some assumptions which are currently being utilized are; all cyanide wastes are environmental problems, no cyanide wastes from the mining industry is an environmental problem, cyanide compounds do not move in the groundwater, and cyanide solutions can be simply neutralized. While these assumptions may hold true in some cases, it is recommended that enough information be developed to support a conclusion, rather than assume there is or is not a problem.

It is also important to recognize that in dealing with high volume waste disposal, cyanide chemistry in the matrix of a mining effluent, geology, geochemistry, and groundwater hydrology there will certainly be some uncertainty. But recognizing this uncertainty, the decision maker, if he is to effectively sort the problems from the nonproblems, must have information on the chemistry of the wastes, degree of containment, fate in the environment, and the hazard posed by release. Only with this type of specific information can regulatory decisions be made which distinguish between wastes which pose no threat to public health and the environment and truly hazardous wastes. In order to accomplish this type of informed decision making, the proponent of a project must provide the type of detailed scientific information necessary to answer the questions. The regulator must then make sure that this information is placed in the proper perspective for the public and the decision maker.

On the broader issues of how cyanide wastes should be regulated in the future, all parties need to work constructively on resolving the real world environmental issues. Detailed information which has been developed for specific sites needs to be examined for general applicability. More specific scientific input is needed in the regulatory development process. Constructive suggestions in the areas of analysis, characterization criteria for determining the degree of hazard, and biological testing are examples. Education for operators, particularly small precious metal operations, and the public on the actual environmental hazards associated with cyanide could help with some common misconceptions and could allow a more focused approach to larger issues. With this type of an approach, a regulatory framework can be developed which protects public health and the environment reasonably and economically, while providing the regulated community a basis for future planning and evaluation. Here in the next several days, individuals with different perspectives on cyanide issues will have an opportunity to discuss ideas and areas that have been addressed and need to be addressed. Continuation of this type of dialogue will go a long way towards providing answers to some of the regulatory dilemma surrounding cyanide.

DISCUSSION

Question (P. Saletta): Concerning NPDES and final discharge upon site abandonment, does EPA have any proposals on how to handle that? You mentioned that NPDES does not require cyanide monitoring in many cases. We (Division of Mined Land Reclamation, State of Colorado) have a couple of sites that may be abandoned in the next 2-3 years, and I believe the waters used in process solutions may have to be discharged.

Answer (R. Walline): Given the way the Clean Water Act is structured, any point source discharge requires an NPDES permit if a discharge of pollutants is involved, so you're getting into a legal grey area. Right now there is no national standard, no effluent guideline for point source discharges after mine abandonment. The legal authority exists to permit it, but the effluent limitations for each permit would be decided on a case-by-case basis, by best professional judgement authority. Mines that were abandoned before the Clean Water Act was passed have not been looked at, and there have not yet been many facilities which have ceased operations after having a permit. However, the consensus, I think, is that there will be permits for inactive and post-operational systems provided there are still point sources.

Question (P. Saletta): Is there any consideration that EPA might utilize or study to determine an allowable controlled discharge at particular times of the year when cyanide could be diluted to non-hazardous levels?

Answer (R. Walline): That type of discharge is possible, particularly on a case-by-case basis. When there is a national effluent guideline--a Best Available Treatment Standard for an active facility--you cannot use dilution to meet that minimum standard. But in cases of meeting water quality standards, or where there is no national standard and you are making decisions on a best professional judgement basis, you can utilize dilution. It has been used in water quality standard permitting where you're trying to meet an in-stream receiving water quality standard which is more stringent than technology can achieve.

CONFERENCE ON CYANIDE AND THE ENVIRONMENT
Tucson, Arizona • December 1984
Published by Geotechnical Engineering Program • Colorado State University • Fort Collins, Colorado 80523

CYANIDES IN THE ENVIRONMENT WITH PARTICULAR ATTENTION TO THE SOIL

by
Wallace H. Fuller[1]

ABSTRACT

The frequency in the identification of groundwater and other environment contamination has placed an additional burden on the already overburdened land in the volume of waste that must be accepted for ultimate disposal. If the soils are not effective in confining the wastes, migration of hazardous constituents into groundwater and food chains will occur. As a result of this vulnerability, the soil as a waste treatment/utilization system must receive special research attention. Cyanide-yielding wastes contain some of the hazardous chemicals demanding immediate attention for this soil treatment/utilization effort.

The purpose of this presentation is to provide information regarding the behavior of cyanide and cyanide-yielding chemicals in soils and the surrounding environment under anaerobic and aerobic conditions. In aerobic soils, the most prominent reactions of environmental concern involve nitrification and, in general, the fate of ammonia, nitrite, nitrate, and nitrogen gas. Under anaerobic soil conditions, the most prominent reactions of environmental concern involve attenuation, precipitation as complexes, denitrification, and transport. This presentation centers on these concerns with respect to utilization of cyanide nitrogen by plants at different loading rates, and considers the factors affect nitrification of cyanamid, dicyanodiamid, guanidine and guanidine nitrate, dicyanodiamidine sulfate (guanylurea sulfate), thiourea, and melamine under different soil conditions. In addition, the mobility of KCN (simple form), $K_3Fe(CN)_6$ (complex form) in aqueous solution, and KCN in natural municipal solid-waste landfill leachate (mixed forms) through five soils of varying physical and chemical properties at rates of 100 and 200 ppm CN^- is described. The soil characteristics that govern the movement of the various cyanide forms in soils are also described and evluated.

INTRODUCTION

New sensitivity toward nature requires us to search for new answers about the environment that surrounds us. A busy area of research, presently, involves the study of toxic wastes in soils. The soil, like the air, is a most abundant natural environmental system

[1] Wallace H. Fuller, Professor, Soils, Water and Engineering, The University of Arizona, Tucson, AZ. 85721.

with which human beings make contact not only directly but indirectly by dust that is breathed, water that infiltrates soil and is pumped for drinking, through food nourished bythe soil, as are plants, and animals nourished in turn by plants. The soil has proven to be an acceptable waste receptacle. Cyanamide as a waste is not an exception. Soils will always play an important part in waste disposal despite trends toward recycling of waste constituents. Moreover, the air, rivers and streams must be recognized as overloaded vehicles of waste transport back to the land. Recent sensitivity to and restrictions on disposal methods used heretofore, such as ocean dumping, serve to emphasize the burden that the land must assume. The threat of contamination in underground water resources and food chains can worsen as disposal volume paces populations and industrial expansion. Control measures must be expanded to lessen the threat of environmental pollution. The soil is a key factor in this control.

The soil is the oldest and most effective chromatographic column in the history of the world. Soil is the unconsolidated outer cover of the earth and represents the weathered product of environmental factors at any specific location. Soils differ in characteristics just as do plants and animals. Thus there are prairie and forest soils; thin soils on steep slopes and thick soils on broad ridges; alluvial, residual, and presoils. Soils differentiate into horizons, A, B, C, with depth. Each horizon is quite different from the other. Soils also differ greatly from one place to another, yet they perform the same unique activities of biodegrading, precipitating, attenuating, sorbing/desorbing, structuring, and integrating every chemical behavior known, or still unknown, to mankind.

To realize the effectiveness of soil in a waste disposal system as a barrier (though a leaky one) to migration, one should begin with an understanding of the soil properties and the way they interact with wastes and their leachates, and specific pollutants such as toxic constituents. There are three major components of the waste disposal environment which interact in any waste that reaches the earth's surface. These must be identified, described, and quantitatively evaluated. They are:

1. The porous medium through which the constituents are transported (e.g. soil, clay, sand, gravel),
2. The vehicle of transport that carries the polluting constituents or is itself the pollutant (e.g. aqueous leachates, organic solvents, oil etc.), and
3. The specific polluting constituent itself (e.g. soluble heavy metal salts, radionucleides, organic compounds, carcinogens, etc.).

All three are important in management of wastes since they are involved in attenuation of the polluting constituents, interact with each other, and change with time.

CYANIDE VERSATILITY

Cyanides appear in a great variety of forms and in a great number of classes of organic and inorganic compounds in nature. Each of the classes contain a cyano group (C=N) as part of its molecule.

Taras (1971) refers to cyanide in industrial waste as all of the CN^- groups present in the cyanide compound that can be determined as cyanide ion, CN^-, by the Liebig distillation method. The CN^- ion is a negatively charged, diatomic species with a sigma bond, two pi bonds, and two empty pi anti-bonding orbitals. These bondings give cyanides unusual properties, particularly in metal-cyanide complexes (Huiatt, et al., 1983).

Cyanides may be classified into four broad groups for this discussion:

1. Free cyanides - CN^- and HCN
   In solution the relationship is highly pH dependent
   $$CN^- + H_2O \rightleftharpoons HCN + OH^-$$
   (Figure 1). The pKa of HCN is at pH 9.367 where the concentrations of CN^- and HCN are equal.
2. Simple cyanides - $A(CN)_x$ where A is an alkali or a metal and x is the valence of A and represents the number of cyano groups present. Cyanide ions are released when alkali cyanides ionize according to:
   $$A(CN)_x \rightleftharpoons A^{+x} + x\ CN^-$$
   $$KCN + H_2O \rightleftharpoons KOH + HCN^-$$
3. Complex cyanides - $A_yM(CN)_x$ where: A is the alkali, y is the number of alkalies (Na, K, NH_4); M is the heavy metal)(Fe^{+++}, Fe^{++}, Cd^{++}, Cu^{++}, Ni^{++}, Ag^{++}, etc.) and x is the number of CN groups equal to the valence of A taken y times plus the valence of the heavy metal. Soluble complex cyanides dissociate into complex ions and not CN groups (e.g.):
   $$A_yM(CN)_x;\ [M(CN)_x]\text{-}yw$$
   W is the oxidation state of A in the original molecule. Further dissociation can take place releasing CN^- ions. Again this reaction is highly pH dependent (Figure 1).

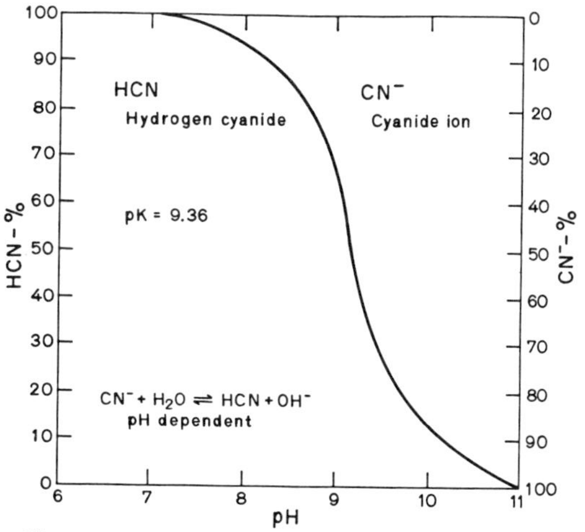

Figure 1. The effect of pH on dissociation of hydrogen cyanide.

4. Organic cyanide-yielders - Represented by cyanogenic (nitriles) glycosides. Glycosides yield one (or more) sugar and one (or more) other compound (e.g. aglycones) when hydrolyzed in vitro by dilute mineral acids or in vivo by enzymes. They are widely distributed in nature.

Cyanides vary in stability in water as illustrated in Table 1 (Scott, 1981). Because of the toxicity of CN^-, the formation of a more stable cyanide has been a significant factor in the activity of biological systems. At the normal pH's and temperatures of streams, the dissociated cyanide ion (CN^-) is toxic to most species of fish at a level of 0.1 mg/liter. Complexed cyanides are far less toxic, and discharge of relatively large concentrations of these compounds to receiving streams is not immediately harmful. Consequently, it has been suggested that cyanide be complexed with metals such as iron, prior to discharge, to reduce toxicity.

CYANIDE DISTRIBUTION IN NATURAL ENVIRONMENTS

PLANTS

Cyanide-yielding organic compounds are introduced naturally into the environment, particularly the soil, by a great number of living systems. One of the most common natural sources originates from plants (Table 2). Over 800 species of plants (70 to 80 families) synthesize cyanogenic glycosides (Knowles, 1976). They are characterized most abundantly by the glycosides that yield hydrocyanic acid (HCN) upon hydrolysis. One of the best known cyanogenetic (or cyanophoric) glycosides occurs in members of the Rosaceae family and are called amygdalin (Kingsbury, 1964). The chemical reaction is diagrammed in Figure 2. The amount of amygdalin glycogen accumulated by a single plant varies between species, depending on environmental conditions--for example, plants that have wilted, frosted, or have been stunted are most suspect in the incidence of HCN rumen poisoning than unstressed plants.

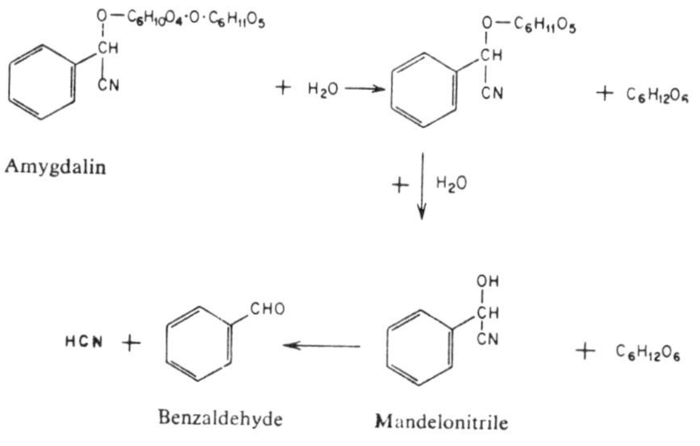

Figure 2. Pathways in the hydrolysis of a cyanogenic glycoside, Amygdalin, yielding HCN

Higher plants have the capacity to metabolize sublethal doses of administered cyanide (Towill, et al., 1978), as have animals. There is belief that all higher plants possess this ability through a reaction between various forms of sulfur (polysulfides and thiosulfate) such as:

$$S_x^{2-} + CN^- \rightleftharpoons [S_{(x-1)}]^{2-} + SCN$$

$$S_2O_3^{2-} + CN^- \rightleftharpoons SO_3^{2-} + SCN^-$$

TABLE 1. Relative stabilities of some common cyanide complexes in water

Stability ratings in water	Examples of cyanides in processing solutions
1. Free cyanide	CN^-, HCN
2. Simple compounds	
a. readily soluble	NaCN, KCN, $Ca(CN)_2$, $Hg(CN)_2$
b. relatively insoluble	$Zn(CN)_2$, CuCN, $Ni(CN)_2$, AgCN
3. Weak complexes	$Zn(CN)_4^{2-}$, $Cd(CN)_3^-$, $Cd(CN)_4^{2-}$
4. Moderately strong complexes	$Cu(CN)_2^-$, $Cu(CN)_3^{2-}$, $Ni(CN)_4^{2-}$, $Ag(CN)_2^-$
5. Strong complexes	$Fe(CN)_6^{4-}$, $Co(CN)_6^{4-}$, $Au(CN)_2^-$

TABLE 2. Selected Plants with Cyanogenic Potential

Species name	Common name
Acacia greggii	catclaw
Bahia opositifolia	bahia
Cercocarpus spp.	mountain mahogany
Florestina tripteris	florestina
Glyceria striata	fowl mannagrass
Holcus lanatus	velvet grass
Hydrangea spp.	hydrangea
Linum spp.	flax
Lotus corniculatus	birdsfoot trefoil
Manihot esculenta	cassava
Phaseolus lunatus	lima bean
Prunus spp.	cherries
Pyrus malus	apple
Sorghum spp.	sudan grass, Johnsongrass, etc.
Stillingia treculeana	queen's delight
Suckleya suckleyana	poison suckleya
Trifolium repens	white clover
Triglochin spp.	arrowgrass
Vicia sativa	vetch seed
Zea mays	maize, corn

MICROORGANISMS

It has been postulated that cyanides accumulate in soils via biological degradation of plants that produce abundant cyanogenic glycosides, such as sorghum (Raugaswami, et al., 1962). Cyanides may also be generated by a great number of soil microorganisms including fungi, bacteria, actinomycetes, and algae. Bach (1956), for example, identified 31 fungal species and many genera that elaborate cyanogenic glycosides. Many well known bacteria possess this capacity (Michael and Corpe, 1965; Knowles, 1976).

When the hypothesis for cyanide accumulation was tested by Strobel (1967) using $^{14}C^{15}N$, he found that the soils most active in utilizing cyanides were those associated with plants that produced cyanogenic glycosides most abundantly. Moreover, nonsterile soil converted cyanide to carbonate and nitrate, whereas sterile soil did not appreciably alter cyanide. Many bacteria, fungi, and algae are capable of utilizing cyanides (Strobel, 1967; Allen and Strobel, 1966; Ware and Painter, 1955; and Towill, et al., 1978, to name a few). Not only is there chemical evidence for cyanide transformation and degradation but there is enzymatic evidence. Cyanides do not accumulate in soils under natural conditions.

SOILS

Cyanides are introduced into the soil from natural sources and through the activities of mankind. The cyanides from natural sources do not persist in the soil. The relatively small amounts produced are readily attached by soil microorganisms and converted to carbonate and ammonia. The soil microorganisms rarely, if ever, leave organic compounds immune to biodegradation. Some cyanide may be released to the atmosphere and dispersed depending on the pH and red/ox of the soil environment. For example, an anaerobic autotrophic actinomycetes species common to sewage, was identified (Ware and Painter, 1955) which grows well on silica gel containing only KCN as a carbon and nitrogen source. The high chemical reactivity of most cyanide also does not permit the accumulation of any significance. Cyanide (CN^-), up to 200 ppm at least, is readily converted to fertilizer nitrogen in the soil (Fuller, et al., 1950a). In fact, levels of many cyanides equivalent to the nitrogen requirements of cultivated crops support plant response, which is almost identical to that from other nitrogen sources such as sodium or ammonium nitrate on an equivalent N basis (Fuller, et al., 1950b).

Cyanide is one of nature's most toxic substances. The level of toxicity of the more stable cyanides depends on the metal present and on the proportion of CN^- groups converted to simpler alkali cyanides. The estimated concentration of cyanide (CN^-) in waste streams of cyanide users, varies from 100 to 50,000 mg/ℓ depending on the efficiency of the manufacturer and process used (Rudolph, 1953). Although the numerous cyanides discharged as wastes differ from each other with respect to their impact on the environment, the loading rate in soil is the paramount factor determining toxicity to microorganisms or hazard for movement into groundwater and food chains. High concentrations in the environment usually are associated with accidental spills or improper waste disposal (Towill et al., 1978).

Because of the high reactivity, low levels do not exist in the soil. Some of the reactions attributed to the low levels of cyanides in soils are:

- Biological dissemination and assimilation
  (metabolism)
- Microbial transformation to CO_2, H_2O, NH_3, and metals
  (hydration and oxidation)
- Dispersion to the atmosphere as gases and/or to water sources
  (translocation, volatilization, and dispersion)
- Complex formations with metals
  (chelation)
- Chemical combination and precipitation
  (precipitation)
- Adsorption to surfaces
  (surface physical chemistry)
- Photodegradation

WATER

Cyanides have not appeared in drinking water sources except for a rare few accidents in history. Nevertheless, threshold limits of drinking water (0.01 HCN/ℓ) have been suggested (U.S. PHS, 1961; U.S. EPA, 1980). Because of the notorious toxicity of cyanide, mining wastes receive treatment before exposure to the surrounding environment. Leaching of mining overburden and gangue does not contribute to cyanide pollution of water. Waters containing leachate from mine tailings where cyanides were used have produced no significant cyanide pollution to surrounding waters. However, during 1980 and 1981 the Public Health Service staff, I am told, became concerned over cyanide-leach-mining that expanded with the high gold and silver prices. Several important references (Resnick et al., 1958; Towill, 1978; and Ecological Analysts, Inc., 1979; Scott, 1981; and Huiatt, 1983) will bring the reader up to date on cyanides in water. Adequate knowledge is available for controlling cyanide pollution in water environments.

AIR

Cyanides find a way into the atmosphere or air primarily from free cyanides in wastewaters collected in lagoons and ponds. Cyanide can enter the atmosphere readily from free-water surfaces. Both HCN and CN^- are in equilibrium in water at a pH of 9.36. HCN is a weak acid with a dissociation constant of 4.365×10^{-10} at 20C and a boiling point of 25.7C. The molecular HCN, therefore, has a high vapor pressure and consequently volatilizes readily into the atmosphere. Factors affecting rate of volatilization include:

- pH value - lower pH levels favor volatilization,
- Temperature - higher temperatures favor volatilization,
- Liquid turbulence - higher turbulences favor volatilization,
- Liquid surface area - higher surface-area ratio to depth of liquid favors volatilization, and
- Concentration of free cyanide - higher solution concentrations favor volatilization.

According to The Chester Engineers (1979) cyanide volatilizes at a rate of 0.021 mg CN/ft^2-hr from still water surfaces containing a concentration range of 0.1 to 0.5 mg/ℓ.

CYANIDE REACTIONS IN THE SOIL

NATURAL SOURCES

The soil as a weathered system does not contain cyanides nor does it generate cyanides, except indirectly in supporting the growth of microorganisms, plants, and other intimate soil life. In fact, soil organic matter inactivates the toxic effects of cyanide as a result of its affinity for combining. Cyanides that enter the soil from the low-level natural sources are rapidly biodegraded and quickly metabolized by soil microorganisms. Strobel (1967) was unable to isolate cyanides from soils growing sorghum, a plant that not only produces cyanogenic glycosides in abundance but grows luxuriously to yield large amounts of plant residue.

PESTICIDES

Pesticides are examples of many cyanides and cyanide-yielding substances that end up in the soil environment over large areas for beneficial use. A list of pesticides, grouped according to six general classes that either contain cyanide radicals or may be metabolized into yielding cyanide radicals, has been compiled in Table 3. Four general groups were identified: dithiocarbamate, triazine, triazol, and pyrethroid. In addition, cyanide capsules and calcium cyanide are used for special purposes. Despite their regular use on agricultural crops and noncrops, cyanides do not accumulate. They biodegrade easily and convert readily to harmless constituents, and some of them even end up becoming valuable nitrogen (HN_4^- and NO_3^-) plant nutrients. The soil microorganisms quickly take advantage of the low levels of readily metabolizable energy sources that reach the soil as a result of pest control applications. Because of this, the compounds listed in Table 3, which represent at least 24 individual marketed pesticides, are considered as among the safest commercial agricultural chemicals used to improve food and fiber production.

FERTILIZERS

Establishment of Cyanides as Fertilizers

The realization that cyanides can be used as fertilizers for agricultural crops is not new. Pioneers of this practical application date back to Miller, 1906; Robine, Lenglen, and LeClere, 1906; Cowie, 1919a,b). And again in 1945a,b. At about this same time, an extensive laboratory and field study was undertaken in Arizona to compare the nitrifying characteristics of some cyanides and cyanide-yielding compounds (Table 4) for commercial fertilizer purposes (Fuller et al., 1950a,b). Calcium cyanamide, dicyanodiamide, guanidine nitrate, guanylurea sulfate, and thiourea were found to nitrify rapidly and compare favorably with the more conventional fertilizers, ammonium sulfate and urea, in Arizona soils when applied at a rate of 100 and

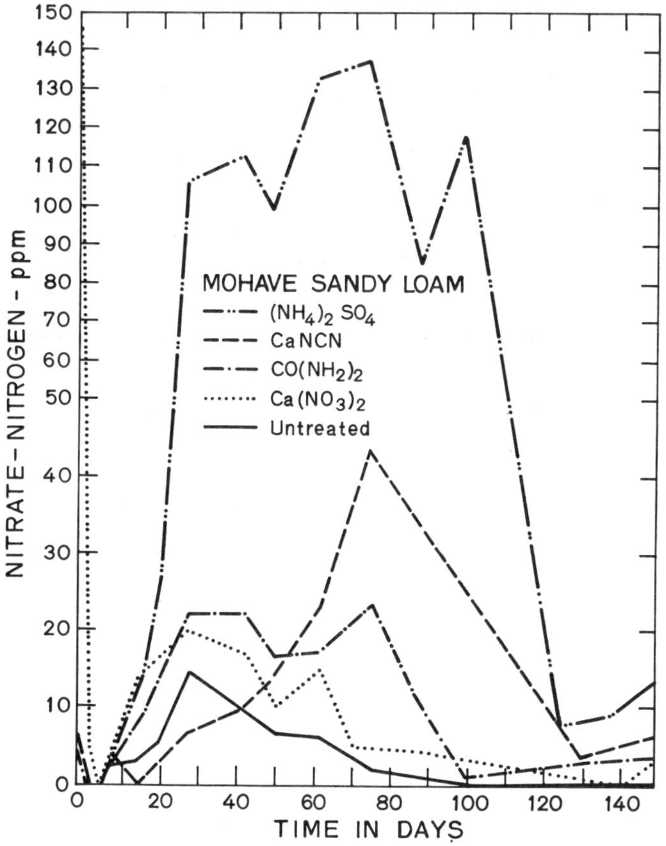

Figure 3. Change with time of nitrate-nitrogen in Mohave sandy loam treated with various nitrogen fertilizers.

TABLE 3. A list of pesticide categories that either contain cyanide radicals or may be metabolized into yielding cyanide radicals.

Chemical Class	Name	Use	Application
1	Dithiocarbamate	fungicide	fruits, melons, grains, vegetables, fiber crops
2	Triazine	herbicide	non-crops, grains, alfalfa, fiber crops
3	Triazine	fungicide	melon, vegetables
4	Triazole	herbicides	non-crops, grains, ornamentals
5	Triazole	fungicides	apples, barley, grapes, wheat
6	Pyrethroid	insecticides	experimental use, cotton, apples, corn, pecans

TABLE 4. Selected nitrogren and/or cyanide yielding compounds that have soil fertilizer value.

Name	Formula
• Ammonium Sulfate	$(NH_4)_2SO_4$
• Cyanamide	$H_2N{-}C{\equiv}N$
• Dicyanodiamide	$NH_2{\cdot}C\begin{smallmatrix}NH\\NH\end{smallmatrix}{\cdot}CN$
• Guanidine Nitrate	$CH_5N_3{\cdot}HNO_3$ $HN{=}C\begin{smallmatrix}NH\\NH\end{smallmatrix}{\cdot}HNO_3$
• Guanylurea Sulfate or Dicyanodiamidine Sulfate	$(NH_2{\cdot}C({=}NH){\cdot}NH{\cdot}C({=}O){\cdot}NH_2){\cdot}H_2SO_4{\cdot}2H_2O$
• Thiourea or Thiocarbamide	$H_2N{\cdot}C({=}S){\cdot}NH_2$
• Melamine or Cyanurotriamide	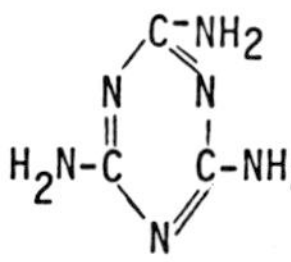
• Uramon or Urea	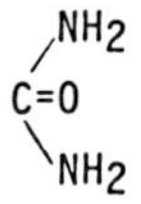

200 ppm N (Tables 5 and 6). Melamine biodegrades so slowly it has questionable value as a fertilizer (Table 5). Calcium cyanamide, added to soil in amounts of 50- to 100 lbs N/A-6 inches under field conditions of wheat and barley production, was also found to be approximately equivalent to conventional commercial fertilizers, Figure 3, (Fuller, et al., 1950a,b). The nitrification rate of calcium cyanamid, for example, compared favorably with urea (Fuller, et al., 1950b; Fuller, 1963; and Volk, 1950). Application of 140 and 250 lbs N/A in the form of calcium cyanamid to Yuma Superstition sand and Mesa Laveen clay loam, supported highly significant barley grain yields over the no-fertilizer control soil (Table 7).

Nitrification Rates of Cyanide-Yielding Compounds

Some inhibition in the rate of conversion from ammonia to nitrate occurred with cyanamide, dicyanodiamide, and thiourea at an application of 200 ppm N but not at the 100-ppm N rate under laboratory conditions. The data clearly revealed that certain cyanogenic compounds were inhibitory to the nitrosomonas and nitrobacter that convert ammonia to nitrate but did not inhibit the microorganisms that transformed the compounds to ammonium (Tables 5 and 6). Since the NO_3^- ion is much more mobile than NH_4^+, the principle of slowing down the nitrification of NH_3 led to the commercial development of compounds that would inhibit nitrate formation from ammonia to delay or reduce fertilizer loss by migration through soils beyond the reach of plant roots. This favorable fertilization principle is demonstrated in the residual effect of nitrogen to the second-season crop from thiourea and cyanamid when applied to barley in field experiments, Table 7 (Fuller et al., 1950a), but this effect did not occur when the fertilizers were ammonium sulfate or urea.

Simple Cyanides as Fertilizers

Sodium cyanide was reported to be only slightly less effective than sodium nitrate as a nitrogen fertilizer for corn, tobacco, and mustard when used on nitrogen-deficient soils (McCool, 1945a,b). Potassium cyanide also has soil fertilizing qualities since it nitrifies rapidly in soils to yield CO_2 and NH_3 (Strobel, 1967). Cyanides may be fixed by soil organisms in several ways. All give rise to some organic nitriles, which in turn yield ammonia with the corresponding organic acids (Strobel, 1967).

Anaerobic Cyanide Reactions

Microbial reactions under anaerobic soil conditions (e.g. waterlogging) are quite different from those under aerobic conditions. Soil microorganisms responsible for degrading cyanide under anaerobic conditions are believed to be more sensitive to the concentrations tolerated under aerobic conditions. The limit of tolerance for effective anaerobic degradation was suggested by Coburn (1949) as 2 ppm. Thus, the opportunity for cyanides to move through soil is expected to be greater under anaerobic than aerobic environmental conditions. Since denitrification of cyanides under anaerobic soil environments is not well known, it is not wise to speculate too freely

Table 5. Changes with time in pH value, ammonium-, nitrite-, and nitrate-nitrogen content of Mohave fine sandy loam receiving various cyanide-yielding organics applied at 200 ppm.

Incubation Period	Ammonium Sulphate 200 p.p.m.* of N				Uramon 200 p.p.m. of N				Cyanamid 200 p.p.m of N				Dicyanodiamid 200 p.p.m. of N				Guanidine Nitrate 200 p.p.m. of N			
	pH	NH_3-N	NO_2-N	NO_3-N	pH	NH_3-N	NO_2-N	NO_3-N	pH	NH_3-N	NO_2-N	NO_3-N	pH	NH_3-N	NO_2-N	NO_3-N	pH	NH_3-N	NO_2-N	NO_3-N
days		ppm*	ppm	ppm		ppm*	ppm	ppm		ppm*	ppm	ppm		ppm*	ppm	ppm		ppm*	ppm	ppm
0	7.5	200	1	0	8.0	20	Trace	1	9.1	16	Trace	†	7.8	8	0	†	7.6	8	Trace	69
5	7.3	186	5	13	7.7	165	4	7	8.4	97	0	0	7.6	15	0	2	7.6	16	1	69
7	7.2	90	78	77	7.3	101	92	56	....	....	....	....	....	....	....	....	....	....	....	....
9	7.3	44	84	93	7.3	59	107	67	8.1	129	Trace	17	7.9	12	0	15	7.6	11	Trace	63
12	7.2	6	2	149	7.0	10	70	109	....	....	....	....	....	....	....	....	....	....	....	....
16	7.4	12	Trace	179	7.4	8	Trace	192	8.1	140	Trace	18	7.9	17	0	18	7.6	10	Trace	81
22	7.6	6	Trace	223	7.7	9	Trace	208	8.2	133	Trace	21	8.0	17	0	23	7.8	10	0	95
29	....	....	....	....	....	....	....	....	8.0	143	Trace	21	....	....	....	....	....	....	....	....
36	....	....	....	....	....	....	....	....	8.1	137	Trace	23	7.9	19	0	24	7.5	7	Trace	153
43	....	....	....	....	....	....	....	....	8.1	128	Trace	24	....	....	....	....	....	....	....	....
57	....	....	....	....	....	....	....	....	8.1	129	0	21	....	....	....	....	....	....	....	....
61	....	....	....	....	....	....	....	....	....	....	....	....	....	....	....	....	....	....	....	....
69	....	....	....	....	....	....	....	....	8.1	133	0	16	8.1	26	0	22	7.6	15	0	157
90	....	....	....	....	....	....	....	....	8.1	109	0	25	8.1	23	0	21	7.5	2	0	224
97	....	....	....	....	....	....	....	....	....	....	....	....	....	....	....	....	....	....	....	....
111	....	....	....	....	....	....	....	....	....	....	....	....	....	....	....	....	....	....	....	....
120	....	....	....	....	....	....	....	....	....	....	....	....	7.9	22	0	15	7.4	1	0	274
159	....	....	....	....	....	....	....	....	....	....	....	....	8.1	36	0	14	....	....	....	....
202	....	....	....	....	....	....	....	....	....	....	....	....	8.2	37	Trace	17	....	....	....	....
248	....	....	....	....	....	....	....	....	....	....	....	....	....	....	....	....	....	....	....	....
370	....	....	....	....	7.5	Trace	Trace	240	....	....	....	....	....	....	....	....	....	....	....	....

*Parts per million on basis of soil.
†Nitrate-nitrogen values were negative for reasons not yet understood.

Incubation Period	Guanylurea Sulphate 200 p.p.m. of N				Thiourea 200 p.p.m. of N				Melamine 200 p.p.m. of N				Untreated			
	pH	NH_3-N	NO_2-N	NO_3-N	pH	NH_3-N	NO_2-N	NO_3-N	pH	NH_3-N	NO_2-N	NO_3-N	pH	NH_3-N	NO_2-N	NO_3-N
days		ppm*	ppm	ppm		ppm*	ppm	ppm		ppm*	ppm	ppm		ppm*	ppm	ppm
0	7.7	9	Trace	3	7.8	10	0	†	7.9	8	Trace	†	7.8	6	Trace	3
5	7.8	18	0	6	8.0	21	0	†	7.7	8	0	8	7.8	6	Trace	6
7	....	....	....	....	....	....	....	....	....	....	....	....	....	....	....	....
9	7.8	12	Trace	20	8.0	25	0	0	7.8	6	0	22	7.8	4	Trace	18
12	....	....	....	....	....	....	....	....	....	....	....	....	....	....	....	....
16	7.8	14	0	23	8.1	39	0	8	7.9	6	0	30	7.8	5	0	21
22	7.8	13	0	31	8.0	50	0	4	8.0	9	0	37	7.9	6	0	37
29	....	....	....	....	7.9	115	0	0	....	....	....	....	....	....	....	....
36	7.9	13	0	37	7.8	68	0	†	7.8	6	0	41	7.8	6	0	41
43	....	....	....	....	7.8	78	0	†	....	....	....	....	....	....	....	....
57	....	....	....	....	7.7	113	0	15	....	....	....	....	....	....	....	....
61	....	....	....	....	7.7	135	0	12	....	....	....	....	....	....	....	....
69	7.8	7	0	39	7.8	136	0	12	7.8	2	0	41	7.8	13	0	33
90	7.4	3	0	128	7.9	160	0	18	7.8	1	0	43	7.8	6	0	44
97	7.4	2	0	179	....	....	....	....	....	....	....	....	7.8	1	0	54
111	7.4	5	0	283	....	....	....	....	....	....	....	....	....	....	....	....
120	7.5	4	0	240	....	....	....	....	7.8	0	0	48	7.6	4	0	54
159	....	....	....	....	....	....	....	....	....	....	....	....	7.7	9	0	59
202	....	....	....	....	....	....	....	....	7.8	6	0	59	....	....	....	....
248	....	....	....	....	....	....	....	....	7.7	4	Trace	56	7.7	9	1	56
370	....	....	....	....	....	....	....	....	7.7	0	Trace	70	7.7	2	Trace	70

*Parts per million on basis of soil.
†Nitrate-nitrogen values were negative for reasons not yet understood.

TABLE 6. Changes with time in pH value, ammonium-, nitrite-, and nitrate-content of Mohave fine sandy loam receiving cyanamide and thiourea applied at 100 ppm.

Incubation Period	Cyanamide 100 p.p.m.* of N				Thiourea 100 p.p.m. of N			
	pH	NH_3-N	NO_2-N	NO_3-N	pH	NH_3-N	NO_2-N	NO_3-N
days		ppm*	ppm	ppm		ppm*	ppm	ppm
0	8.7	28	Trace	15	8.0	11	Trace	†
4	8.1	79	Trace	15	8.0	3	0	†
11	8.2	76	2	17	8.0	39	0	†
14	8.0	73	Trace	23	8.0	48	0	†
18	8.1	62	1	20	8.0	57	0	4
39	7.9	58	0	37	7.9	87	Trace	18
61	....	......	......	......	....	......	......	....
70	7.6	1	0	104	7.5	45	8	24
79	7.7	10	0	100	7.5	36	Trace	64
90	....	......	......	......	....	......	......	.....
125	....	......	......	......	....	......	......	.....
152	....	......	......	......	....	......	......	.....
198	....	......	......	......	....	......	......	.....
322	....	......	......	......	....	......	......	.....

*Parts per million on basis of soil.
†Nitrate-nitrogen values were negative for reasons not yet understood.

TABLE 7. The influence of some cyanogenic fertilizers on barley grain yields from two calcareous soils.

Material Added	Increase in Barley Due to Nitrogen Application: Laveen clay loam	Superstition sand
	%	%
None	...	...
Dicyanodiamide	3.1	...
Guanylurea sulfate	7.5	...
Guanidine nitrate	27.8*	0.5
Ureaform N-20	30.6*	8.0
Ammonium sulfate	32.6*	38.8*
Ureaform N-40	40.3*	20.8*
Cyanamide	45.3*	52.4*
Thiourea	62.3*	62.4*

*Highly significant increase, 1% level.

and interpret significance much beyond what is actually known. But there is evidence that the denitrification process does occur in certain soluble cyanides and that it yields N_2 gas, probably through nitrates under limited free O_2 conditions, and particularly, where sulfur compounds are available (Huiatt, 1983, Ch.2).

LANDFILLS

Untreated cyanide disposals to landfills are not allowed under the present regulations. However, cyanide wastes that have been placedin drums during some former period may pollute the soil environment through leakage. Should such occur, remedial procedures must be initiated to confine the chemical (Tolman et al., 1978). The real problem centers around toxicity since concentrations may be expected to be higher than just discussed with soil fertilization. Microbial degradation rates and the attenuation capacity of the soil could be exceeded.

LAGOONS, PONDS, AND WASTE WATERS

One of the oldest methods of confining mining and plating cyanides, preventing their movement to the surrounding environment, is the establishment of shallow earth lagoons and ponds. Such facilities designed for deep soils of fine textures, clay-lined and deep watertables, have been quite successful in confining cyanides. Shallow ponds of low-level cyanides exchange gases readily with no appreciable limitation of oxygen sufficient to convert cyanides readily to nitrates. In fact, the accumulation of nitrates may pose a greater problem to underground water quality than cyanides. Fortunately, another mechanism is available in properly designed mining lagoons and ponds that is centered in the clay lining and acts as an anerobic denitrifying barrier to underground flow similar to that in a rice paddy. The nitrates denitrify at this low red/ox juncture in the bottom of the pond with the discharge of harmless N^2 gas into the atmosphere.

The threshold limit of CN^- toxicity on biological activity of aqueous systems varies widely with such environmental factors as water quality, temperature, type and size of the organism. Thus, definite effects cannot be established except in terms of the nature of the effects. For example, Lockette and Griffiths (1947) report that 5.0 ppm of CN^- in sewage treated by the activated process had a marked depression effect on the purification process, whereas Ludzack et al. (1951) found inhibition effects as low as 0.3 ppm under certain other conditions. In concentrations of 6% CN^-, all waters studied were purified up to 50% or more of the control within 10 days of incubation.

Of particular interest because of its toxicity to the cytochrome system is the utilization of cyanide by specific microorganisms found in wastewaters. Ware and Painter (1955) isolated an aerobic autotrophic actinomycete from sewage which is capable of growing on silica containing only KCN as a source of carbon and nitrogen. This organism can utilize concentrations of CN^- up to 15 mgm/100 ml but grows more favorably at 4 mgm/100 ml concentrations. The rate of utilization in colony culture approached a maximum of 0.5 mgm CN/day. Presumably the general reaction proceeds as follows:

$$2KCN + 4H_2 + 3O_2 \rightarrow 2KOH + 2NH_3 + 2CO_2$$

Other examples of specific microbial assimilation and transformation of CN^- in synthetic media (not soil) are those given by Reynolds (1924), Strobel (1964), and Allen and Strobel (1966).

CYANIDE MOVEMENT IN THE SOIL

SCOPE

Since many of the cyanide wastestreams, waste ponds, lagoons, and leachates end in an anoxic soil environment, a fundamental research program was undertaken to study cyanides under anaerobic soil conditions with specific objectives:

. To study the rate of degradation of simple and complex cyanide under saturated and unsaturated (70% of field water-holding capacity) soil conditions.

. To evaluate the influence of different organic energy sources on the rate of degradation or transformation of cyanides.

. To study the mobility of certain cyanides, in water and municipal landfill leachate, through soils with distinctly different chemical and physical properties, in order to statistically relate soil parameters to observed attenuation and degradation.

SATURATED ANAEROBIC SOIL CONDITIONS

Experimental

Three sets of four different soils (Table 8) were packed in a pvc column 5 cm in diameter and 12 cm long to a specified bulk density (Fuller, 1982; Fuller and Warrick, 1984a,b). Each set was connected to one of three constant head devices and each one contained a different cyanide solution. Solution #1 contained potassium cyanide in water; solution #2 contained potassium cyanide in a landfill leachate, and solution #3 contained a complex form of cyanide in deionized water alone, Table 9 (Alesii, 1976; Alesii and Fuller, 1976).

TABLE 8. Reference Soils Used in the Cyanide Movement Research

Series* Soil	Order Soil	Clay	Silt	Free Iron Oxides	Soil Paste pH	Cation Exch. Capacity	Elec. Cond.of Extract	Bulk Density
		%	%	%		meg/100g	μmhos/cm	g/cm^3
Molokai	Oxisol	52	25	23.0	6.2	14	1262	1.44
Nicholson	Alfisol	49	47	5.6	6.7	37	176	1.56
Mohave(Ca)	Aridisol	40	28	2.5	7.8	12	510	1.54
Ava	Alfisol	31		4.0	4.5	19	157	1.44

*Oriented on basis of clay content.

The flow of the solution was regulated to provide approximately one pore volume of displacement each day. The displacements were continued until 20 pore-space volumes were collected. The effluent was collected each day in a 125 ml bottle containing 5 ml of 1N sodium hydroxide. The sodium hydroxide was necessary to keep the cyanide that comes through with the solution from volatilizing. The solution collected was analyzed for total cyanide by the Liebig distillation method according to Taras (1971).

The distillation of the sample was required to convert all the complex cyanide in the sample into simple cyanide ions. The sample was then easily analyzed by the Liebig titration method using silver nitrate and Rhodanin indicator (when the concentration was above 1 ppm). When the concentration was below 1 ppm, the Liebig colorimetric method involving pyridine-pyrazalene was used.

TABLE 9. Characteristics of Cyanide Solution Used in the Movement Research

Cyanide solution	pH of solution	Concentration of cyanide in solution	Type of ion present
		mg/L	
KCN in deionized water	10.0	97	$CN^{\ominus}$
$K_3Fe(CN)_6$ in deionized water	8.5	98	$Fe(CN)_6^{\ominus}$
KCN in landfill leachate	5.4	80	Unknown (mixed)

Discussion

The relative mobility of the three cyanide solutions is best illustrated in Mohave (Ca) clay loam and Kalkaska sand (Figure 4). All data are plotted as pore volume versus C/C_{max}, where C/C_{max} is the ratio of effluent concentration to influent concentration. KCN and $K_3Fe(CN)_6$ in deionized water were both found to be very mobile in soils, while KCN in landfill leachate was the least mobile of the three solutions.

The effect of soil type on the movement of the three cyanide solutions is illustrated in Figure 5, showing the amount of KCN in deionized water that was leached through four soils. The $CN^{\ominus}$ was retained most by soils having a high concentration of Mn and hydrous oxides of Fe (Nicholson silty clay and Molokai clay). Korte et al. (1975) found similar results working with the anion forms of As, Cr, Se, and V. This conclusion is further supported by data from Berg and Thomas (1959). They found $Cl^{\ominus}$, which is similar to $CN^{\ominus}$ in its adsorption behavior, attenuated in soils having a high percentage of kaolin clay and iron and aluminum oxides. Schofield (1939) also reports that soils high in these oxides have a high anion exchange capacity. Kamprath (1956) found good retention of SO_4^{2-} by an acidic soil high in oxides and kaolin, whereas the 3-layer minerals appeared to have relatively poor retention for SO_4^{2-}. The acidic soil (Ava silty clay loam) in this study proved, on the contrary, to be a poor attenuator of $CN^{\ominus}$. Texture seems to have little measurable effect on the attenuation of KCN. Free iron oxide and $CaCO_3$ seem to have a greater influence on the movement of KCN in water than either soil pH or texture.

Figure 5 illustrates the movement of $K_3Fe(CN)_6$ in deionized water through four soils (Mohave (Ca) clay loam, Ava silty clay loam, Nicholson silty clay loam, and Kalkaska sandy loam). The ferricyanide ion also migrated most rapidly through soils having a high pH and in the presence of free $CaCO_3$ (Mohave (Ca) clay loam) for the same reason as KCN in water. Ferricyanide moved slowest in soils having a low pH (Ava silty clay loam and Kalkaska sandy loam). A low pH would indicate the clay surface to have a high percentage of positive exchange sites which would attract the $Fe(CN)_6^{3-}$ ion and retain it. Texture seems to play a more important role in this case.

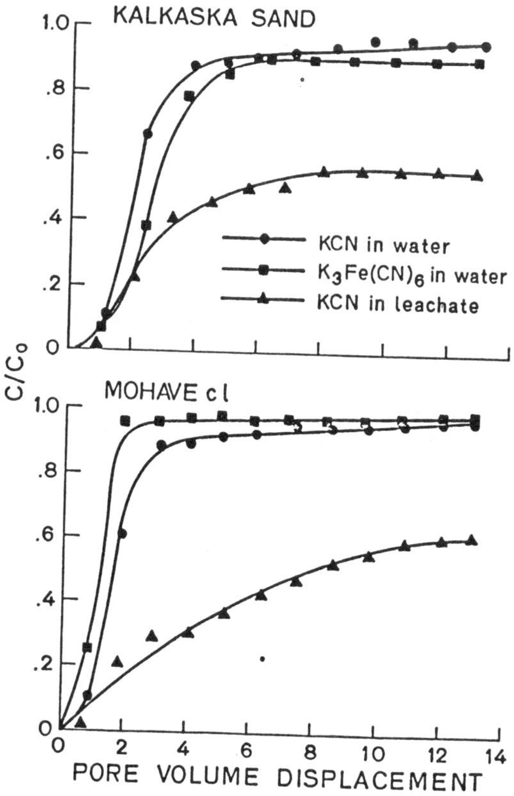

Figure 4. Relative mobility of three cyanide solutions (water and leachate) through Kalkaska sandy loam and Mohave (Ca) clay loam.

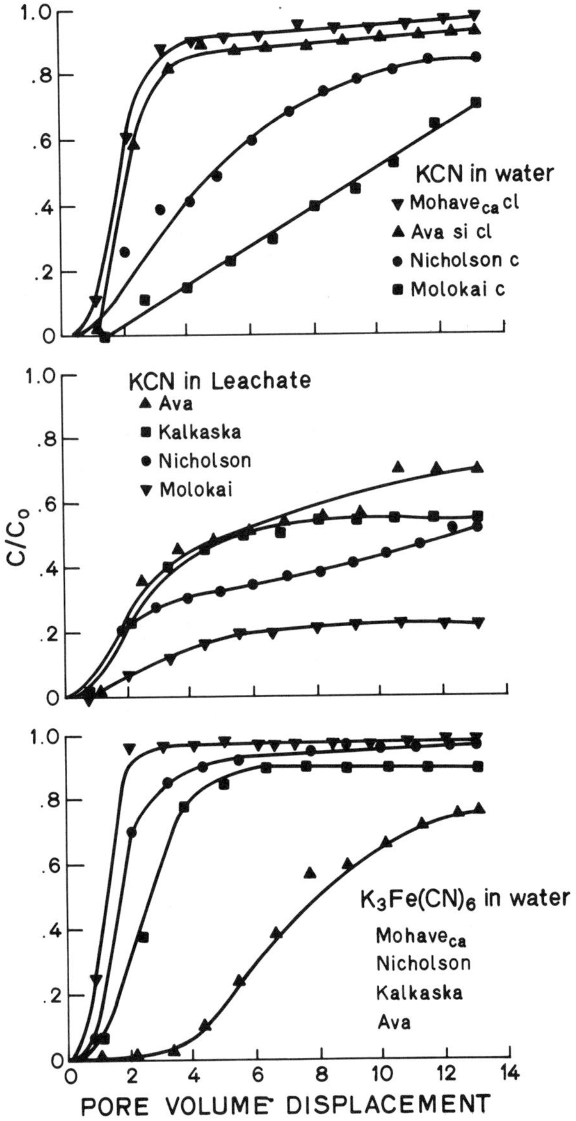

Figure 5. Effects of soil type on the mobility of KCN in water and leachate and $K_3Fe(CN)_6$ in water

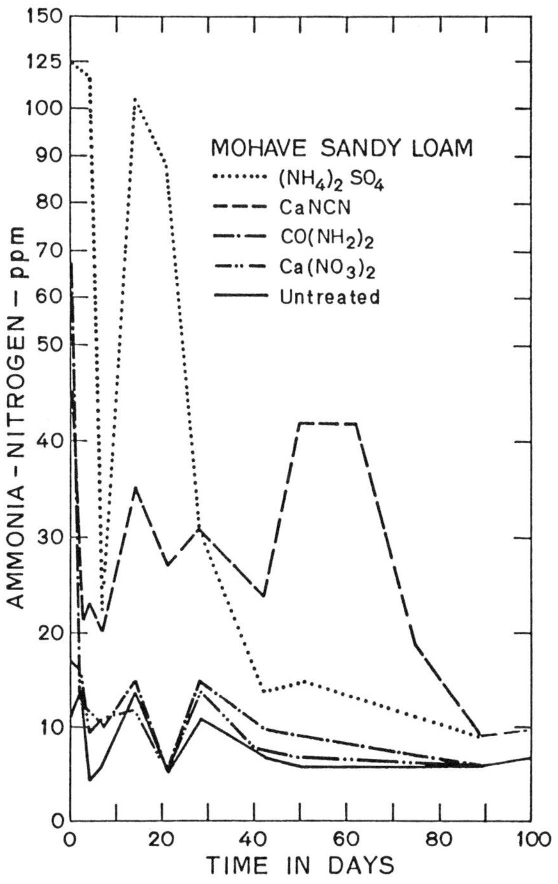

Figure 6. Change with time of ammonia-nitrogen in Mohave sandy loam treated with various nitrogen fertilizers

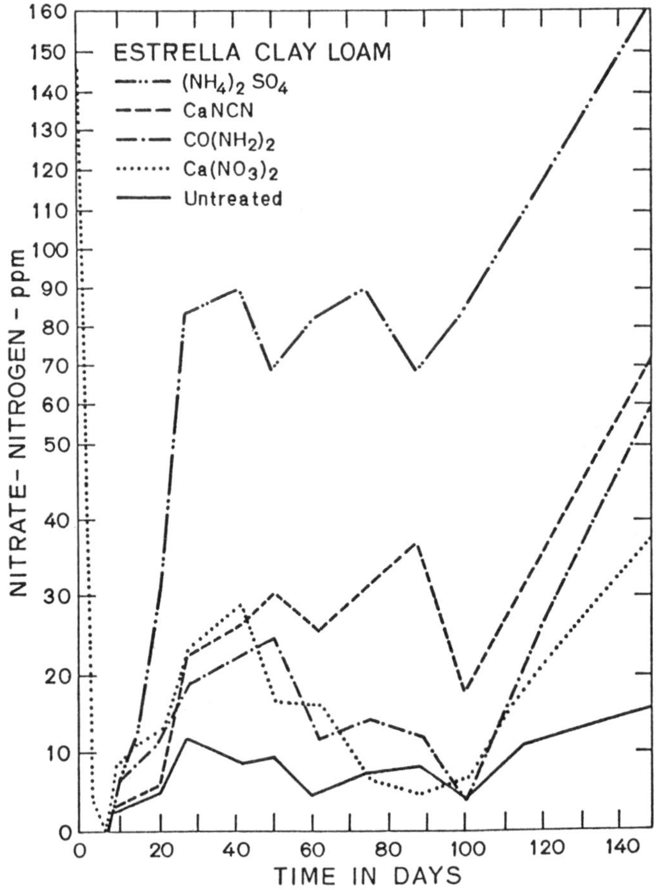

Figure 7. Changes with time of nitrate-nitrogen in Estrella clay loam treated with various nitrogen fertilizers

The high clay content soil (Ava silty clay loam) retained more of the $Fe(CN_6)^{3-}$ than the sandier soil of similar pH (Kalkaska sandy loam). Although iron-oxide seemed to have some affinity for $Fe(CN)_6^{3-}$, its presence was not as effective as soil pH in governing the movement of this form of cyanide.

KCN in MSW landfill leachates migrating through the four soils moved through those with the lowest pH (Ava silty clay loam and Kalkaska sandy loam). Cyanide was retained most extensively by soils having a high concentraton of iron-oxide (Figure 5).

Of the three cyanide solutions, KCN in MSW leachate was found to move through the soils most slowly. This can be explained partly by the precipitation of Prussian blue when KCN was added to the leachate (Robine et al., 1906). This blue precipitate was found infiltrating the top 4 cm of the soil columns. The accumulation indicates that Prussian blue may be quite immobile in soils. The cyanide that came through the soil was the CN^- that did not react with the Fe in solution to form Prussian blue.

The anaerobic state of the soil columns inhibited microbial degradation of cyanide. Microorganisms responsible for degrading cyanide under anaerobic conditions are very sensitive to an elevated concentration of this compound. The limit for effective anaerobic degradation of cyanide was found by Coburn (1949) to be 2 ppm in the wastestream, a concentration much lower than the approximate 100 ppm that passed through the soil columns. The incubation studies, therefore, were negative with respect to cyanide degradation, i.e. degradation did not occur significantly in the water-saturated, anaerobic soil. Nitrate, nitrite, and ammonium were not found as a result of possible CN^- transformation; but there was no measurement of N_2 gas for the detection of denitrification.

UNSATURATED, AEROBIC SOIL CONDITIONS

The cyanides react quite differently under aerobic than anaerobic soil conditions. The differences are apparent by comparing migration or movement in anaerobic soil columns with the same soils under field conditions where cyanide-yielding compounds rapidly ammonify and nitrify. Calcium cyanamide, for example, ammonifies more rapidly than urea and nitrifies comparably to ammonium sulfate and more rapidly than urea in Mohave sandy loam under field conditions (Figures 3 and 6). Nitrification of calcium cyanamide also progresses well in Estrella clay loam (Figure 7). Cyanide was not detected in soil deeper than 20 cm (8 in) or beyond the layer of cyanide incororation. Soils in Mesa and Yuma, Arizona, also were sampled every 10 days throughout the barley growing season for detection of the original material, cyanide, or cyanide-related comounds (Table 5). None of these were found within or below the incorporation layer, except for the traces from the original substances (cyanamide, dicyandiamide, guanylurea sulfate, guanidine nitrate, thiourea) in the 8-inch incorporation layer only, found immediately after being applied. However, nitrate-nitrogen, attributable to the application of fertilizers and cyanides, was detected to a depth of about 30 cm (12 in) after the first irrigation.

Certain conditions in the field, compared with those in soil columns, also delegate against cyanide movement through the soil; such as,

- Molecular oxygen availability is greater in the field,
- Wetting and drying is more prominent in the field,
- Soil microorganisms are more active under natural conditions,
- Photochemical activity is greater in the field,
- Fluctuation in soil moisture levels is greater in the field.

CONCLUDING KEYNOTE STATEMENT

1. Cyanides and cyanide-yielding componds are found well distributed in the total earth surface environment.

2. Cyanides from widespread natural sources of plants, micororganisms, animals, and infrequently identified in soil, water, and air, originating from biological sources, offer little hazard to the inhabitants of the earth surface environment.

3. Low levels of free cyanides in nature do not persist in soils due to many highly reactive indigenous chemical and enzymatic transformations and degradation processes.

4. Cyanide toxicity originating from natural sources through plant consumption by rumens has occurred but proper management of feeding and grazing appears to minimize this hazard.

5. Commercial sources of cyanides have proved useful to agricultural crop production as exemplified by pesticides and fertilizers both of which are readily converted to plant nutrient sources such as ammonia and nitrate. Cyanides used for these purposes do not persist in the soil.

6. Free cyanide is one of nature's most toxic substances. Free cyanide, also, is a very reactive ion readily forming insoluble and very slowly soluble complex compounds. The loading rate in soils, therefore, is the paramount factor in determining the hazard for biological systems and movement to ground waters. Simple cyanides have been applied at rates of 280 kgN/ha to aerobic soils as fertilizers with no hazardous effects. In anaerobic soils the "safe" level drops to a few ppm.

7. Adequate knowledge exists for controlling cyanide poolution in soil, water, and air environments.

8. The soil is the first and main line of defense for accidental cyanide spills and inadvertant overloading of disposal areas.

9. The soil factors most responsible for control of cyanides in the environment are: (a) clay content, (b) depth of soil, (c) hydrous oxides of iron, manganese, aluminum and other metals, (d) pH, (e) aerobic conditions, and (f) presence of soil organic matter.

REFERENCES

Allen, J. and G. A. Strobel. 1966. The assimilation of $H^{14}CN$ by a variety of fungi. Can. J. Microbiol. 12:414-416.

Alesii, B. A. 1976. Cyanide mobility in soils. M.S. Thesis, University of Arizona Library, Tucson, AZ.

Alesii, B. A. and W. H. Fuller. 1976. The mobility of three cyanide forms in soils. In "Residual Management by Land Disposal." Proc. of the Hazardous Waste Res. Symp., Feb. 2-4, 1976. Tucson, AZ (ed) W. H. Fuller. EPA-600/9-76-015, U. S. Environmental Protection Agency. Cincinnati, OH. 280 pp.

Bach, E. 1956. The Agaric Phaliota aurea: Physiology and Ecology. Dansk Botan, Arkiv., 16: Hefte 3.

Berg, W. A. and G. W. Thomas. 1959. Anion elution patterns from soils and soil clays. J. Soil Sci. Soc. of Amer. Proc. 23:348-350.

Cowie, G. A. 1919a. Decomposition of cyanamide and dicyanodiamide in the soil. J. Agr. Sci. 9:113-127.

Cowie, G. A. 1919b. The mechanism of the decomposition of cyanamide in the soil. J. Agr. Sci. 10:163-176.

Coburn, S. E. 1949. Limits of toxic waste in sewage treatment. Sewage Works J. 2:522.

Ecological Analysts, Inc. 1979. Cyanide. An overview and analysis of the literature on chemistry, fate, toxicity, and detection in surface waters. Prepared for the Inter-Industry Cyanide group.

Fuller, W. H. 1963. Reactions of nitrogenous fertilizers in calcareous soils. Agric. Food Chem. 11:188-193.

Fuller, W. H. 1978. Investigation of landfill leachate pollutant attenuation by soils. U. S. Environmental Protection Agency. MERL EPA-600/2-78-158. Cincinnati, OH. pp. 218.

Fuller, W. H. 1982. Methods for conducting soil column tests to predict pollutant movement. In Land Disposal: Hazardous Waste. Proc. Eighth Ann. Res. Symp., March 16-18. Cincinnati, OH. David Shultz, ed. U. S. EPA-600/9-82-002 MERL. U. S. Environmental Protection Agency, Cincinnati, OH. 45268.

Fuller, W. H., B. A. Alesii, and G. E. Carter. 1979. Behavior of municipal solid waste leachate: I. Composition variations. J. Environ. Sci. Health, A14(6):461-485.

Fuller, W. H., A. B. Caster, and W. T. McGeorge. 1950. Behavior of nitrogenous fertilizers in alkaline calcareous soils. I. Nitrifying characteristics of some organic compounds under controlled conditions. Univ. Ariz. Tech. Bull. 120, Ariz. Agric. Expt. Sta., Tucson,. AZ 85721. 451-467.

Fuller, W. H., W. H. Martin, and W. T. McGeorge. 1950b. Behavior of nitrogenous fertilizers in alkaline calcareous soils. II. Field experiments with organic and inorganic nitrogenous materials. Univ. Ariz. Agr. Expt. Sta. Tech. Bull. 121.

Fuller, W. H. and A. W. Warrick. 1984a. Soil in waste treatment and utilization. Vol. I. Land Treatment. Chemical Rubber Co. Press, Inc., Boca Raton, FL. pp. 263.

Fuller, W. H. and A. W. Warrick. 1984b. Soil in waste treatment and utilization. Vol. II. Pollutant Containment, Monitoring, and Closure. Chemical Rubber Co. Press, Inc., Boca Raton, FL. pp. 245.

Fry, W. E. and R. Millar. 1972. Cyanide degradation by an enzyme from Stemphylium lati. Archiv. Biochem. Biophys. 151:468-474.

Howe, R. H. L. and J. E. Howe. 1966. Cyanide degradation products soluble end products. Ind. Waste Tret. p. 51-54.

Huiatt, J. L. 1984. Synopsis of a workshop on cyanide from mineral processing. TMS-AIME Ann. Meet. Feb.-Mar. 2, 1984. Los Angeles, CA.

Huiatt, J. L., J. E. Kerrigan, F. A. Olson, and G. L. Potter. 1983. Cyanide from mineral processing. Proceedings of workshop. Salt Lake City, UT, February 1983. Utah Mining and Mineral Resources Research Institute, Salt Lake City, UT, Ch. 4.

Jacob, K. D., F. E. Allison, and J. M. Braham. 1924. Chemical and biological studies with cyanamid and some of its transformation products. J. Agr. Res., 28:37-68.

Kamprath, E. J., W. L. Nelson, and J. W. Fitts. 1956. The effect of pH, sulfate and phosphate concentration on the absorption of sulfate in soils. J. Soil Sci. Soc. Amer. Proc. 20:463-466.

Kingsbury, J. M. 1964. Poisonous plants of the United States and Canada. Prentice-Hall, Inc., Englewood Cliffs, NJ. pp. 626.

Knowles, C. J. 1976. Microorganisms and cyanide. Bacterial. Rev. 40:652-680.

Korte, N. E., J. Skopp, W. H. Fuller, E. E. Niebla, and B. A. Alesii. 1976. Trace element movement in soils: Influence of soil physical and chemical properties. Soil Sci. 622:350-359.

Lockett, W.T., and Griffiths, J. 1947. Cyanides in trade effluents and their effect on the bacterial purification of sewage. Jour. and Proc. Inst. Sew. Purif., Part 2, p 121.

Ludzack, F. J., W. A. Moore, H. L. Krieger, and C. C. Ruchhoft. 1951. Effect of cyanide on biochemical oxidation in sewage and polluted water. Sewage and Ind. Wastes, 23:1298-1307.

McCool, M. M. 1945a. Agronomic relationships of sodium cyanide. Contrib. Boyce Thompson Inst. 13:455-561.

McCool, M. M. 1945b. Fertilizer value of sodium cyanide. Contrib. Boyce Thompson Inst. 13:479-485.

Michaels, R. and W. A. Copre. 1965. Cyanide formation by _Chromabacterium violaceum._ J. Bacterio. 89:106-112.

Miller, A. A. 1906. The Cyanide Process. John Wiley and Sons Publishing Co. p. 12-34. New York, NY.

Ragaswami, G. and A. Balasubramanian. 1962. Studies of the rhizosphere microflora of sorghum in relation to hydrocyanic acid content of roots. Canadian J. Microbial. 9:719-725.

Resnick, J. D., W. A. Moore, and M. B. Ettinger. 1958. Behavior of cyanates in polluted water. Inc. Eng. Chem. 50(1):71-72.

Reynolds, E. S. 1924. Some relations of _Fusarium lini_ and potassium cyanide. Am. J. Botany, 11:215-217.

Robine, R., M. Lenglen, and J. S. LeClere. 1906. The cyanide industry theoretically and practically considered. John Wiley and Sons Publishing Co. pp. 1-84. New York, NY.

Rudolph, W. 1953. Industrial Wastes, Their Disposal and Treatment. Reinhold Publishing Corp., New York, NY.

Scott, J. S. 1981. Removal of cyanide from gold mill effluents. Cyanide in Gold Mining Industry: A Technical Seminar Sponsored by Environmental Canada and Canadian Mineral Processors, Jan. 22-23, 1981. Environ. Canada.

Strobel, A. G. 1964. Hydrocyanic acid assimilation by a Psychrophilic basidiomycete. Can. J. Biochem. 42:1637-1639.

Strobel, G. A. 1967. Cyanide utilization in soil. Soil Science. 103(4):299-302.

Taras, M. J. 1971. Cyanide. (ed) In Standard Methods for the Examination of Water and Waste Water. 13th Ed. Am. Pub. Health Assoc., New York. pp. 397-406.

The Chester Engineers. 1977. Report on the lower Monongahela River study - Water quality conditions. Point and non-point source wastes loads and waste load allocation. Vol. 1 and 2. Prepared for the U. S. Steel Corp., Coraopolis, PA.

Tolman, A. L., A. P. Bellestero, Jr., W. W. Beck, G. H. Emrich. Guidance manual for minimizing pollution from waste disposal sites. MERL, U. S. Environmental Protection Agency EPA-600/2-78-42. Cincinnati, OH. p. 83.

Towill, L. E., J. S. Drury, B. L. Whitfield, E. B. Lewis, E. L. Galyan, and A. S. Hammons. 1978. Reivews of the environmental effects of pollutants: V. Cyanides. Interagency Rept. Oak Ridge Natl. Lab. Rept. No. ORNL/EIS-81 and Environmental Protection Agency Rept. No. EPA-600/76-027.

U. S. EPA. 1980. Ambient water quality criteria for cyanide. U. S. Environmental Protection Agency EPA-440/5-80-00.

U. S. PHS. Advisory Committee on Revision of U. S. PHS. August 1961. 1946 Drinking Water Standards 1961. J. Am. Water Works Assoc. 53:935.

Volk, Gaylord, M. 1950. Factors determining efficiency of cyanamid and uramon for weed control in tobacco plant beds. Soil Sci., 69:377-390.

Ware, G. C. and H. A. Painter. 1955. Bacterial utilization of cyanide, Nature. 175:99.

DISCUSSION

Comment (W. Fuller): One item I did not bring to your attention, but which is very important, is that as cyanide is used and oxidized, nitrate builds up. Nitrate is a mobile anion, as you know, and the hazard may not be cyanide, but nitrate.

Question (F. DeVries): It seems to me that the levels of cyanide we deal with in disposal problems are an order of magnitude or so less than the hazardous level of nitrates. Is that not correct?

Answer (W. Fuller): I have seen ponds with 500 ppm nitrate in the water, and that is a little high for water to be used as recharge.

Question (F. DeVries): We usually talk about cyanide concentrations in water effluents under a part per million, perhaps less than one tenth of a part per million. My understanding is that nitrate concentrations allowable in potable water approach 10 ppm.

Answer (W. Fuller): That's right, but some of these ponds are continually fed and the nitrate concentration builds up.

Question (P. Saletta): Dr. Fuller, concerning the replacement of soils in the final reclamation of cyanide tailings disposal sites, have there been any studies, that you know of, of possible effects on those replaced soils from the solid waste disposal of cyanide tailings?

Answer (W. Fuller): No, but I'm glad you asked that question. One of the important things about this conference is that, although the soil scientists, the biochemists and the civil engineers are most often located in different buildings and often don't cross-inoculate, here we have finally come to the conclusion that we need to work as a team.

Question: Dr. Fuller, would you say there are any naturally-occurring cyanides in lakes or other water bodies that would build up to toxic levels? If so is that taken into consideration in assessing possible spills?

Answer (W. Fuller): None that I know of.

Comment (R. Walline): I have seen detectable levels of 'natural cyanide', but not toxic levels. So in comparison to a spill, it's usually negligible compared to the industrial component.

Question: Dr. Fuller, theoretically speaking, could it occur?

Answer (W. Fuller): I don't see a great possibility for it. Remember that the high reactivity of cyanides, the biological attack on them and so forth, really limits their accumulation in natural environments. On the other hand, I refer you to Dr. Reed's talk on animals which may eat plants that have high amounts of glycosides.

Question: If bacteria exist which can decompose cyanide, is it possible that artificial culture of these bacteria might be an eventual solution to the problem of getting rid of cyanide in our tailings ponds?

Answer (W. Fuller): That is a very important item, but there are problems with inoculation. First, the environmental conditions must be specific for that one organism. I gave you an example of an actinomyces that grows in sewage under anaerobic conditions and will grow on potassium cyanide alone. However, if we have the idea of finding that organism and putting it in other sewage, we have to remember that sewages vary considerably. Nevertheless, it's a good point and I'd like to see more research done on it. We have found in biological pure-culture work that it takes a lot of effort and money to support that kind of work, but I would not rule out the possibility. If I find one, I'm going to patent it.

Comment (R. Walline): To follow up on that, later in the week, Terry Mudder from Homestake Mining Company will be speaking. Homestake Mine is using a biological system--a specific bacteria--to treat mining effluent specifically for cyanide, so there is now a system in place doing just what you suggest.

CONFERENCE ON CYANIDE AND THE ENVIRONMENT
Tucson, Arizona • December 1984
Published by Geotechnical Engineering Program • Colorado State University • Fort Collins, Colorado 80523

CYANIDE COMPOUNDS IN PLANTS AND THEIR EFFECTS ON ANIMALS

by
Raymond E. Reed[1]

ABSTRACT

Varieties of native and cultivated plants consumed by herbivores produce cyanogenic glycosides which release hydrocyanic acid (HCN) upon hydrolysis. HCN is toxic to both plants and animals. In animals it poisons the enzyme cytochrome oxidase, producing cell-level asphyxiation. The presence of HCN in plant tissue or ingesta is detected by a simple qualitative test, and there is an effective antidote applicable in cases recognized in time for treatment.

Consumption of plants of the genus Lathyrus by humans or animals is associated with nervous system degeneration and abnormal bone and joint development, attributed to toxic compounds containing the CN radicle. Observation of similar effects in animals poisoned by lupine and locoweed has prompted an association with lathyrism and the identification of toxic CN compounds in those plants. Finally, observation of lower spinal cord neuron degeneration with stumbling, urinary bladder paralysis and chronic cystitis in horses grazing hybrid sudan grass, has led to speculation that still another disease may be caused by CN-containing substances other than HCN.

REPORT

In the spectrum of health problems affecting animals, infectious diseases are prominent, other causes such as intoxications receiving relatively much less attention. A trend away from this obscurity began with the public's increasing apprehension of toxic substances in the environment. Concern about chemical spills and uncontrolled dumping has prepared the public to recognize and worry about chemical contamination of their food and water supply and to read with alarm about the threat of chemicals contaminating animal feed. In the same category is concern over adverse effects on the consumer of substances fed to animals to promote growth and control disease. Most of us are aware that the Food and Drug Administration is becoming increasingly restrictive in regulating exposure of food animals to antibiotics, hormones, carcinogens, teratogenic substances and other substances potentially hazardous to the consumer. We are less aware that another and far more significant source of intoxicants to both humans and other animals has probably been with us since life began, injuring, killing, producing fetal monsters and leading to cancer, and this source, poisons produced by plants, is subject to no control whatever.

[1] Raymond E. Reed, Professor and Diagnostic Pathologist, Department of Veterinary Science, University of Arizona, Tucson, Arizona.

Not all cyanide compounds are generated in factories or laboratories. It is quite possible that most life threatening cyanide intoxications occur because grazing animals consume plants that have generated cyanogenic glycosides. Such plants are found all over the world in at least 800 plant species representing 70 to 80 families (Smolenski, 1981), including the Leguminosae, some of the most valuable food and forage plants that we cultivate. When liberated from plant tissue as hydrocyanic acid by hydrolysis, cyanide interferes with intracellular oxidation by poisoning the cytochrome oxidase system. Although ample oxygen reaches the cells, it cannot be utilized. The blood remains bright red while the poisoned host dies of cell-level suffocation (Kingsbury, 1964).

Plant species well known for their cyanogenic potential are listed by Kingsbury as follows:

Acacia spp.	catclaw, whitehorn
Bahia oppositifolia	bahia
Cercocarpus spp.	mountain mahogany
Florestina tripteris	florestina
Glyceria striata	fowl mannagrass
Holcus lanatus	velvet grass
Hydrangea spp.	hydrangea
Linum spp.	flax
Lotus corniculatus	birdsfoot trefoil
Manihot esculenta	cassava
Phaseolus lunatus	lima bean
Prunus spp.	cherries
Pyrus malus	apple
Sorghum spp.	Sudan grass, Johnsongrass, etc.
Stillingia treculeana	queen's delight
Suckleya suckleyana	poison suckleya
Trifolium repens	white clover
Triglochin spp.	arrowgrass
Vicia sativa	vetch seed
Zea mays	maize, corn

In addition, Heteromeles arbutifolia (Christmas-berry) is known to be cyanogenic in California.

A second mechanism for intoxication involving compounds containing the CN radicle is less clear-cut, but is associated with the ancient disease of man and animals known as lathyrism after the genus Lathyrus. Poisoning is associated with human consumption of large quantities of peas during times of food shortage or with animals grazing species of plants belonging to the genus Lathyrus, specifically, L. hirsutus, L. incanus, L. pusillus, and L. sylvestris (Kingsbury, 1964). Nervous degeneration and a distortion of the skeleton are associated with intoxication, the mechanism involving interference with the cross-linking of collagen molecules (Smolenski, 1981). Also of interest is the suggested inclusion of locoism and lupinosis in this category of plant poisonings (Keeler, 1967, Shupe, 1967). To the above list of plants we may add:

Astragalus spp.	locoweeds
Lathyrus spp.	peas, vetch
Lupinus spp.	lupine

Clinical manifestation of hydrocyanic acid intoxication depends on the concentration of the substance in plant tissue, the size of the animal, the amount of plant consumed within a given time period and the rate of release after consumption. Cyanide is more likely to be present in and rapidly liberated from plants subject to drought or other cause of wilting or to freezing. It is released with greater speed and in greater quantity in ruminants than in monogastric animals, presumably due to degradation of plant cells by bacterial enzymes. Animals have an impressive ability to detoxify and excrete cyanide (Kingsbury, 1964). Cyanide may react with substances present in rumen contents, creating compounds that aren't absorbed. If all the potential safeguards fail and something in excess of 2 mg HCN per pound of animal is absorbed per hour, death follows within a few minutes to a few hours. When early signs of intoxication go unobserved, owners report animals dropping in their tracks, but usually there is time to observe rapid breathing changing to labored breathing, excitement, disorientation, staggering, prostration, coma and death.

If the owner is present and recognizes the cause of the problem, it is possible to administer an antidote consisting of 1 percent sodium nitrite and 25 percent sodium thiosulfate by vein in 75 - 150 ml. quantities, care being taken to avoid overdosing and producing nitrite poisoning.

The presence of HCN in plant tissue or fresh rumen contents is detected by a simple test. Filter paper strips are dipped in a mixture of 5 percent Na_2CO_3 and 0.5 percent picric acid, allowed to almost dry and then placed in test tubes filled with crushed sample to which a few drops of chloroform have been added. A brick red color develops on the paper within a few to 10 minutes if there is significant cyanide present. Field collection of cyanide-containing plants or rumen contents may lead to false negative tests due to volatility of the substance. Quantitative measurement is seldom made, but plants containing 20 mg HCN per 100 grams are considered at least potentially dangerous (Kingsbury, 1964).

Locoweed poisoning is part of western folklore. The toxic principle was presumed to be an alkaloid in most cases, although some species of the plant were recognized selenium converters. Animals may develop a selective appetite for locoweed, seeking it out even when safe forage is abundant. Locoism is characterized by depression, stupor, abnormal gait, violent behavior, circling, head pressing and falling. Abortion is a common sequel in pregnant females, and fetuses surviving to term may have abnormal skeletal and joint development. Cellular degeneration involves many tissues, and the observation of irreversible nerve cell damage and the production of fetal skeletal defects led to the association with lathyrism (Keeler, 1967). Lathyrism is characterized by nervous degeneration and abnormalities of the skeletal system attributed with fair agreement to substances elaborated from B-cyano-L-alanine (Ressler, 1962).

Consumption of species of lupine by sheep or cattle during certain stages of pregnancy leads to the production of deformed offspring (Shupe, 1967). Alkaloids isolated from lupine were held to be the toxins that produced both nervous disorders and teratogenic effects until it was found that the plants contained the lathyrogenic compound, aminoacetonitrite. This compound has also been identified in locoweed (Keeler, 1967).

A degenerative disease of horses known as sorghum cystitis may also be a result of exposure to cyanide-containing substances occurring in hybrid Sudan grass, and possibly other Sorghum spp. Although plants of this genus produce toxic amounts of HCN, the problem in horses grazing them is characterized by degenerative changes occurring in the lower spinal cord manifest as rear leg ataxia, bladder paralysis and subsequent cystitis. Classical HCN intoxication isn't evident. The cause of the nervous tissue degeneration has been suggested to be lathyrogenic B-cyanoalanine.

There are no antidotes for poisonings attributable to lathyrogenic compounds, and no simple tests to substantiate diagnosis.

The mechanism of cyanogenic glycoside toxicity has been accepted beyond question and the plants producing the phytotoxin are widely recognized. Proof that other compounds containing the CN radicle account for nervous, skeletal and teratogenic disorders associated with lathyrism, locoism, lupinosis and sorghum cystitis remains somewhat tenuous, perhaps because research progress in the field of plant poisonings is slow.

REFERENCES

Keeler, R. F., James, L. F., Binns, W., and Shupe, J. L.: Apparent Relationships Between Locoism and Lathyrism. Canadian J. Comp. Med. and Vet. Sci., 31:334-341, 1967.

Kingsbury, J. M.: Poisonous Plants of the United States and Canada. Prentice-Hall, Inc., Englewood, Cliffs, NJ, 1964.

Ressler, C.: Isolation and Identification From Common Vetch of the Neurotoxin B-cyano-L-alanine, a Possible Factor in Neurolathyrism. J. Biol. Chem., 237:733-735, 1962.

Shupe, J. L., Binns, W., James, L. F., and Keeler, R. F.: Lupine, A Cause of Crooked Calf Disease. J. Am. Vet. Med. Assoc., 151:198-203, 1967.

Smolenski, S. J., Kinghorn, A. D., and Balandrin, M. F.: Toxic Constituents of Legume Forage Plants. Economic Botany, 35:321-355, 1981.

CONFERENCE ON CYANIDE AND THE ENVIRONMENT
Tucson, Arizona • December 1984
Published by Geotechnical Engineering Program • Colorado State University • Fort Collins, Colorado 80523

Role of Cyanide in Gold and Silver Recovery

by

Hans von Michaelis[1]

In December 1884 a group of Americans were excited about progress that they had made in their plans to open a new university, the University of Arizona here in Tucson, which opened its doors to students in 1885. On 12 December 1884, the famous London firm of Johnson Matthey & Co. completed an assay of four samples of ore submitted by three American explorers from a sunbleached patch of veld in the Transvaal - which could then be reached by an almost 1000 mile trek through the desert from Cape Town or 400 miles from Durban through lion infested terrain and inhabited by hostile Zulus. At that time there was no university at all in the whole of continent of Africa. The rock samples assayed over one ounce of gold per ton and resulted in the Struben brothers announcing to President Kruger and the Transvaal Volksraad that a major gold discovery had been made on the Witwatersrand. On 12 December 1885, exactly one year later they started up a battery of stamps purchased from the English firm called Sandcroft financed by a loan of $5,000 from the Transvaal government. The Strubens were mining the Confidence Reef - a quartz vein just north of where the Witwatersrand conglomerates outcropped. In 1884 one of the Struben brothers had tested some Banket rock and found it to be barren. Although they had not found the Witwatersrand reefs their excited claims followed by the first gold production in the area led to an outbreak of gold fever which resulted in the discovery only a year later of the first of the true Witwatersrand ore deposits.

According to ROSENTHALL (1970) more than half the gold reserve of the whole world, 25,000 tons, worth over a quarter of a trillion dollars has been mined during the last hundred years from this small patch of veld in southern Africa. This astonishing area, the richest on the globe, does not owe its wealth to spectacular gold bonanza type deposits, but to the amazing uniformity and size of the deposits laid down 2000 million years ago.

On this unique Rand goldfield, which within human memory was a parched wilderness of rock and grass, has grown the city of Johannesburg with its 1.5 million inhabitants and about twice that many in the region which has become the industrial and financial heartland of South Africa.

Gold and wealth from the Witwatersrand helped to revolutionize the world economy a hundred years ago, during a period like the one we know today when there was such a dearth of exchange media that a financial breakdown was considered a serious possibility.

[1] Hans von Michaelis, Randol International Ltd.,
21578 Mountsfield Drive, Golden, CO 80401, (303) 526-1626.

Although located 10,000 miles across the sea, the Rand influenced American politics in a way that few appreciate today. ROSENTHALL (1970) wrote how it tipped the scale in presidential elections and put an end to the once mighty campaign for bimetallism and "free silver".

The enormous wealth of the Rand embroiled this patch of bush in the international intrigues which led to the Anglo Boer War - in which Baden-Powell invented Boy Scouting, and also in which trench and guerilla warfare and concentration camps were introduced to the world. The importance of this gold resource made the Transvaal one of the colonial prizes which were undoubtedly a contributory cause of the First World War and which today still make this area a focal point of world political economics, but which has also elevated it from third world status.

What does all this have to do with cyanide and its role in gold and silver recovery? Without the discovery and development of the cyanidation process most of the gold of the Witwatersrand would likely never have been recoverable. Cyanide made it possible to treat the deeper unoxidized Witwatersrand ores and those of lower grade. Today four of the forty odd mining complexes on the Witwatersrand individually produce more gold than the USA and Canada combined.

HISTORY OF CYANIDATION

Almost exactly at the same moment as the Strubens began mining the Confidence Reef, another pair of brothers entered into a partnership with important results. Two doctors, Robert and William Forrest joined forces with a self-taught chemist, John S. MacArthur to seek an improved process for recovering gold from "complex" ores (those that did not yield to mercury amalgamation). They experimented for years in a room behind the Forrest brothers' surgery in a Glasgow suburb.

As far back as the 1840's British and other chemists had experimented with the reactions of gold and silver and potassium cyanide, which was already successfully used in silver plating. L. Elsner had published the basic idea of leaching gold in cyanide solution and oxygen in 1846.

$$2Au + 4KCN + O + H_2O \quad = \quad 2AuK\ (CN)_2 + 2KOH$$

Michael Faraday demonstrated the dissolution of gold metal before the Royal Institute in London. In 1867 Julius Ray and Simpson were granted a patent in Washington for "an improved method of treating auriferous and argentiferous ores" which used potassium cyanide.

Not until 1887 did MacArthur discover the secret that made the process work. To achieve practical results the pulp had to be agitated in the presence of air and gold could then be recovered by precipitation with zinc from a separated gold-cyanide solution. For the first time an efficient process existed and in October 1887 British patent No. 14,174 was issued to MacArthur and the Forrests, and another, No. 10,223, on the use of alkali and alkali earth hydroxides for pH modification of the pulp and fine zinc dust for precipitation of gold from cyanide solution immediately thereafter.

Almost immediately the Cassel Gold Extracting Company acquired the rights to the process and placed MacArthur in charge of its metallurgical department. With new financial backing, representatives of the firm went to New Zealand, USA, Chile, British Columbia, India, Mexico, the Straits Settlements and, as it happens, last of all to the Transvaal. According to SHOEMAKER (1984) the first use of cyanide for gold extraction was at the Small Crown Mine in New Zealand in 1889, although the first works on a commercial scale seem to have been at Karangahaki in the same year. It was first applied in the USA at Consolidated Mercur in Utah in 1891.

According to ROSENTHALL (1970) hardly any results flowed from the earlier expeditions, and MacArthur confessed that at first they met with a very chilly response, particularly in America. Only in 1889 did Alfred James of the Cassel Company arrive on the Witwatersrand where he was followed in 1890 by "the Ringleader of the Inventors" as he was jocularly referred to, MacArthur himself. Soon thereafter the Salisbury Gold Mining Company, anxious to outdo its rival, the Robinson Mine, which had a new chlorination plant, placed its mill at his disposal. The results were an immediate success and by the end of that year the Robinson Mine had installed a commercial plant too. Between 1890 and 1893 the production of gold recovered by cyanidation increased by a thousand times to 10 tons per year - and has grown subsequently to around 700 tons per year today.

Meanwhile in 1887 Dr. Werner von Siemens, an eminent electrician from Berlin, while experimenting with electroplating noticed that gold anodes lost weight when immersed in a cyanide liquor without current flowing through the bath. This gave him the idea of using cyanide to leach gold followed by direct electorwinning of gold from the solution. Four large Siemens-Halske plants were installed on the Witwatersrand in direct competition with the MacArthur process which used zinc precipitation after cyanidation. However, steadily the MacArthur cyanidation and zinc precipitation process proved its superior practicability. In 1889 the world consumption of cyanide was less than 50 tons per year. In 1905 consumption was about 10,000 tons of which the Transvaal gold fields took about one-third.

Leaders of the gold industry in• the Transvaal decided to challenge the validity of patents No. 47 and 74 issued in Pretoria on which rested the MacArthur Forrest claims to royalties. Without going into details of what until recently was the most expensive and drawn out legal battle in South African history, the result was that in 1896 the MacArthur-Forrest patents were disallowed and the inventors not only lost all rights to royalties, but were saddled with costs of litigation estimated at about $1 million. MacArthur died a poor man in 1920. Long after his role has been summed up by leading South African chemists: "Though he was deprived of the material prosperity that should have been his, through the agency of the law courts, yet his service was one of merit. The greater part of new developments in metallurgy destined to increase the world's stock of gold, is to recover gold from ores of poorer, and yet poorer value. There would have been no known method of working these low grade ores but for the discovery of the cyanide process in Glasgow in 1887 by John Stewart MacArthur and the brothers Forrest."

This statement could not be more true today as we see the expansion that is taking place in the exploitation of low grade surface gold and silver deposits in North America and abroad. Very low grade disseminated deposits are made into profitable ventures by the new heap leaching process. Although there have been many attempts, I know of no process other than cyanidation which is more applicable to heap leaching. Ores with 1 part per million (0.03 oz/st) and less are economical using the cyanide leach process, and a huge new horizon has been opened up for the creation of new wealth in many parts of the world.

At the end of the last century when the realm of chemical processes was scoured to find a better way to recover gold from "refractory" ores, none was found that came close to being as suitable as cyanidation. In those days "refractory" meant refractory to amalgamation - and a whole string of technologies were tested. The deeper Witwatersrand ore associated with pyrite yielded only about 30% of its gold to amalgamation. The chlorination process was an improvement yielding 60% or so recovery. Cyanidation today recovers about 97-98%. In those days the incentive to find a better process was first to find a way to treat the deeper ores and then to find a way around the expensive royalties demanded for the MacArthur-Forrest cyanidation process.

CYANIDE AND THE ENVIRONMENT

Today, the search for better non-cyanide processes goes on. Now the incentive is to find ways to recover gold from "refractory" gold and silver ores - but the meaning has changed - "Refractory" today means not amenable to cyanidation, a process which has become standard practice. Another "incentive" lies in the misplaced perception of environmental objections to the use of cyanide which are the subject of this symposium and which threaten to become part of regulatory limitations. I say "misplaced" because the impact of mineral processing on the environment comes in two kinds with greatly different consequences. There are some aspects of mining and mineral processing which can sometimes have long term impact on the environment. Acid mine drainage is one such problem where technology is needed to avoid the need for perpetual treatment. However other aspects of mineral processing are at worst temporary in nature - when the operation ceases, so the environment quickly repairs itself leaving no permanent scars. The use of cyanide which is biodegradable belongs to this category. Although every effort must be taken to prevent damage to aquatic life, where applicable, during the life of cyanidation operations, it is clear that there are far more serious environmental problems that need to be addressed before becoming concerned about the cyanide non-problem which is to be discussed in detail at this symposium.

From Table 1 it is seen that about 41% of the cyanide consumed in gold and silver recovery is consumed in South Africa where about two thirds of the "free" world gold is produced. In South Africa all this cyanide consumption takes place in a few localized, highly concentrated mining areas on the fringes of the Witwatersrand basin - by perhaps 40 mining operations. Several of these are located in periurban environments and some of the older operations in fact were right on Main Street, Johannesburg where the conglomerate ore outcropped.

Numerous large tailings piles are to be seen in the environs of Johannesburg and other more recent Witwatersrand cities such as Welkom, Stilfontein and Klerksdorp. A recent trend has been to treat these dumps - some for the second time - in order to recover more gold and uranium as well as the real estate. It could be expected that with so much cyanide consumed in such a concentrated area that this would be a good place to examine for environmental impact. It is interesting to note that when the reworking of the Johannesburg dumps was first proposed a society was formed for the preservation of mill tailings which had become excellent wildlife refuges and which provided some relief to an otherwise featureless terrain.

Although mining and mineral processing may contribute to the deterioration in quality of Johannesburg's water supply, the problem lies in dissolved salt buildup e.g., calcium sulfate which can only be removed by expensive desalination processes. Cyanide in the Witwatersrand environment is not considered a major problem. It is true that the Witwatersrand climate may have a lot to do with this as will be discussed in more detail later in these sessions.

Water Management and Treatment technologies for cyanide are discussed at length later in this symposium and by RANDOL (1985).

TABLE I

Approximate Consumption of Cyanide in Gold and Silver Recovery

	Tons/d Ore Treated	Kg Cyanide/t	Tons Cyanide/year
Canada (1985 est.)	35,000	0.45	5,800
South Africa	300,000	0.28	30,800
Total "Free" World		0.40 est.	75,000

CYANIDE AND OPERATOR SAFETY

Although cyanide is lethal to humans if misused it is also relatively easy to handle safely. This reagent is routinely used in metallurgical operations in all the major gold mining camps of the world without a history of accidents, even where unskilled labor is employed. The fine safety record of gold and silver mines with respect to cyanide speaks for itself, although it is a reagent which must be treated with respect. Vendors are always happy to provide informed training sessions such as the one that was provided here yesterday.

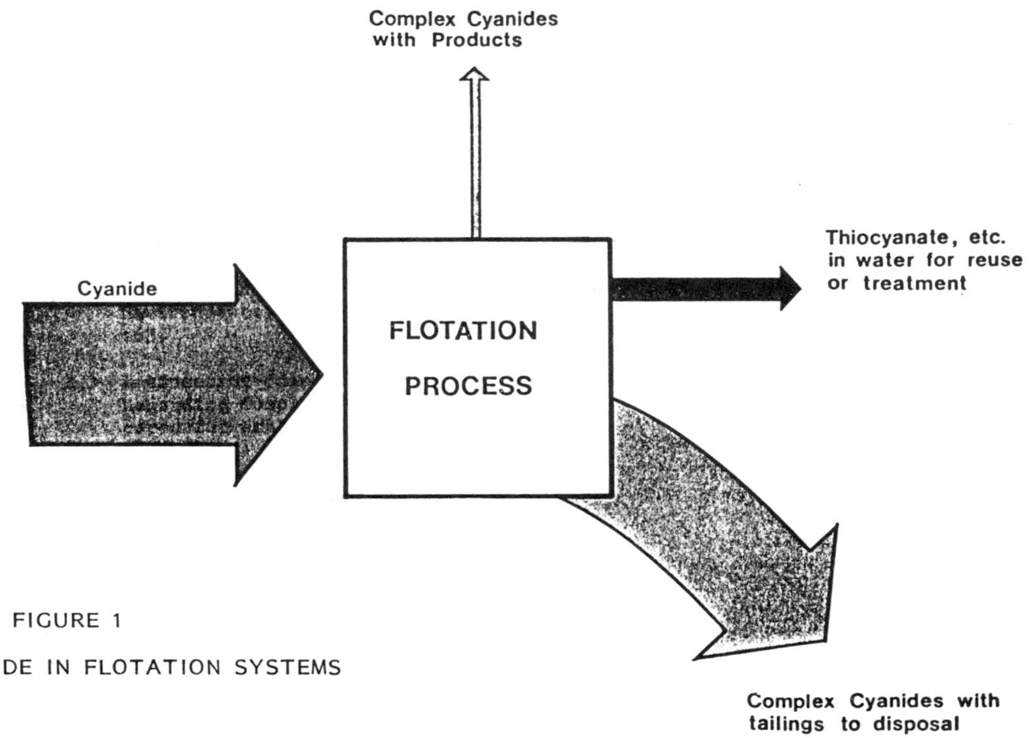

FIGURE 1

FATE OF CYANIDE IN FLOTATION SYSTEMS

Source: AMAX OF CANADA (1980)

TABLE 2

ESTIMATED MAXIMUM PROBABLE
CONCENTRATION OF CYANIDE TAILINGS

Plant No.	Mine Type	Cyanide Added lb/ton	Ore Processed tons/day	Probable Concentration of Cyanide in Tailings ppm
A	Cu/Mo	0	60,000	0
B	Cu/Mo/Ag	0	92,000	0
C	Cu	0	50,000	0
D	Cu	0	42,000	0
E[2]				
F[2]	Cu/Mo/Others	0.02	105,000	5
G[2]				
H[4]	Lead/Zinc/Cu	0.05	5,000	10
I[4]	Lead/Zinc/Cu	0.05	7,500	10
J[4]	Lead/Zinc/Cu	0.05	5,000	10
K[4]	Lead/Zinc/Cu	0.05	2,500	10
L	Lead/Zinc/Cu	0.02	4,200	1
M	Lead/Zinc	0.01	6,500	5
N	Zinc/Copper	0.1	7,000	35
O[3]	Zinc	0.0-0.02	6,500	5
P[3]	Zinc	0.0-0.02	3,200	5
Q[3]	Zinc	0.0-0.02	1,900	10

1. Data from US EPA Contract No. 68-03-2552.
2. Plants E, F and G reported as one facility
3. Intermittent usage; estimated using ore feed as tailings estimate since ore: Tailings ratio is approximately 1:1.
4. Suppress zinc and iron; zinc recovered due to intermittent iron suppression.

Source: AMAX ESI (1980)

FIGURE 2 CYANIDE CONTENT OF VARIOUS MATERIALS

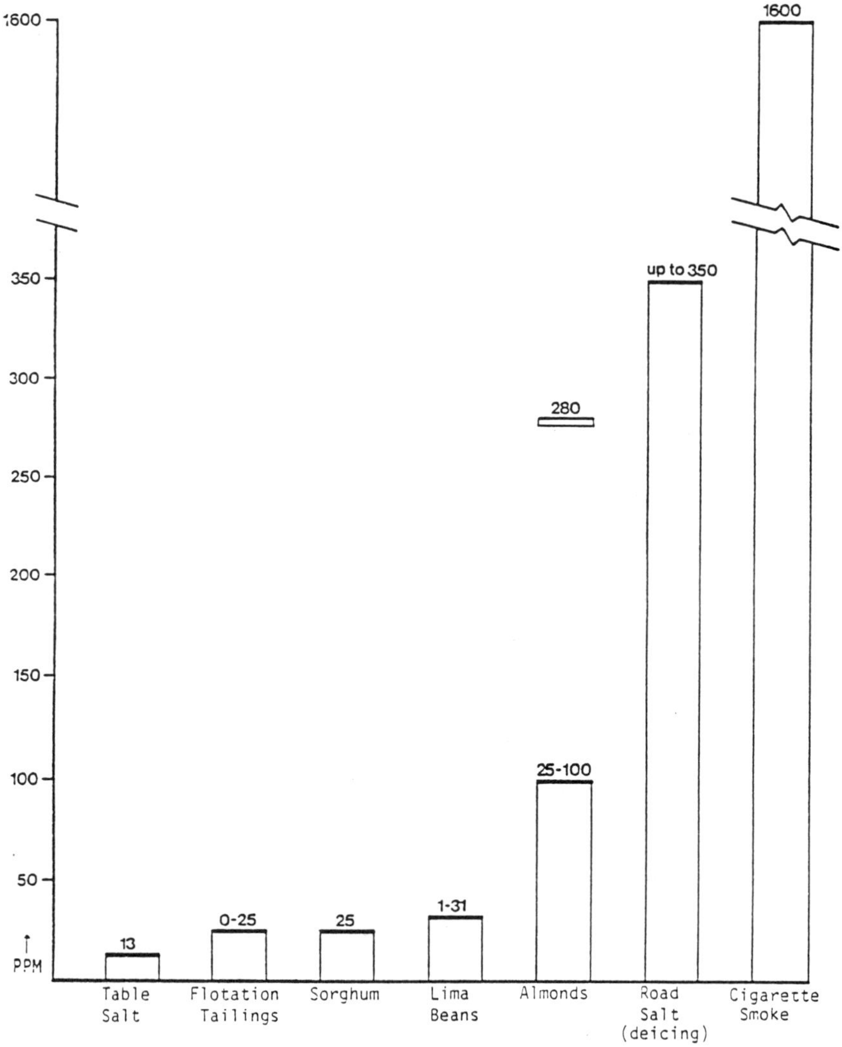

Source: AMAX OF CANADA (1980)

CYANIDE APPLICATIONS IN GOLD AND SILVER RECOVERY

Flotation

In addition to its use as a lixiviant for gold and silver from ores, cyanide is also used in flotation plants where low level additions allow pyrite to be effectively depressed while other sulfide minerals are floated. It is also an excellent depressant in the separation of copper and molybdenum sulfides, however in this paper on the role of cyanide in the recovery of gold and silver, it is the use of cyanide in the recovery and separation of metal concentrates from complex sulfides containing silver which is of interest. Very much more silver is recovered with flotation concentrates of base metals copper, lead and zinc than by primary recovery processes such as cyanide leaching.

AMAX OF CANADA LTD. (1980) and AMAX ENVIRONMENTAL SERVICES INC. (1980) reviewed information of the concentration of complex cyanides in such flotation tailings. Table 2 presents a summary of their findings.

In order to place this concentration in perspective, a complex cyanide (sodium ferrocyanide) is approved for use in table salt at a level of 13 ppm and road salts spread on highways as deicers contain up to 350 parts per million of complex cyanides (sodium ferrocyanide and ferric ammonium cyanide).

Since cyanide used in selective flotation processes is carefully controlled by metering in weak solutions to selectively react with the surface of a small portion of the ore, it is improbable that concentrations of complex cyanides would vary significantly from those indicated in Table 2. Furthermore, since some cyanides are converted in the flotation circuit by oxidation to cyanates or thiocyanates and may not report to the tailings, and due to other factors, these estimates are likely to be high.

Figure 2 shows the relative concentration of cyanide in common materials as a method of gauging the relative concentration in flotation tailings which this author considers also to be a non-problem.

Gold and Silver Cyanide Leaching

There are three main approaches to gold and silver cyanidation. Conventional, CIP/CIL and Heap Leaching are schematically portrayed in Fig. 3. There are numerous pitfalls and innovations involved in recovering gold and silver from different ore-types; these are discussed in great detail by RANDOL (1982,1985).

The older process still referred to as the "conventional" approach uses an alkaline cyanide agitation leach followed by a solid-liquid step (filtration or CCD) to recover a gold and silver cyanide pregnant solution. The pregnant solution is then vacuum de-aerated and gold and silver are recovered by zinc precipitation followed by filtration. The filtrate after gold and silver recovery is referred to as "barren solution" and since it still contains valuable cyanide and lime values it is usually recycled to the leaching and filter wash steps of the process.

1. CONVENTIONAL LEACH-MERRILL CROWE Zn PRECIPITATION

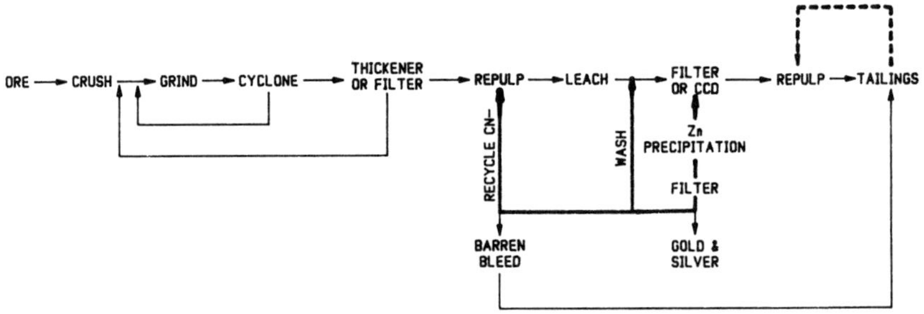

2. CARBON-IN-PULP

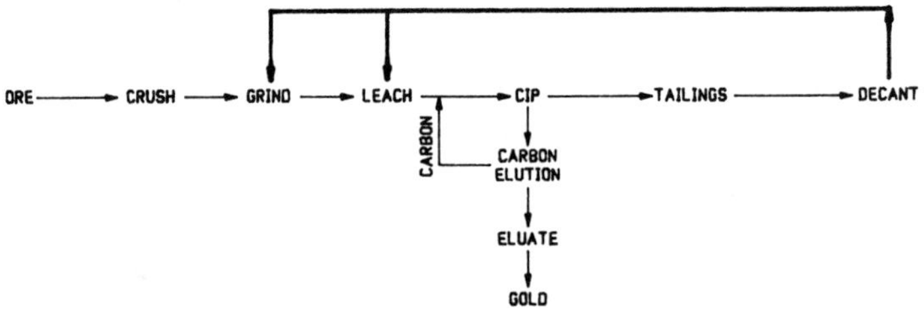

3. HEAP LEACHING

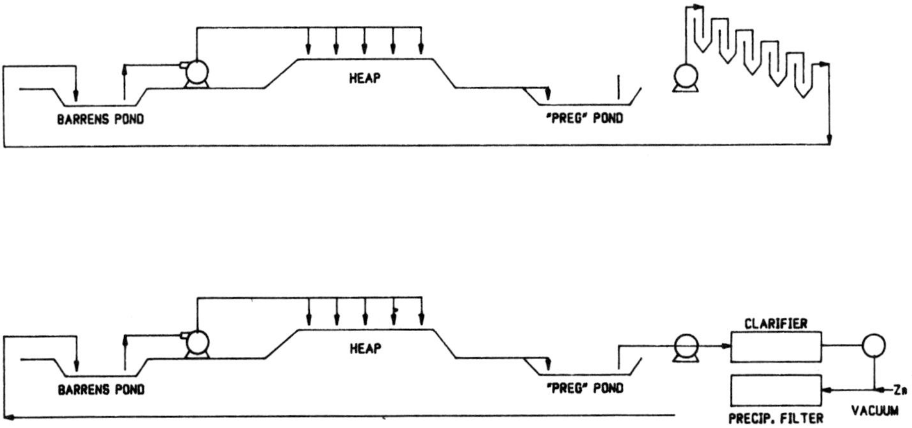

FIGURE 3

The tailings are repulped in fresh or tailings reclaim water and pumped to a tailings impoundment. In this process arrangement most of the cyanide is usually recycled to the process which means that very little reaches the tailings pond. However, since base metals also dissolve in the cyanide leach solution, if these are present in the ore in cyanide soluble form then their levels build up in the recirculated cyanide solutions until they might interfere with leaching and precipitation of gold and silver to a point where a barren bleed must be discarded. In a conventional process arrangement typical water consumption is around 0.75 m^3 new water per ton ore, but this varies up or down depending on impurities in the ore and the availabilty of water.

Silver ores are still most often treated by the "conventional" process and gold ores are now more often than not treated by the newer carbon-in-pulp or carbon-in-leach process.

Carbon-in-pulp/Carbon-in-leach

CIP and CIL are more applicable to gold recovery than to most silver ore treatment arrangements. In CIP ore is agitation leached in cyanide solution followed by recovery of gold by adsorption onto activated charcoal. In CIL the leaching and carbon adsorption steps are performed in the same agitated tanks usually because the ore contains a preg-robbing species. In CIP and CIL arrangements there is a major difference as far as cyanide management is concerned in that there is no solid liquid separation step to recover a barren solution to be recycled. All cyanide in the pulp leaving the CIP or CIL circuit goes to the tailings pond with the tailings. Only after decantation in the pond is reclaim water recovered and reused. During the residence time of the solution in the tailings pond generally more cyanide values will be lost through natural degradation in the pond than in the conventional process. For this reason CIP consumption of cyanide is generally considerably more than in the conventional process.

Heap Leaching

In heap leaching cyanide is either added to a crushed ore during the agglomeration stage or it is added in a dilute solution that is irrigated over the heaps.

The crushed (and often agglomerated) ore is leached over an impermeable leach pad which serves to collect the pregnant solution containing gold and silver values which are collected in a "preg pond" and recovered either by carbon adsorption in columns or by zinc precipitation after clarification and deaeration of the pregnant solution.

Heap leaching is generally more water efficient than the other processes and also uses less cyanide, but it takes a lot longer. The fate of cyanide in leached heaps is a separate topic to be discussed at this symposium.

The processes by which gold and silver are leached by cyanide are well known and appear in several texts on cyanidation such as JULIAN & SMART (1909), CLENNELL (1915), HAMILTON (1920), DORR (1936), KING(1949) and ADAMSON (1972). They are not repeated here.

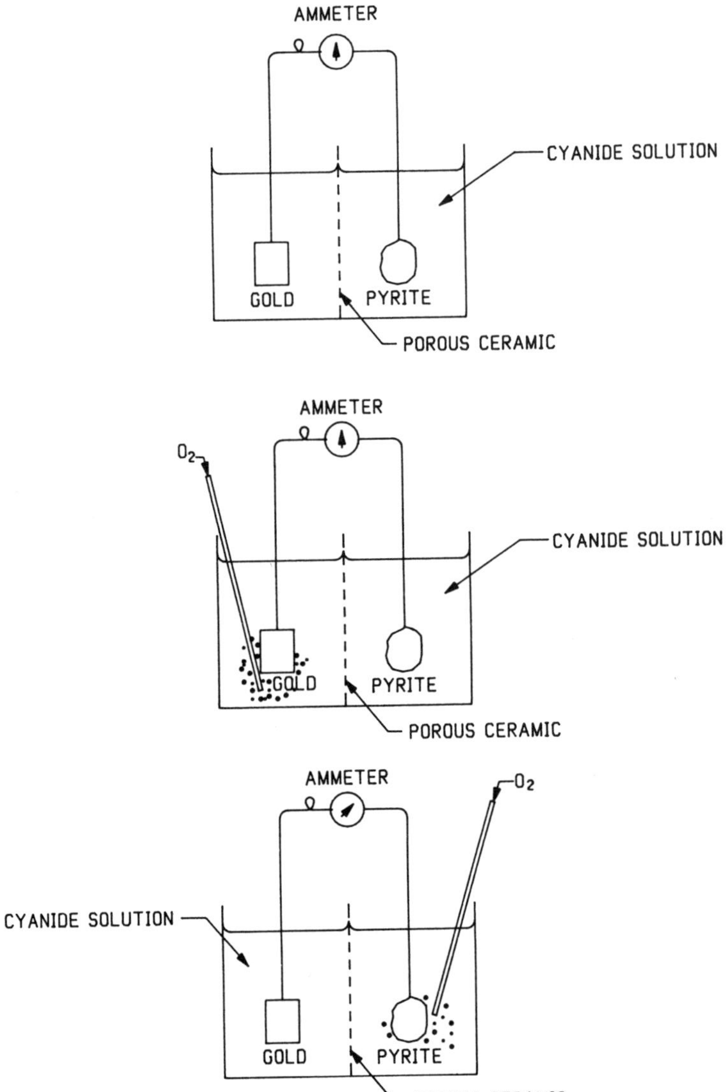
AMMETER
CYANIDE SOLUTION
GOLD
PYRITE
POROUS CERAMIC
AMMETER
O_2
CYANIDE SOLUTION
GOLD
PYRITE
POROUS CERAMIC
AMMETER
O_2
CYANIDE SOLUTION
GOLD
PYRITE
POROUS CERAMIC

FIGURE 4

An interesting observation of the mechanism of cyanidation however was described by JULIAN and SMART (1915) in which a particle of gold and one of pyrite are submerged in a cyanide solution but separated by a porous membrane. The two particles are connected by an electrical conduit as shown in Fig. 4 into which an ammeter is inserted. The ammeter immediately shows that the gold is leaching by indicating the flow of electrons through the conductor, but the needle soon returns to neutral indicating that the reaction has ceased. By introducing a flow of oxygen beneath the gold particle, the reaction does not start again as might be expected from Elsner's equation. However, if the oxygen stream is directed to flow past the pyrite particle, the reaction immediately starts again. Clearly there is more to leaching gold by cyanide than meets the eye. A simple explanation for this phenomenon is provided by RANDOL (1982) which also provides a possible explanation of enhanced leach rates sometimes observed in the sonic leach process.

CONCLUSIONS

Just as the University of Arizona looks forward to another 100 years of good service to the community and mankind, so will cyanide remain the preferred reagent for gold recovery. Long after the gold reserves of the Witwatersrand and other present day mines have been depleted, cyanidation will be in use in gold and silver recovery.

In many parts of the world, particularly where zero discharge of effluents cannot be achieved because rainfall exceeds evaporation, in colder climates where natural degradation is slow, it is becoming mandatory to destroy cyanide in effluents before they can be discharged. There are relatively high costs associated with the destruction of cyanide in such cases. Although it is likely that less costly ways will be developed to destroy cyanide in effluents, the added cost of cyanide destruction adds to the incentive to find ways of recovering it for reuse, or to control its addition carefully in the first place.

There is a moral to the historical account of the role of cyanide in gold and silver recovery. That is, if one happens to be tempted to develop and patent a metallurgical process, make sure that the royalties requested from users are modest and not large enough to justify too extensive a search into the past, because almost invariably it will be found that someone had the same idea before you.

JULIAN and SMART (1909) produced what is probably the most interesting book on gold cyanidation ever written to describe numerous detailed experiments that they performed with cyanide. One of them was run over by a bus and the other, Smart, had the misfortune of being murdered by an African mineworker not long thereafter. Both died prematurely before they could complete their life's work. Somehow I've always felt that the unfortunate story of Julian and Smart holds a special message for this symposium.

REFERENCES

ADAMSON, R. J. Ed. (1972) Gold Metallurgy in South Africa, Chamber of Mines of South Africa.

AMAX ENVIRONMENTAL SERVICES, INC. (1980) A Compilation of Pertinent Information Regarding Complexed Cyanides in Mineral Flotation Tailings, July 1980.

AMAX OF CANADA, LTD. (1980) Background Information of Cyanide/Mining/Environment. Data presented in support of permit application for a mine-mill complex in British Columbia.

CLENNELL, J. (1915) The Cyanide Handbook, McGraw Hill, New York.

DORR, J. & BOSQUI, F. L. (1936) Cyanidation and Concentration of Gold and Silver Ores. McGraw Hill, New York.

HAMILTON, E. (1920) Manual of Cyanidation, McGraw Hill, New York.

KING, A. Ed. (1949) Gold Metallurgy on the Witwatersrand, Transvaal Chamber of Mines.

JULIAN, H. F. & SMART, E. (1909) Cyaniding Gold and Silver Ores.

RANDOL INTERNATIONAL LTD. (1982) Innovations in Gold and Silver Recovery Phase II, Multi-Client Report.

RANDOL INTERNATIONAL LTD. (1985) Water Management and Treatment Technology for Mining and Metallurgical Operations, Multi-client study in final stages.

RANDOL INTERNATIONAL LTD. (1985) Innovations in Gold and Silver Recovery Phase III, Multi-client report in preparation. Randol International Ltd., 21578 Mountsfield Drive, Golden, CO 80401, (303) 526-1626.

ROSENTHALL, ERIC (1970) "Gold! The Johannesburg Gold Rush," McMillan Co., New York.

SHOEMAKER, R. S. (1984) Gold. Proc. of Conference on Precious Metals: Mining, Extraction and Processing, Ed. Kudryk, N. et al., Metallurgical Society of AIME, Los Angeles, 27-29 February 1984.

CONFERENCE ON CYANIDE AND THE ENVIRONMENT
Tucson, Arizona • December 1984
Published by Geotechnical Engineering Program • Colorado State University • Fort Collins, Colorado 80523

CYANIDE FROM MINERAL PROCESSING: PROBLEMS AND RESEARCH NEEDS

By J. L. Huiatt[1]

ABSTRACT

Lack of reliable technical information on the use of, and possible hazards associated with, cyanide in precious metal processing and mineral froth flotation processes is of concern to the mining industry, regulatory agencies, and the general public. Technical representatives from the mining community, Government research groups, regulatory agencies, and academia participated in a workshop to help resolve this problem. The workshop identified problems and research needs, discussed the state of technology, and provided information pertinent to cyanide use in the mineral industry. The areas where more technical information and study are needed include (1) the analytical chemistry of cyanide as it relates to the mining industry, (2) laboratory, field, and literature investigations on the ultimate disposition of cyanide compounds to aid in decisionmaking on environmental control and regulation, (3) the toxic nature of cyanide-bearing compounds, other than free cyanides, formed through mining and milling operations, and (4) the toxic nature of the total effluent from mineral processing operations.

This paper reviews the current status of the identified problems and research efforts associated with the use of cyanide in the mining industry.

INTRODUCTION

When one considers the extensive use of cyanides by the U. S. industry, particularly the mining industry, and then reads reports that have preconceived notions that cyanide by definition is bad, one is hard-pressed to explain the small number of incidents of adverse impact on the environment. Many chemicals that are used today and find their way into the environment have received little study. Cyanide and its numerous compounds and reaction products are among the possible environmental pollutants about which insufficient scientific information is known.

To help resolve the problem, a workshop on cyanide use in mineral processing was held in Salt Lake City, UT, on February 2-3, 1982. The workshop was sponsored by the mineral industry, supporting industries, the Interior Department's Bureau of Mines, and the National Science

[1] Research supervisor, Salt Lake City Research Center, Bureau of Mines, U. S. Department of the Interior, Salt Lake City, UT.

Foundation through the Utah Mining and Mineral Resources Research Institute, College of Mines, University of Utah. The National Science Foundation and the Bureau of Mines provided the basic grant for the support of the workshop. The participants were technical representatives from the mining community, Government research groups, Government regulatory agencies, and academia.

The workshop focused on use of cyanide as it relates to the gold and silver mining industry and froth flotation processes employed by mineral mining companies. Its intent was to discuss state of technology and provide information pertinent to the use of cyanide in the mineral industry. No attempt was made to advocate regulatory limits or set policy governing the use of cyanide. The principal topics of discussion were (1) the chemistry and use of cyanides, (2) control and treatment of cyanide mining wastes, (3) toxicity of mining wastes, (4) fate of cyanide in the environment, and (5) the analytical chemistry of cyanide.

From the workshop discussions, the problems associated with cyanide use in the mining industry and areas where technical information is insufficient were identified. Research required to understand and resolve possible adverse environmental problems was also identified. A proceedings of the workshop was published (Huiatt et al., 1983).

CYANIDE IN MINING RESIDUES

The principal uses of cyanide in the mining industry occur in gold and silver cyanidation processing and froth flotation processing.

CYANIDATION

The most common method used in milling of gold is cyanidation. The basic principle of cyanidation is that the cyanide ion forms very stable complexes with gold, silver, and other metals. Gold dissolution occurs in an aqueous solution by the ionic reaction

$$4Au + 8CN^{-} + O_2 + 2H_2O \rightleftharpoons 4Au(CN)_2^{-} + 4OH^{-}.$$

The rate of dissolution depends on cyanide concentration, oxygen availability, and solution pH. Optimum cyanide concentration is about 0.05 pct, and optimum pH is 10.3. The most efficient leaching occurs when the ore contains clean free fine-sized gold particles and no cyanicide impurities that may destroy cyanide or inhibit its reaction. Cyanidation is applied in (1) heap leaching of low-grade ores, (2) standard countercurrent decantation (CCD), leaching, and (3) carbon-in-pulp (CIP) leaching.

Many gold mining companies design their processes to use recycled waste solutions and thus avoid discharging the wastes, whereas others design their processes to discharge treated wastes. Two principal cyanide-containing streams are discharged from conventional gold mills: waste barren solutions and leached tailings slurry. As a result of tailings backfill operations, some mine waters may also contain sufficient cyanide to be a concern if discharged. The waste streams may contain free cyanide and metal cyanide complexes of copper, iron, nickel, and zinc, as well as reaction products of sulfur (from sulfide minerals) and cyanide, e.g., S^{2-}, $S_2O_3^{2-}$, SCN^-, CNO^-, NH_3, etc. Other compounds soluble in alkaline solutions (arsenic, antimony, silica, etc.) may also be present.

FLOTATION

In the flotation of base metal sulfide ores, cyanide and cyanide complexes are often added as depressants. In lead-zinc separations, cyanide is added to prevent the activation of sphalerite while galena is being floated. Similarly, cyanide is used to prevent sphalerite flotation in copper-zinc mineral separations. In copper-lead separations, copper minerals are depressed with cyanide. In copper-molybdenum separations, chalcocite is depressed with ferrocyanide and cyanide. Cyanide is added to leach residual copper from molybdenum concentrates. In copper-iron separations, pyrite depression is achieved at high pH through cyanide additions.

The principal cyanide-bearing waste from froth flotation processing is the final tailing slurry. The aqueous phase of the slurry may contain free cyanide and complex metal-cyanide compounds and other chemicals, such as reaction products of sulfur and cyanide and mineral dissolution products. The solid phase of the slurry may contain physically and chemically adsorbed cyanide compounds. The aqueous phase is of some concern if it is discharged.

FORM OF CYANIDE IN MINING WASTES

A large variety of cyanide compounds and their derivatives are present in barren solutions and waste effluents. They can be broadly classified as free cyanides, simple cyanides, and complex cyanides. Scott (1981) distinguishes these compounds as free cyanide, simple compounds (readily soluble and relatively insoluble), weak complexes, moderately strong complexes, and strong complexes.

Free cyanide in solution is the total concentration of CN^- and HCN. The relative amounts of CN^- and HCN in solution are predicted by the relationship

$$CN^- + H_2O \rightleftharpoons HCN + OH^-.$$

The relationship is strongly dependent on solution pH. At pH 9.36, which is equal to the pKa of HCN, the concentration of HCN and CN^- are equal. At pH values below pH 9.36, most of the free cyanide occurs as HCN. In natural waters HCN is the dominant species.

Simple cyanides are represented by the formula $A(CN)_x$, where A is an alkali or a metal and x, the valence of A, represents the number of cyano groups present. The alkali cyanides ionize to release cyanide ions according to the reaction

$$A(CN)_x \rightleftharpoons A^{+x} + xCN^-.$$

Solubility is influenced by pH. Upon hydrolysis of cyanide ion, subsequent behavior would be the same as for HCN.

The complex alkali-metallic cyanides can be represented by the formula $A_yM(CN)_x$, where A is the alkali, y is the number of alkalies, M is the heavy metal (ferric or ferrous iron, cadmium, copper, nickel, silver, etc.), and x is the number of CN groups. The value of x is equal to the valence of A taken y times plus the valence of the heavy metal. The soluble complex cyanides dissociate into the complex ion $M(CN)_x$ rather than the CN group by the reaction

$$A_yM(CN)_x \rightleftharpoons yA^{+x} + [M(CN)_x]^{-yw},$$

where w is the oxidation state of A in the original molecule. The complex ion may undergo further dissociation, releasing cyanide ion.

Although a simple equation may be written to describe the dissociation of a complex cyanide ion, the actual process involves a number of intermediate reactions which may be important. A rate limiting reaction among the intermediates may prevent rapid dissociation in water. Two factors influencing dissociation rate are pH and concentration of other reactants.

The relative stabilities of metal cyanide complexes are shown in table 1. The complexes are listed in relative increasing order of stability. As cyanide complexes become more stable, less "free" cyanide is formed in aqueous wastes. However, if total cyanide must be reduced in final wastes, treatment becomes a serious and expensive problem due to extreme stability of strong complexes such as $Fe(CN)_6^{4-}$, and $Co(CN)_6^{4-}$.

TABLE 1. - Relative stabilities of cyanide complexes in water

Term	Examples present in gold and silver processing solutions
1. Free cyanide	CN^-, HCN
2. Simple compounds	
a. Readily soluble	NaCN, KCN, $Ca(CN)_2$, $Hg(CN)_2$
b. Relatively insoluble	$Zn(CN)_2$, CuCN, $Ni(CN)_2$, AgCN
3. Weak complexes	$Zn(CN)_4^{2-}$, $Cd(CN)_3^-$, $Cd(CN)_4^{2-}$
4. Moderately strong complexes	$Cu(CN)_2^-$, $Cu(CN)_3^{2-}$, $Ni(CN)_4^{2-}$, $Ag(CN)_2^-$
5. Strong complexes	$Fe(CN)_6^{4-}$, $Co(CN)_6^{4-}$, $Au(CN)_2^-$

Source: Adapted from Scott 1981

The form in which cyanide occurs in flotation and cyanidation process tailings impoundments is not well defined. The cyanide may be chemically or physically adsorbed on tailing gangue mineral surfaces and/or it may have reacted with metallic and nonmetallic constituents in tailings to produce cyano complexes and cyanates at the mineral surfaces or in the interstitial solutions. Each cyanide form influences or changes the environmental impact in different ways, and the treatment methods to mitigate environmental problems vary accordingly.

CONTROL AND TREATMENT

IN-PROCESS CONTROL

In-process control methods can reduce cyanide concentrations in mining effluents and thus mitigate the potential for adverse environmental impacts and treatment costs to the operator. Methods for reducing the amount of cyanide to be treated include (1) decrease the waste volume, (2) control process conditions tightly to minimize cyanide additions, and (3) control and reduce other process stream constituents that may consume reagents that eliminate cyanide and its derivatives.

Reduction in volume of water to be treated may be achieved by segregating waste streams and rerouting process solutions within the mill facility. Ingles and Scott (1981) recommend that as far as possible, untreated barren solutions should be recycled to cyanidation and treated barren solutions should be used for washing filter cakes, repulping tailings, and floor washing. Total recycle of all solutions is not possible in all cases because impurity levels build up and inhibit mill processes.

The cyanide content of the effluent water can be reduced by improved feeding and monitoring of cyanide in both cyanidation and flotation processes. Adding excessive amounts of reagents is a common occurrence in many milling operations, particularly small operations where control instrumentation is inadequate and reagent additions are "eye-balled." The practice reduces product grade and recovery and increases production and water treatment costs.

Polysulfides and polythionates (produced by oxidation of sulfide minerals present in base metal and precious metal ores) may react with free cyanide to form thiocyanate according to the reactions:

$$S_x^{2-} + CN^- \rightleftharpoons [S_{x-1}]^{2-} + SCN^- \quad \text{and}$$

$$S_2O_3^{2-} + CN^- \rightleftharpoons SO_3^{2-} + SCN^-.$$

Minimizing thiocyanate formation is particularly important because it consumes greater quantities of reagents used in oxidative treatment of cyanide wastes, reduces the gold dissolution rate (McCreedy et al. 1961), and increases cyanide consumption. Ammonium ion also consumes reagents used in the oxidative destruction of cyanide and must be removed.

ALTERNATE REAGENTS

Obviously, substitution of alternate depressants in flotation or alternate lixiviants for precious metal recovery would reduce waste water treatment costs. However, because of economical and technical problems, only limited use has been made of these substitutes.

Mezey and Neuerdorf (1981) evaluated 14 pyrite depressants, including heavy metals, reducing agents, oxidizing agents, and a lignin derivative. The reagents were tested by bench-scale flotation of chalcopyrite, copper-lead-zinc, and zinc ores. The three most promising depressants, with respect to environmental effects, flotation selectivity, stage of development, and costs, were sodium sulfide, sodium thiosulfate, and sodium sulfite. Reagent consumptions for the sulfide, thiosulfate, and sulfite are generally higher than for cyanide depressants. Also cyanide reagents still may have to be added to achieve optimum flotation selectivity and product grade. Consequently, the cost effectiveness of using non-cyanide-type depressants in selected sulfide mineral separations is still very much open to debate.

Notwithstanding waste water treatment problems, sodium cyanide is the most cost effective lixiviant for gold and silver. Leaching gold and silver ores with substitute reagents, such as thiourea and thiosulfate, produces excellent metal recoveries; however, reagent consumptions and costs are considerably higher. When treatment of cyanide-bearing effluents becomes too costly, these substitute reagents can be applied. Thiourea and thiosulfate reagents are being tested in pilot operations in the United States, South Africa, and Canada, but results of these tests are unavailable. A small gold mine in British Columbia is building a mill that will use thiourea for leaching. Juneau Mining Company, Juneau, AK, will leach precious metals from old tailings and ores using thiourea.

TREATMENT OF CYANIDE MINING WASTES

A literature review describing mine effluent treatment techniques and cyanide removal was done by Ingles and Scott (1981) and Homestake Mining Company. The information is also summarized in the Proceedings of the Workshop-Cyanide From Mineral Processing by Huiatt et al. (1983). The methods are organized into seven categories: (1) natural degradation, (2) oxidation processes, (3) acidification-volatilization-reneutralization, (4) adsorption processes, (5) electrolytic processes, (6) conversion to less toxic forms, and (7) biological treatment. Natural degradation, oxidation, and biological treatment are of particular interest.

Natural Degradation

Schmidt, Simovic, and Shannon (1981) of Environment Canada reported on the natural degradation of cyanide in a waste barren pond. Barren solution from mill tailings was bled into a holding pond from October to March. The cyanide, pH, thiocyanate, cyanate, temperature, and suspended solids were monitored from March through August. Total cyanide, weakly dissociated cyanide, and free cyanide methods, as described by Conn (1981), were used to analyze cyanides. The results of the monitoring program follow: (1) Cyanide content decreased from 65 ppm in March to 0.05 ppm in August, (2) pH dropped from 10.5 to 7.0, (3) pH drop was due to natural carbonation and hydrolysis of thiocyanate,

(4) over 90 pct of the cyanide decrease was attributed to volatilization of molecular HCN, and (5) some photodecomposition of ferrocyanides occurred. The results are extremely important because they show that cyanide does not persist in the environment; consequently, long-term environmental problems may be negligible.

Oxidation Processes

Alkaline chlorination is the most highly developed of all techniques for treating cyanide wastes. The method has some serious disadvantages, namely, (1) reagent costs are high, (2) toxic chlorine derivatives can form, (3) cyanide is not recovered, (4) hexacyanoferrates are not decomposed, (5) metals are not recovered, and (6) residual excess chlorine can be toxic to aquatic species.

Many methods under development are designed to prevent problems that may occur when using chlorination. One such method is the INCO process recently developed by the International Nickel Company (Devuyst, Ettel, and Borbely, 1982). The method rapidly removes cyanide and metal-cyanide species by oxidation of effluents using a mixture of SO_2 in air (2.5 pct) at pH 9 in the presence of a small amount of copper catalyst. Iron cyanide is removed by precipitation as copper or zinc ferrocyanides. Thiocyanate, which is relatively nontoxic, does not decompose; consequently, it is not removed. The method is now being used successfully to treat cyanides from waste pulps at the Scotty Gold Mine near Stewart, British Columbia (Scott, 1983). Because of its successful use at the Scotty Mine and in several pilot operations, the method is gaining acceptance. The Caroline Gold Mine is scheduled to start treating barren solution from a 1,500-t/d gold mill using the Inco process. Several gold mines in British Columbia, two in Quebec, and two in Ontario are seriously considering the process. Inco's Queenston Mine in Ontario will be on stream using this cyanide treatment process. The process is reported to be more cost effective than alkaline chlorination because thiocyanate does not degrade (thiocyanate degradation by alkaline chlorination requires about six times more reagent).

Other methods, such as ozonation and peroxidation, are also employed. Ozonation rapidly destroys CN, HCN, SCN, and weakly dissociable metallo-cyanide, but does not destroy iron cyanides. Peroxidation by the Kastone process or by a copper catalyst reaction destroys CN, HCN, and weakly dissociable metallo-cyanides but does not destroy SCN nor iron cyanides; however, the iron cyanides are precipitated.

Schiller (1983) devised a method which uses hydrogen peroxide and thiosulfate to convert free and weakly complexed cyanide to nontoxic thiocyanate. Steryldimethylbenzylammoniumchloride is added to precipitate ferrocyanide, and ferric sulfate is added to remove heavy metals. Cyanide concentrations can be reduced from 30 to 0.02 mg/L. The method has not been evaluated on a commercial scale.

Biodegradation

Homestake Mining Company (Mudder, 1984) has developed a biological filtering method for removing cyanide and metal ions from effluents. The method involves filtering 10 ppm CN - 70 ppm SCN solution through biological contactors that are colonized by microorganisms. Total CN was reduced to 0.1 ppm, and metals content was reduced to less than 0.1 ppm. The method required addition of nutrients to sustain biological activity. High free-cyanide concentrations can destroy bacteria.

A commercial unit has been constructed at Homestake and should be completely operational this year. Homestake Co. is working under site-specific discharge limits as agreed upon with EPA. An important aspect of this agreement is that the discharge standard is based on bioassaying rather than chemical assaying. This appears to be a trend as State agencies are following the EPA procedure.

PROBLEMS

Many small mining operations in the Western United States use heap leaching in recovery of precious metals. Each waste represents a unique problem with respect to environmental control and monitoring. Many of the processes used to treat effluents to remove cyanide require considerable retention times and may not be practical or applicable to the small operator. Additionally, the actual discharge limits are in a "gray" area so the operators have problems in selecting the proper treatment process. Studies are needed to improve technology so that it can be used by small, as well as large, operations.

The problem of cyanide effluent can be mitigated through in-process control methods which can reduce the amount of cyanides within the effluents to be treated. The principal diffficulties are in delineating the cyanide species to be treated and in adapting a treatment process to meet discharge criteria without compounding the waste disposal problem by creating new species that are incompatible with the environment. Many methods are being used or have been proposed for eliminating, destroying, or reducing the cyanide content in process waste water. Operation limits of most of these treatment methods have not been clearly defined. Research still needs to be performed to determine (1) where and when the methods can be applied, (2) toxic side effects from treatment, (3) processing problems caused by recycling treated cyanide waste streams, and (4) types of cyanide compounds being treated.

TOXICITY OF CYANIDES IN MINING WASTES

A toxicant is a chemical or physical agent which acts upon a living organism producing a harmful effect. Any substance or agent, e.g., sodium chloride, aspirin, sunlight, sound, etc., can be toxic depending on the amount received. The level of administration of an agent, not its innate nature, determines toxicity.

TOXICITY OF FREE CYANIDES

Free-cyanide toxicity in man, mammals, and aquatic species is well documented (Doudoroff 1976; Ecological Analysts 1979; Towill et al. 1978). The lethal doses reported for human adults are (1) 1 to 3 mg/kg body weight if ingested, (2) 100 to 300 ppm if inhaled, and (3) 100 mg/kg of body weight if adsorbed. Acute toxicity of free cyanide to freshwater invertebrates ranges from 0.028 to 2.295 mg/L, depending on species and test conditions. Generally, free-cyanide concentrations greater than 0.1 mg/L are expected to kill sensitive species in freshwater or marine environments (Doudoroff 1976; Cardwell et al. 1976). Several variables can affect the degree of free-cyanide toxicity: pH, water exchange, temperature, oxygen content of water, ionic strength, species acclimation, and body size. A summary of these variables was reported by Huiatt et al. (1983).

TOXICITY OF OTHER CYANIDES AND RELATED COMPOUNDS

Metallocyanide Complexes

Complexed cyanides, especially those associated with flotation tailings, are reportedly less toxic than free cyanides. However, complexed cyanides undergo varying degrees of dissociation when in solution and release free cyanide (Caruso 1975). The degree of toxicity of solutions of complexed cyanides is dependent upon the amount of free cyanide present (Doudoroff 1976; Smith et al. 1979). Certain complexes that are readily dissociated in aqueous solution (zinc-cyanide, cadmium-cyanide) are highly toxic because of the availability of free cyanide. Doudoroff et al. (1966), by comparing the median survival time (MST) and the free cyanide levels in simple cyanide solutions (NaCN) and in complex cyanide solutions, identified the active component(s) responsible for mortality of bluegill fish. The toxicity of metallocyanide complexes was attributable almost solely to the concentration of free cyanide in equilibrium with the complex. The concentration of free cyanide depends markedly on pH because pH strongly influences dissociation of the metallocyanide complex.

A case is reported in which disposal of cyanide wastes in a gravel pit near Cologne, Germany, resulted in ground water contamination by potassium hexacyanoferrate; however, tests revealed that the complexed cyanide was relatively innocuous, so the water supply was not shut down (Effenberger 1964). In another case reported by Scheidt (1967), highway salt contaminated a drinking water supply. Tastes and odors resulted and were attributed to the presence of sodium ferrocyanide used in an anticaking agent. Recommendations were made that amounts of sodium ferrocyanide mixed with the road deicing salt be reduced from 250 to 50 mg/L, and that suitable covering be provided for the storage piles to minimize salt penetration into the ground water.

Conflicting opinion regarding the hazards associated with the iron-cyanide complexes exists because of their tendency to undergo photodecomposition in the presence of ultraviolet radiation and release free cyanide. Photodecomposition of iron-cyanide complexes may be negligible in deep, turbid, or shaded waters, and slowly liberated free cyanide may decay, react and complex again, or escape as rapidly as it is released. This position is corroborated by Doudoroff (1976).

Thurston (1984) reported that solutions of ferrocyanide and ferricyanide proved to be more acutely toxic to rainbow trout when tested under light than when tested in total darkness. His work also indicated that free cyanide formed by photodecomposition of iron cyanide compounds was not the sole toxic agent under the conditions examined. Additionally, Thurston indicated that the chemical assay method (Method C of ASTM) was not the true measure of concentration of free cyanide.

Within flotation tailings, the more stable iron-cyanide complexes predominate because of operational practices associated with ore extraction procedures and also because of thermodynamic equilibrium considerations associated with the competing metallic ions. Thus, the complexed cyanides associated with flotation tailings, in addition to being present in low concentrations, are generally nonhazardous due to their stability. Information regarding mineral process tailings toxicity is scant. A survey conducted by Engineering Science (1980) found no reported incidence of flotation tailings resulting in damage to human health or the environment.

Thiocyanate

Compared to cyanide, thiocyanate is relatively harmless; however, it should not be treated as an innocuous compound. Thiocyanate is a common cyanide reaction product found in mill effluents where cyanide is used in processing. Also, thiocyanate is a metabolic byproduct of cyanide. Very little attention seems to have been given to thiocyanate toxicity; however, Thurston, Montana State University, is now doing research to determine toxicity of thiocyanate to aquatic animals. His data have not been published.

PROBLEMS

The scope of the problem of cyanide toxicity cannot be limited to free cyanide in the broad perspective, although this may be the specific criterion of immediate interest. Interactive compounds, compounds resulting from waste water treatment, downstream toxic effects, long-term life-cycle effects, and many other factors enter into the ultimate question of toxicity in real environmental settings. To resolve the problems, cyanide species in effluent must be identified and their toxicity determined. The toxicity of whole effluents, the toxic components of the effluent, and concentration limits must also be determined.

FATE OF CYANIDE IN THE ENVIRONMENT

MIGRATION OF CYANIDE

An EPA study (USEPA 1976) revealed that some cyanide compounds are quite immobile in different soils while others are mobile. Ferric ammonium hexacyanoferrate mobility was very slow, whereas mobility of cyanide as $Fe(CN)_6^{3-}$ and CN^- was high. Soil properties such as low pH, percent free-iron oxide, and the presence of kaolin-, chlorite-, and gibbsite-type clays tended to decrease mobility. High pH, free carbonate, low clay content, and the presence of montmorillonite clay tend to increase mobility of certain cyanides. Towill et al. (1978) concluded from a review of the environmental effects of cyanide that the movement of cyanide in soil is usually limited because it is either complexed by trace metals or metabolized by various microorganisms. High concentrations of cyanide in the soil can usually be attributed to improper waste management procedures.

ENVIRONMENTAL PERSISTENCE AND DEGRADATION

Conversion to Thiocyanate

Free cyanide rarely occurs in nature because the molecule has a high reactivity. In small concentrations, free cyanide reacts with various forms of sulfur from pyrite and other mineral constituents to form thiocyanate, which is relatively nontoxic. Thiocyanate has been shown to be an intermediate compound which is produced during biodegradation and detoxification of free cyanide in living systems.

Complexation With Metal Ions

Cyanide will also complex trace metals to increase or decrease mobility. According to Ford-Smith (1964), about 28 elements can form complexes with cyanides to produce about 72 metallocyanide complexes. The most important metal complexes in effluents from gold mining are iron, copper, zinc, nickel, cobalt, and cadmium. Gold and silver complexes are excluded because they are present in minute amounts. Complex metallocyanides, such as those associated with flotation tailings, exhibit varying degrees of persistence in the environment, depending on whether they remain in a solid or an aqueous phase. In an aqueous phase, pH, dissolved oxygen concentration, ultraviolet radiation, and availability of other complexing agents affect persistence and mobility. In the solid phase, most complexes associated with flotation tailings remain inert. However, one complexed iron species (ferric ferricyanide) degrades in the solid phase and releases CO_2, N_2, and traces of other compounds. Complexes associated with flotation tailings are usually tightly bound, thermodynamically stable compounds, such as metal hexacyanoferrates, which do not dissociate readily (Walker and Watkins 1968). In an iron-rich medium containing excess ferric, ferrous, and copper ions, an almost totally insoluble metal hexacyanoferrate precipitates. Because the cyanide compounds are present in very low concentrations (low parts per million range) in such tailings, confirmation of their presence or absence is difficult or impossible by current analytical technology.

Hendricks (1984) initiated work to determine the disposition of cyanide compounds in old mill tailings and leach spoils. Preliminary results indicate the presence of some unidentified cyanide complexes in subsurface tailings solids. Hendricks is using ASTM standard procedures for total cyanide analysis.

Photochemical Degradation

The major environmental concern regarding persistence of ferrocyanide and ferricyanide involves the photochemical degradation of these ions under ultraviolet light to form free cyanide. This problem is not important in solid mine tailing wastes because of lack of exposure to ultraviolet light except at the surface of the waste.

Photodegradation could become important if complex cyanide ions leach into ground or surface waters.

Free cyanide can be oxidized to cyanate and ultimately to ammonia and carbon dioxide by ozone produced from ultraviolet irradiation (Owerbach 1978). Whether this conversion reaction can occur nonbiochemically is not clear.

PROBLEMS

Natural oxidants, sunlight, bacteria, organic and inorganic materials, type of soils, water chemistry, mineral constituents of tailings, permeabilities of soils and tailings, type of cyanide compound, concentration of the cyanide compound, rate of migration of cyanides, and materials of construction and design of leach pads and tailings ponds all affect the ultimate fate of cyanide in the environment. Accurate knowledge of cyanide disposition is necessary if meaningful practical regulations are to be established for monitoring or controlling mineral process effluents. Nearly all regulations are now handled on a site-specific basis. Any information concerning fate of cyanides and related compounds would be of considerable value to the mine operator and to the monitoring agency.

PROCEDURES FOR ANALYZING CYANIDE

Because more concern is given to understanding the impact of cyanide compounds released to the environment, the need to determine cyanide species in a wide variety of water matrices has resulted in a profusion of analytical methods. These methods are frequently both complex and cumbersome to use routinely. Some general problems associated with chemical analyses of cyanides include (1) commonly used methods require high skill to produce consistent acceptable data, (2) different matrices require alternate methodologies, (3) sample preparation and preservation techniques are specific for the matrices and methodologies, and (4) techniques for preservation of samples containing particulates are not defined.

ANALYTICAL METHODS

From an analytical viewpoint, four methods of measuring cyanide are described: (1) total cyanide, (2) cyanide amenable to chlorination, (3) weak-acid-dissociable cyanide, and (4) free cyanide.

Total Cyanide

Total cyanide may be defined as the amount measured by the reflux mineral acid distillation method. The amount includes complex iron cyanides, weak-acid-dissociable cyanide, free cyanide, and most other inorganic complex cyanides except gold, cobalt, and some platinum complexes. The most common method is an acid reflux-distillation in which a catalytic agent is used to facilitate breakdown of metallo-cyanide complexes. Hydrogen cyanide that is liberated and distilled is collected in an alkaline absorbing solution and is usually measured by titration, colorimetry, or specific ion electrodes, depending on concentration.

Over the years, modified versions of the standard methods have been published, but many laboratories are still using procedures inadequate for their samples. This, together with interferences from thiocyanate and reduced sulfur compounds, has led to great difficulties in comparing data produced by the mining industry.

Knechtel and Conn (1981) reported a modified version of the acid distillation technique for determining low level cyanide in presence of thiocyanate. The method, referred to as the Wastewater Technology Center (WTC) method, uses hydrochloric acid and hydroxylamine hydrochloride as decomposition agents. Cadmium chloride is added to precipitate sulfides that distill. The method was reported to be successfully applied in a number of laboratories and mill locations to measure cyanide in mine process water.

Distillation methods are relatively time consuming and inadequate for routine analysis of a large number of samples. The method can be accelerated by decomposing with ultraviolet irradiation; however, thiocyanate also decomposes and gives positive results. Pohlandt, Jones, and Lee (1983) in their review of a number of procedures felt that the combination of ion chromatography, which is recommended for determining ionic cyanide, and irradiation could give a fast and sensitive method for total cyanide.

Cyanide Amenable to Chlorination

This method is particularly important to mining operations that chlorinate cyanide effluents. The method is based on the difference between total cyanide determinations in a sample both before and after chlorination. One portion of a sample is analyzed for total cyanide; another portion is treated with sodium hypochlorite at an alkaline pH for 1 h, the chlorine residual is removed, and the solution is analyzed by the total cyanide procedure. Alkaline chlorination oxidizes most cyanides as well as thiocyanate and other oxidizable compounds. Iron cyanides are not oxidized. The difference between the two total cyanide values is the cyanide amenable to chlorination.

Although the procedure is accepted as standard by ASTM and several other agencies, it obviously is only as good as the original total cyanide value before chlorination. If the method for total cyanide is unsuitable or if interferences such as thiocyanate are not considered, then a totally wrong value for cyanide amenable to chlorination is obtained.

Weak-Acid-Dissociable Cyanides

The method for analyzing weak-acid-dissociable cyanide will determine a number of cyanide species including cyanide ion, hydrogen cyanide, and complex cadmium, copper, nickel, silver, and zinc. The method now accepted by ASTM (1981) as a standard method is a variation of one proposed by Roberts and and Jackson (1971). It is often referred to as Method C. The distillation is performed in a similar manner as the total cyanide distillation procedure, except different reagents are introduced. The reagents are zinc acetate and an acetic acid-sodium acetate solution of pH 4.5. Zinc acetate prevents ferrocyanide decomposition. No cyanide recovery from ferro, ferri, and cobalt complexes has been reported; however, test work reported by Conn (1981) at the Wastewater Technology Center in Canada suggested that 2 pct breakdown of ferrocyanide could occur. Thiocyanate does not interfere with this method.

Free Cyanide

Free cyanide at pH 8 or lower will be molecular HCN and can be determined by either solvent extraction or sparging the HCN from solution and collecting it for subsequent analysis. Free cyanide can also be determined by gas dialysis, microdiffusion, or measuring gaseous HCN in equilibrium with the aqueous phase. The methodologies for free cyanide (HCN and CN^-) are primarily research tools. They are not applicable, or have not been tested, for routine determination of cyanide in mine effluents. ASTM has not published results of any interlaboratory testing of free cyanide methods.

Direct determination of free cyanide in solution using titrimetic, colorimetric, and electrochemical (specific ion electrode) methods are liable to interferences from ionizable metal cyanide complexes, e.g., zinc cyanide. Thiocyanates, sulfides, oxidizing agents, nitrates, urea, and other organic compounds may interfere depending on the procedure. Obviously, direct determination of free cyanides can only be accomplished if interferences are removed.

PROBLEMS

Obtaining reproducible analytical data on cyanide in mineral processing waste streams appears to be a general problem for mining companies, consulting laboratories, and/or Government laboratories. Data discrepancies can be attributed to a lack of adequate techniques for sampling and preserving mine process samples and a lack of satisfactory laboratory methodology to routinely measure free cyanides.

Sampling of mine process waters is difficult because particulates are not uniformly distributed throughout the streams. These particulates may act as gatherers or sinks for cyanide-bearing molecules, thus reducing the cyanide content of the water. Consequently, homogeneity of the waste stream must be assured before sampling. The relative concentration of cyanide species in effluent water is dependent on time and preservation techniques; consequently, water analyzed immediately after sampling could have an entirely different chemical profile from water preserved and analyzed several days later.

The methods used to analyze the various cyanide compounds vary considerably and are subject to many interferences. Most accepted methods involve sophisticated procedures to compensate for the interfering variables. The methods appear to work well in carefully controlled laboratory conditions; however, in field situations such as may be encountered in a mineral processing operation, the precision and accuracy of the methods suffer significantly. Round-robin analyses of control samples have demonstrated that the methods are marginally reliable at low concentrations. Because decisions involving toxicity levels, control, processing, and fate of cyanides hinge upon reliable analytical results, concerted effort is needed to investigate the variables that interfere with the analyses of free or total cyanides and methods for analyzing other cyanide species such as metallo-cyanides and cyanide chemical oxidation products such as cyanates.

SUMMARY AND CONCLUSIONS

Although general information on cyanide chemistry and toxicity is available, specific knowledge of cyanide as it relates to the environmental aspects of mineral processing needs to be expanded. The information is needed to identify and mitigate potential problems associated with its use. Based on the overall response of the participants of the Workshop on Cyanide From Mineral Processing, one of the most pressing needs is research into the analytical chemistry of cyanides as it relates to the mining industry. Reliable analytical techniques are necessary if subsequent research is to be credible. Another concern is that the lack of information on the fate of cyanides, cyano complexes, and cyanide oxidation products (cyanates) in a mineral processing system has made decisions on proper environmental control and regulation difficult; consequently, literature, laboratory, and field investigations are needed to provide more information. Almost all toxicological studies have been directed toward measuring the effect of free cyanide on aquatic organisms. Additional studies are needed to determine the toxic nature of cyanide-bearing compounds, other than free cyanides, that are introduced or formed through mining and milling operations and to examine toxicity associated with total effluent.

REFERENCES

1. ASTM. 1981. Proposed Revision of Standard Methods of Test for Cyanide in Water. Standard D-2036-81, American Society for Testing and Materials.

2. Cardwell, R. D., D. G. Foreman, T. R. Payne, and D. J. Wilber. 1976. Acute Toxicity of Selected Toxicants to Six Species of Fish. EPA 600/3-76- 008. U.S. Environ. Protect. Agency. Duluth, MN, 116 pp.

3. Caruso, S. C. 1975. The Chemistry of Cyanide Compounds and Their Behaviorism in the Aquatic Environment. Carnegie-Mellon Institute of Research. Mellon Institute.

4. Conn, K. 1981. Cyanide Analysis in Mine Effluents. In Cyanide and the Gold Mining Industry: A Technical Seminar. Sponsored by Environment Canada and Canadian Mineral Processors.

5. Devuyst, E. A., V. A. Ettel, and G. J. Borbely. 1982. New Method for Cyanide Destruction in Gold Mill Effluents and Tailing Slurries. Inco Metals Company, Process Research, 14 pp.

6. Doudoroff, P. 1976. Toxicity to Fish of Cyanides and Related Compounds. A Review. Environmental Protection Agency Report No. EPA-600/3- 76-038.

7. Doudoroff, P., G. Leduc, and C. R. Schneider. 1966. Acute Toxicity to Fish of Solutions Containing Complex Metal Cyanides in Relation to Concentrations of Molecular Hydrocyanic Acid. Trans. Am. Fish Soc. 95:6-22.

8. Ecological Analysts, Inc. 1979. Cyanide, An Overview and Analysis of the Literature on Chemistry, Fate, Toxicity, and Detection in Surface Waters. Prepared for the Inter-Industry Cyanide Group.

9. Effenberger, V. E. 1964. Verunveinigung Eines Grundwasserdurch Cyanid (Continuation of Ground Water Through Cyanide). Arch. Hyg. Bakteriol. (Munich) 148:271-287.

10. Engineering Science. 1980. A Compilation of Pertinent Information Regarding Complexed Cyanides in Mineral Flotation Tailings. Prepared for AMAX Environmental Services, Inc., Denver, CO.

11. Ford-Smith, H. M. 1964. The Chemistry of Complex Cyanides: A Literature Survey. London, Her Majesty's Stationery Office.

12. Hendricks, J. L. 1984. University of Nevada. Personal Communication.

13. Huiatt, J. L., J. E. Kerrigan, F. A. Olson, and G. L. Potter (eds.). 1983. Workshop: Cyanide From Mineral Processing. Printed by Utah Mining and Mineral Resources Research Institute, College of Mines and Minerals Industries, Salt Lake City, UT, Feb. 1983, 143 pp.

14. Ingles, J. C., and J. S. Scott. 1981. Overview of Cyanide Treatment Methods. Cyanide in Gold Mining Seminar, Ottawa, Ontario.

15. Knechtel, R. J., and K. Conn. 1981. Determination of Cyanide in Wastewater -A New Approach. Environment Canada, Wastewater Technology Center, Burlington, Ontario.

16. McCreedy, H., C. C. Clark, and W. A. Gow. 1961. The Use of the Gold-Leaf Test To Check the Effects of Certain Possible Contaminants of Cyanide Solutions. Mines Branch Extraction Metallurgy Division. Investigation Report IR 61-25.

17. Mezey, E. J., and D. W. Neuerdorf. 1981. Alternatives to Sodium Cyanide for Flotation Control. Prepared for Industrial Environmental Research Laboratory. USEPA Contract Report No. 68-03-2552, T2008.

18. Mudder, T. I., and J. L. Whitlock. 1984. Biological Treatment of Cyanidation Wastewaters. Presentation at SME-AIME Annual Meeting, Los Angeles, CA. February 26 - March 1, 1984. Preprint No. 84-37.

19. Owerbach, D. 1978. The Instability of Free Cyanide in Photographic Processing Effluents. J. App. Photo. Eng. 4:72-76.

20. Pohlandt, C., E. A. Jones, and A. F. Lee. 1983. A Critical Evaluation of Methods Applicable to the Determination of Cyanides. Journal of the South Affican Institute of Mining and Metallurgy, January 1983, pp. 11-19.

21. Roberts, R. J., and B. Jackson. 1971. The Determination of Small Amounts of Cyanide in the Presence of Ferrocyanide by Distillation Under Reduced Pressure. Analyst, Lond. v 96, pp. 209-212.

22. Scheidt, M. E. 1967. Environmental Effects of Highways. J. Sanitary Engineers Division, Proceedings of the American Society of Civil Engineers 93, No. SA5 Paper No. 5509, pp. 17-25.

23. Schiller, J. E. 1983. Removal of Cyanide and Metals From Mineral Processing Wastes. Bureau of Mines Report of Investigations 8836, pp. 8.

24. Schmidt, J. W., L. Simovic, and E. Shannon. 1981. Natural Degradation of Cyanides in Gold Milling Effluents, A Progress Report. Environment Canada, Wastewater Technology Center, Burlington, Ont. Presented at the Cyanide and Gold Mining Industry Seminar, Ottawa, Ont., Jan. 22-23, 1981.

25. Scott, J. S. 1981. Removal of Cyanide From Gold Mill Effluents. Cyanide and the Gold Mining Industry: A Technical Seminar. Sponsored by Environment Canada and Canadian Mineral Processors, Jan. 22-23, 1981.

26. Scott, J. S. 1983. Water Pollution Control Directorate. Environment Canada. Personal Communication.

27. Smith, Jr., L. L., S. J. Broderius, D. M. Oseid, G. L. Kimball, W. M. Koenst, and D. T. Lind. 1979. Acute and Chronic Toxicity of HCN to Fish and Invertebrates. Environmental Protection Agency Report No. EPA-600/3-79-009.

28. Thurston, R. V. 1984. Fisheries Bioassay Laboratory. Montata State University. Personal Communication.

29. Towill, L. E., J. S. Drury, B. L. Whitfield, E. B. Lewis, E. L. Galyan, and A. S. Hammons. 1978. Reviews of the Environmental Effects of Pollutants: V. Cyanides. Interagency Report. Oak Ridge National Laboratory Report No. ORNL/EIS-81 and Environmental Protection Agency Report No. EPA 600/1-78-027.

30. USEPA. 1976. Water Pollution Caused by Inactive Ore and Mineral Mines. U.S. Environmental Protection Agency EPA 600/2-76-298.

31. Walker, R. G., and K. O. Watkins. 1968. A Study of the Kinetics of Complex Formation Between Hexacyanoferrate (III) Ions and Iron (III) to Form $FeFe(CN)_6$ (Prussian Brown). Inorganic Chemistry, 7(5):885-889.

Analytical/Toxicity Aspects

CONFERENCE ON CYANIDE AND THE ENVIRONMENT
Tucson, Arizona • December 1984
Published by Geotechnical Engineering Program • Colorado State University • Fort Collins, Colorado 80523

PHYSIOLOGICAL AND TOXIC EFFECTS OF CYANIDES TO FISHES: A REVIEW AND RECENT ADVANCES

by

Thomas A. Heming[1] and Robert V. Thurston[2]

INTRODUCTION

Toxicity of Cyanide

The acute and chronic effects of cyanide, and the effect levels, have been extensively studied in most groups of animals including fishes. This information is reviewed and summarized by Doudoroff (1976), Towill et al. (1978), Vennesland et al. (1981), and Huiatt et al. (1983). Generally, concentrations exceeding 0.1 mg/liter as HCN have been found to kill sensitive fish species. Debilitating sublethal effects have been reported to occur at concentrations several orders of magnitude lower. Kimball et al. (1978), for example, report that 0.005 mg/liter HCN comletely inhibited spawning of the bluegill sunfish, Lepomis macrochirus. The U.S. Environmental Protection Agency has adopted a freshwater aquatic life criterion for free cyanide of 3.5 ug/liter for any 24-hour average, and of 52 ug/liter, not to be exceeded at any time (US EPA 1980).

Cyanide can be introduced into fish by ingestion, and by absorption across the skin and gills. Once introduced, cyanide enters the bloodstream and is distributed to other body tissues. Cyanide is virtually un-ionized (Izatt 1962) within the physiological pH range of fish blood and, consequently, is transported in blood primarily as HCN. It has long been recognized that HCN is more toxic than the ionized moiety, CN^- (Wuhrmann and Woker 1948), because of the easier penetration of HCN through biological membranes including the gill epithelium.

The effects of cyanides arise primarily from the formation of CN^- complexes with metalloporphyrins and disulfide bond

[1]Aquatic Toxicology Section, Alberta Environmental Centre, Vegreville, Alberta T0B 4L0, Canada

[2]Fisheries Bioassay Laboratory, Montana State University, Bozeman, Montana 59717, USA

molecules of protein, and subsequent inhibition of protein function. In vertebrates, cytochrome oxidase is one of the proteins most sensitive to cyanide; complete inhibition of the enzyme occurs at 10 nM cyanide, 0.26 ug/liter (for review see Towill et al. 1978, Vennesland et al. 1981). Cyanide thus inhibits oxidative phosphorylation at the level of the mitochondria and produces histotoxic hypoxia. Death results from depression of the central nervous system (CNS), the tissue most sensitive to hypoxia. Fatal doses initially produce CNS stimulation, followed rapidly by CNS depression, hypoxic convulsions, and death.

The major pathway for detoxification of cyanide is via the conversion of cyanide to the less toxic thiocyanate (SCN^-). This reaction is catalyzed by the enzyme rhodanase (thiosulfate sulfur transferase) found intracellularly in liver, gill, and other tissues (see Westley 1973, Vennesland et al. 1981). A number of minor routes for cyanide detoxification also exist, including reactions with methemoglobin, vitamin B_{12}, and cystine to form cyanomethemoglobin, cyanocobalamine, and beta-thiocyanoalanine. Cyanomethemoglobin is subsequently metabolized to release thiocyanate. Thiocyanate and the other end products of cyanide metabolism are excreted via the urinary tract and gill.

<u>Toxicity of Thiocyanate</u>

Thiocyanate enters the aquatic biosphere directly as SCN^- and indirectly as a product of the metabolism of cyanide. The fact that endogenous conversion of cyanide to thiocyanate is the principal pathway for cyanide detoxification in many animals does not infer that thiocyanate is not toxic. Thiocyanate inhibits transport of halides in the thyroid (Wolff 1964), stomach (Davenport 1940, Davies 1951), cornea (Zadunaisky et al. 1971), and gills (Epstein et al. 1973, 1975), and also inhibits various enzymes such as carbonic anhydrase (Davenport 1940), succinic dehydrogenase (Solomon et al. 1973), and moieties of ATPase (Katz and Epstein 1971, Solomon et al. 1973).

Thiocyanate has been used therapeutically in the treatment of hypertension in humans, occasionally with unpredictable and fatal consequences (Garvin 1939, Goodman and Gilman 1970). Toxic effects to humans are due to an action of SCN^- on the central nervous system and include irritability, nervousness, hallucinations, psychosis, mania, delirium, and convulsions (Barnett et al. 1951). Evidence of the conversion of inorganic and organic thiocyanates to cyanide has been found in mammals (Boxer and Rickards 1952a, 1952b, Goldstein and Reiders 1951, Pines and Crymble 1952) and in fish (Heming et al. 1985). It has been proposed that these conversions involve a red cell enzyme, thiocyanate oxidase (Goldstein and Reiders 1953), and the enzyme glutathione-S-transferase (Habig et al. 1975).

Information on the toxicity of thiocyanate to aquatic life forms is scant and contains conflicting results (see Doudoroff 1976, Huiatt et al. 1983, Towill et al. 1978). Doudoroff (1976), for example, noted effect levels under various conditions to occur at concentrations ranging from 29 to 5,000 mg/liter SCN^-; he concluded that "thiocyanate is somewhat toxic". APHA et al. (1980) have dismissed the toxicity of thiocyanate as being relatively unimportant unless subsequent chlorination, which would produce cyanogen chloride, is anticipated. The U.S. Environmental Protection Agency (U.S. EPA 1980) does not list a criterion for thiocyanate. Further examination of the aquatic toxicity of thiocyanate is timely because of the recent development of the INCO SO_2/air process for cyanide removal from industrial effluents. This process selectively oxidizes cyanide and metal cyanide complexes, but has little effect on thiocyanate (Devuyst et al. 1982, Huiatt et al. 1983).

Toxicity of Metallocyanide Complexes

The toxicity of complexed cyanides in the aquatic environment is dependent upon the degree to which these complexes dissociate to release free cyanide (Doudoroff 1976, Huiatt et al. 1983). Certain complexes readily dissociate in aqueous solution and are highly toxic (e.g. zinc-cyanide, cadmium-cyanide), certain others exhibit moderate degrees of dissociation and are less toxic (e.g. copper-cyanide, nickel-cyanide, silver-cyanide), and still others are tightly bound together and have been considered non-toxic (e.g. iron-cyanide, cobalt-cyanide) (see Caruso 1975).

Ferrocyanide $[Fe(CN)_6^{4-}]$ and ferricyanide $[Fe(CN)_6^{3-}]$ are byproducts of the cyanidation process employed in the extraction of gold and silver from ore. Both complexes are frequently present in ore mine effluents. Environmental concerns about these iron cyanide complexes generally center around their photodegradation to free cyanide. Light of wavelength less than 420 nm is active in the decomposition of ferrocyanide, and of less than 480 nm in the decomposition of ferricyanide (Broderius and Smith, 1980). Light source and intensity, therefore, are critical in any toxicity testing with these two anions. Free cyanide concentration, as well as total cyanide concentration, is important in interpreting test results. Although quality and intensity of light appear to be the most important factors in the decomposition process, temperature, pH, and dissolved oxygen also play significant roles.

RECENT RESEARCH

In this presentation, we will discuss the results of recent research at Fisheries Bioassay Laboratory (FBL) on the acute toxicity to fishes of both iron cyanide complexes and thiocyanate. The toxicants we tested were reagent grade potassium ferrocyanide, potassium ferricyanide, and potassium thiocyanate. The test fish were hatchery-reared rainbow trout (Salmo gairdneri) and brook trout (Salvelinus fontinalis). Chemical analyses were conducted according to methods prescribed by APHA et al. (1980), ASTM (1981), and U.S. EPA (1974). Fish were tested using diluters either of the design of Benoit (1982) or Mount and Brungs (1967). Each diluter delivered water to one control tank and five test tanks; each of the test tanks was maintained at a different concentration of toxicant. Except as noted, ten fish were tested in each tank. Median lethal concentration (LC50) values were determined according to the Trimmed Spearman-Karber method (Hamilton et al. 1977). More complete details of the testing methods have been reported elsewhere (Meyn et al. 1984, Heming et al. 1985).

Iron-Cyanide Toxicity Tests - Procedures

A series of 96-hour flow-through toxicity tests was conducted on rainbow trout to determine the toxicity of ferrocyanide and of ferricyanide under two light regimes: total darkness, and a cycle of 18 hours light/6 hours darkness. A minimum of two tests was run with each chemical under each light regime. Four additional tests, two each on ferrocyanide and ferricyanide, were conducted at an elevated temperature under a cyclic regime of 18 hours light/6 hours darkness. The tanks were glass aquaria with glass covers, and had a water volume of approximately 14 liters. The diluters had a flow rate of 30 ml/minute and the turnover time was approximately 8 hours. Tests were started with the test concentrations already establish in the tanks. Fish for a given test were from a single pool, and were distributed at random among the control and test tanks. The tests were conducted in a room equipped with wide-spectrum bulbs (Spectralite, Long-Life Lighting Products) that were reported to produce a spectral energy distribution similar to daylight. For tests conducted in total darkness, a red bulb was used for illumination during the collection of water samples and during mortality checks.

In designing the experiment, it was assumed there might be marked differences in photodecomposition of the toxicants between a test regime of total darkness and one that provided light during a simulated daytime period. It was further assumed that at relatively low light intensities (as compared with the intensity of bright sunlight), modest differences in intensity between tanks would not significantly affect test results. As a consequence, no special attempt was made to ensure that light intensities at the water surface of the different tanks in each test were identical. Two sets of test tanks were used; the range of light intensity at the tank water surface for one of these was 230-400 lux (mean 330 lux) and for the other was 550-780 lux (mean 680 lux). It subsequently developed that these light intensity differences most probably played a far greater role in determining the test results than originally anticipated; these differences may have been sufficient to mask differences in results attributable to temperature within the range tested (9-16 C).

Water samples for cyanide analysis were collected from the effluent of each tank three times during each test. Sodium hydroxide was added to each sample to raise the pH to 12; samples were then refrigerated and shipped to Homestake Mining Company at Lead, South Dakota, for analysis. Total cyanide (total CN^-) was determined using a modified acid reflux/distillation method (ASTM 1981), and "weak acid dissociable cyanides" were determined by

"Method-C" (ASTM 1982). Under our test conditions using FBL water, which contained only insignificant quantities of metals (Meyn et al. 1984), "weak acid dissociable cyanides" was essentially free cyanide. Results for all tests were reported in terms of total CN^-; results for two tests in the dark and all tests in the light also were reported in terms of Method-C CN^-. All other water measurements were made at FBL, and included dissolved oxygen, temperature, pH, alkalinity, and hardness (Meyn et al. 1984).

It should be noted that solutions of ferricyanide ion are distinctly yellow. The intensity of color increases with increasing concentrations and was almost orange at the highest concentrations tested. By contrast, ferrocyanide ion imparts only a pale yellow color to its solutions, even at very high concentrations. The presence of iron interfered with alkalinity and hardness determinations in all but the control tanks. Light intensity measurements were made with a Gossen Panlux Electronic Foot-Lambert meter, recorded as foot-candles and converted to lux.

The LC50 values derived in terms of either total CN^- or Method-C CN^- should be considered valid only under the conditions of testing, i.e., total darkness or 18-hour day, and at the specified temperature and concentration of dissolved oxygen. The LC50 values expressed in terms of Method-C CN^- are further restricted by being computed from the means of concentrations that increased during some of the tests.

<u>Iron-Cyanide</u> <u>Toxicity</u> <u>Tests</u> - <u>Results</u>

Comparison of the results of the ferrocyanide tests conducted in total darkness (Tests 1074, 1077, 1078) and those under an intermittent light regime of either 330 lux (Tests 1088, 1090) or 680 lux (Tests 1080, 1083) shows the fish were more sensitive to the test water in those tests conducted under light (Table 1). Comparison of results of the tests conducted under light further shows that the fish were more sensitive to the test water at 680 lux than at 330 lux. A variable introduced in this second comparison, however, is that the 330-lux tests were conducted at a higher temperature (15-16 C) than those at 680 lux (9-10 C).

Comparison of the results of the ferricyanide tests conducted in total darkness (Tests 1075, 1076, 1079) with those conducted under an intermittent light regime of 680 lux (Tests 1085, 1087, 1089) shows markedly greater toxicity under light (Table 2). Of the three tests conducted at 680 lux, one was conducted at 10 C (Test 1085) and the other two at 16 C (Tests 1087, 1089). Results show a slight increase in toxicity at the higher temperature, but the overlap in LC50 confidence intervals for these tests suggests that this finding is not conclusive.

To see whether there are additional conclusions that might be drawn from these data, we combined the results of all tests and made the assumption that differences in toxicity, if any, resulting from temperature differences were over-ridden by other factors. We

Table 1. Ferrocyanide toxicity tests - Summary of test conditions and 96-hour LC50 values obtained. (Ten fish/tank).

Test No.	Light regime, hours of light/dark	Mean light intensity, lux	Mean pH (range)	Mean temperature, °C (range)	Mean D.O., mg/liter (range)	Method-C CN^- 96-h LC50, mg/liter (95% C.I.)	Total CN^- 96-h LC50, mg/liter (95% C.I.)
1074	0/24	0	-	9.4 (9.4-9.5)	8.44 (7.03-8.85)	-	752 (474-1190)
1074	0/24	0	-	-	-	-	> 867
1078	0/24	0	7.95 (7.89-8.01)	9.4 (9.4-9.5)	8.83 (8.76-8.97)	1.10 (0.99-1.23)	939 (828-1064)
1088	18/6	330	7.77 (7.66-7.94)	15.7 (15.4-16.1)	8.22 (8.01-8.49)	0.79 (0.63-1.0)	220 (184-261)
1090	18/6	330	7.83 (7.75-7.95)	15.2 (15.2-15.4)	7.85 (7.64-8.11)	0.71 (0.51-0.98)	232 (178-302)
1080	18/6	680	7.33 (7.30-7.34)	9.6 (9.6-9.7)	7.93 (7.77-8.17)	0.15 (0.13-1.17)	33.0 (28.7-37.9)
1083	18/6	680	7.55 (7.50-7.57)	9.5 (9.5-9.6)	8.37 (8.16-8.58)	0.17 (-)a/	37.4 (-)a/

a/ Confidence interval not calculable by method used.

Table 2. Ferricyanide toxicity tests - Summary of test conditions and 96-hour LC50 values obtained. (Ten fish/tank).

Test No.	Light regime, hours of light/dark	Mean light intensity, lux	Mean pH (range)	Mean temperature, °C (range)	Mean D.O., mg/liter (range)	Method-C CN^-, 96-h LC50 mg/liter (95% C.I.)	Total CN^- 96-h LC50, mg/liter (95% C.I.)
1075	0/24	0	7.87 (7.46-8.23)	9.3 (9.1-9.4)	8.18 (7.03-8.85)	-	1210 (1060-1380)
1076	0/24	0	7.96 (7.75-8.17)	9.3 (9.2-9.4)	8.88 (8.70-9.01)	-	869 (680-1110)
1079	0/24	0	-	-	-	> 1.14	> 877
1081	18/6	330	7.33 (7.30-7.34)	9.6 (9.5-9.7)	7.91 (7.61-8.11)	0.24 (0.23-0.26)	69.6 (54.7-88.5)
1082	18/6	330	7.56 (7.53-7.58)	9.6 (9.5-9.7)	8.28 (8.09-8.43)	> 0.50	> 541
1084	18/6	330	-	-	-	> 0.61	> 731
1085	18/6	680	7.78 (7.76-7.80)	10.3 (10.1-10.7)	8.26 (8.13-8.34)	0.42 (0.36-0.50)	44.2 (38.2-51.0)
1087	18/6	680	7.96 (7.89-8.06)	16.0 (15.8-16.1)	8.69 (8.58-8.83)	0.40 (0.36-0.43)	38.8 (25.0-60.2)
1089	18/6	680	7.89 (7.79-8.10)	16.0 (15.5-16.4)	8.16 (8.05-8.37)	0.31 (0.30-0.32)	10.8 (8.96-13.1)

looked at all the data for each test, and from each we selected the tank with the highest Method-C CN^- concentration at which no more than 10% mortality occurred (Table 3). For two of the ferricyanide tests, more than 10% of the fish died at even the lowest concentration tested. These were Test 1087 with 40% mortality in Tank 2, and Test 1089 with 30% mortality in Tank 2. To include these tests in our data pool it was necessary to use these tanks with > 10% mortality; presumably $\leq$ 10% mortality would have occurred at a lower Method-C CN^- concentration. We then plotted the measured light intensity for each of these test tanks versus its measured Method-C CN^- concentration, using the highest single measuremment of Method-C CN^- in each tank as opposed to the mean of three measurements. The rationale for selecting the highest measured Method-C CN^- value was that the toxic action of cyanide is rather rapid, and the fish that died were probably most affected by that highest concentration, rather than by a 96-hour average.

The results of this plot (Figure 1) are revealing. The estimated curves for both sets of tests (ferrocyanide and ferricyanide) are similar, and one may conjecture that there may not be a significant difference between them. The implications are that the toxicity of Method-C CN^- is light dependent, i.e., there is a correlation between the toxicity of Method-C CN^- and light intensity.

The behaviour and distress symptoms of fish in the ferrocyanide and ferricyanide acute toxicity tests were similar to, but less dramatic than, those that we also observed during acute toxicity tests on thiocyanate. These symptoms included flaring of the gills, gaping of the mouth, erratic and sudden movement, and immediate stiffness of the body when the fish died. The symptoms were particularly noticeable at the termination of a test when all remaining fish were anesthetised with tricainemethanesulfonate prior to weighing and measuring. The degree to which these symptoms were evident was directly related to toxicant concentration; at the lowest concentrations tested, and in the control tanks, fish did not evidence these symptoms.

<u>Thiocyanate Toxicity Tests - Procedures</u>

Acute (96-hour) toxicity tests were conducted on both brook trout and rainbow trout under continuous-flow conditions as described above, except that these tests were started at zero toxicant concentration, and full test toxicant concentrations were effectively reached within 18 hours. Tests were conducted under two conditions: an ambient photoperiod with fish visually exposed to normal laboratory traffic and activities and controlled photoperiods with fish isolated from these activities by curtains. Controlled photoperiods were 24-hours white light (223 lux), 12-hours light/12-hours dark, and 24-hours dim red light (0.2 lux). Effects of stress on thiocyanate toxicity were assessed in tests in which fish were forced to swim vigorously for 30 seconds, by inserting a hand-held dip net into the tank water and moving it around taking care not to touch the fish.

Table 3. Light intensity in tanks with highest Method-C CN^- concentration at which no greater than 10% mortality occurred.

Test no.	Tank with ≤10% mortality: Highest measured Method-C CN^-, mg/liter	Light intensity, lux
	Ferrocyanide Tests	
1074	1.15	0
1078	1.13	0
1080	0.13	780
1083	0.14	590
1088	0.35	250
1090	0.49	310
	Ferricyanide Tests	
1079	1.30	0
1081	0.22	310
1082	0.64	400
1084	0.58	390
1085	0.46	780
1087	0.47[a/]	780
1089	0.33[b/]	780

[a/] Test tank reported is that with lowest mortality (40%). [See text]

[b/] Test tank reported is that with lowest mortality (30%). [See text]

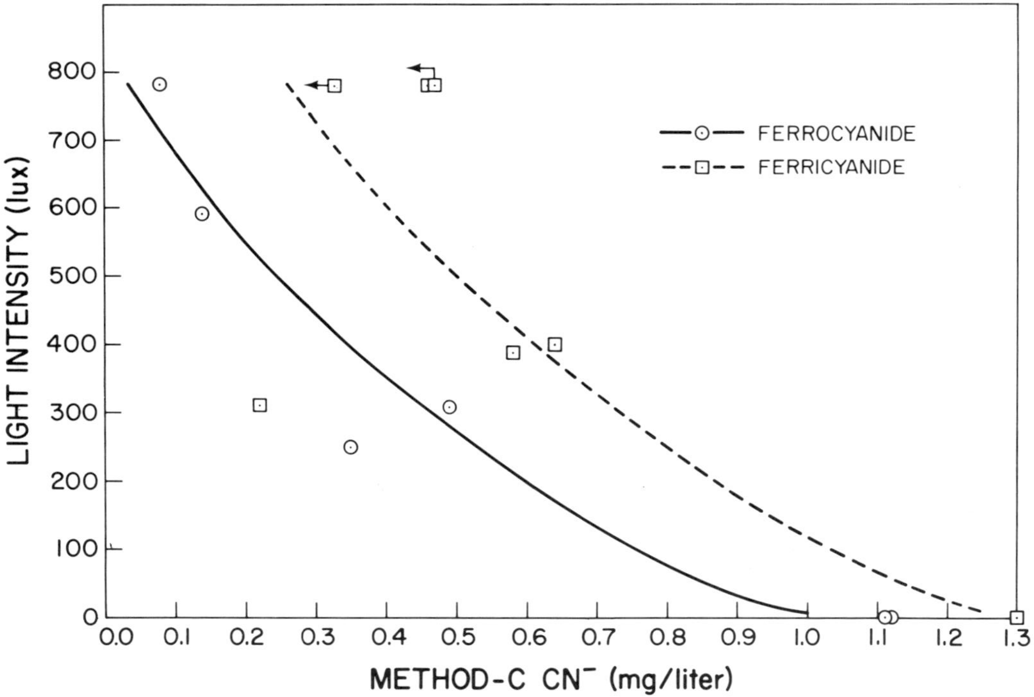

Figure 1. Test tank concentrations with ≤ 10% mortality vs. light intensity. (Ferricyanide data points with arrows indicate > 10% mortality.)

Thiocyanate Toxicity Tests - Results

In conducting our initial thiocyanate acute toxicity tests on brook trout, we observed that, although there was an overall dose response correlation, some fish survived the 96-hour test period at thiocyanate concentrations an order of magnitude greater than those that caused a high percentage of mortality to others (Table 4). We also observed that the death of fish frequently would be sudden, i.e. fish that evidenced little or no sign of distress at the time of routine scheduled mortality observations were under distress or dead shortly thereafter. We further observed that when we were removing the fish from the tank at the end of the test, some of the seemingly healthy fish died in the dip net. These mortalities in the tank or upon removal were characterized by sudden rapid movement, onset of tonic convulsions, loss of equilibrium and buoyancy, gasping, flaring of the operculae, darkening of the skin epithelia, and finally cessation of ventilation and extreme rigor. We termed this occurrence "sudden death syndrome" (SDS).

To test the hypothesis that SDS was related to the fish being distressed by activity near the test area, two 96-hour acute toxicity tests, one each on brook trout (Test 658) and rainbow trout (Test 723), were conducted during which activity near the test area was reduced to a necessary minimum. At the close of the standard 96-hour test periods the fish were stressed with a dip net. Mortality counts taken 15 minutes later (Test 658) and 75 minutes lates (Test 723) showed a dramatic increase over those taken at 96 hours (Table 5). Two additional 96-hour tests on brook trout (Tests 657 and 659) were conducted during which the fish (10 fish per tank) were stressed with a dip net at 24, 48, 72, and 95 hours. Fish size and measured water chemistry variables for these tests were similar to those reported for Test 658. The 96-hour LC50 for Test 657 was 13.8 mg/liter SCN^- and that for Test 659 was 13.3 mg/liter SCN^-.

To determine whether the toxicity of thiocyanate might differ with different photoperiods, duplicate 96-hour tests were conducted on rainbow trout under each of three different light regimes: continuous exposure under red light, a daily regime of 12 hours white light and 12 hours in the dark, and continuous exposure to white light. The fish appeared to be least sensitive to thiocyanate toxicity under red light, more so under the alternate light/dark regime, and most sensitive under continuous exposure to white light (Table 6). At the end of the 96-hour test periods, the fish tested under continuous red light were briefly exposed to white light, and the light was briefly turned off on the fish tested continuously under white light; mortality counts were taken again 45 minutes later for each of these tests. Although not as dramatic as in the tests with trout subjected to stress at the close of the 96-hour test period (Table 5), there was an increase in mortality in three out of four of these tests following the sudden change in light regime.

The persistence of SDS was tested by stressing (dip net method) separate groups of juvenile rainbow trout (8-10 fish per group) at 0,

Table 4. Percent mortality of brook trout[a] in each test tank during 96-hour acute toxicity tests on thiocyanate[b] (Tests 651, 652, 653, 655).

Test No.-Tank No.	Exposure concentration, mg/liter SCN^-	No. of fish	Percent mortality at 96 h
651-6	517	10	90
651-5	375	10	90
651-4	298	10	80
651-3	232	10	80
652-6	198	10	90
651-2	163	10	80
652-5	148	10	70
652-4	115	10	90
653-6	96.4	15	73
652-3	90.8	10	90
653-5	72.1	15	47
652-2	65.4	9	56
653-4	56.1	15	73
653-3	44.3	15	53
653-2	31.6	15	47
655-6	31.3	10	50
655-5	24.1	10	70
655-4	18.5	10	30
655-3	14.8	10	20
655-2	10.5	10	0
All tests-1	0.0	45	0

[a] Mean fish size (and range): 6.7(5.56-7.94) g, 8.2(6.1-10.2) cm.

[b] Other measured water variables, mean values and ranges for all tanks: temperature 15.1(12.9-17.3) C; dissolved oxygen 7.70(6.38-8.31) mg/liter; pH 7.88(7.83-7.90); alkalinity 176(167-181) mg/liter as $CaCO_3$; hardness 203(195-208) m/liter as $CaCO_3$.

Table 5. Percent mortality before and after stress of fish exposed to thiocyanate[a] (Ten fish/tank).

	Brook trout[b] (Test 658)			Rainbow trout[c] (Test 723)		
		Percent mortality			Percent mortality	
Tank No.	Exposure concentration, mg/liter SCN^-	96h	96.25h	Exposure concentration, mg/liter SCN^-	96h	97.25h
1	0.00	0	0	0.02	0	0
2	5.52	0	10	7.70	0	100
3	8.00	10	70	9.90	0	100
4	9.99	10	70	11.8	30	80
5	13.0	0	80	15.3	0	100
6	16.7	10	100	20.8	50	90

[a]Other measured water chemistry variables, mean values (and ranges) for all tanks: Test 658 - temperature 16.3(15.9-16.7) C, dissolved oxygen 7.54(7.20-7.93) mg/liter, pH 7.86(7.83-7.95), alkalinity 164 mg/liter as $CaCO_3$ (all measurements), hardness 194(194-195) mg/liter as $CaCO_3$; Test 723 - temperature 11.8(11.3-12.5) C, dissolved oxygen 9.35(9.20-9.78) mg/liter, pH 7.95(7.92-8.00), alkalinity 175(172-178) mg/liter as $CaCO_3$, hardness 202(198-206) mg/liter as $CaCO_3$.

[b]Mean fish size (and range)· 8.9 g, 9.1(7.8-10.7) cm; 96-h LC50 > 16.7 mg/liter SCN^-, 96.25-h LC50 7.79 mg/liter SCN^- (95% C.I. 6.62-9.16).

[c]Mean fish size (and range) 0.72(0.32-1.42) g, 4.16(3.15-5.25) cm; 96-h LC50 20.8 mg/liter SCN^- (95% C.I. not calculable by method used), 97.25-h LC50 < 7.70 mg/liter SCN^-.

Table 6. Acute toxicity of thiocyanate to rainbow trout[a] during tests[b] with different light regimes. (Ten fish/tank).

Test No.	Light regime	LC50 mg/liter SCN^- (95% C.I.) 96-h		96.75-h	
721	Continuous red light	159	(119-213)	76.3	(48.7-120)
725	Continuous red light	64.6	(13.2-316)	64.6	(13.2-316)
727	12h white light/12h dark	83.5	--[c]		
728	12h white light/12h dark	55.7	(39.0-79.6)		
720	Continuous white light	48.3	(34.6-67.5)	38.7	(25.7-58.3)
724	Continuous white light	44.9	(30.0-67.2)	41.4	(27.4-62.5)

[a]Mean fish size (and range) 0.83(0.28-1.79) g, 4.42(3.10-5.55) cm.

[b]Other measured water variables, mean values and ranges for all tanks: temperature 13.0(12.2-13.5) C, dissolved oxygen 8.96(8.66-9.30) mg/liter, pH 7.93(7.77-8.87), alkalinity 174(168-206) mg/liter as $CaCO_3$, hardness 202(200-206) mg/liter as $CaCO_3$.

[c]Confidence intervals not calculable by method used.

4, 12, 24, and 48 hours after exposure to 6.7-8.0 mg/liter SCN^- for 96 hours under flow-through conditions; a single control group was stressed at each of these time periods. After the 96-hour exposure period, thiocyanate addition to the incoming water to each test tank was discontinued; concentrations in the test tanks at 4 hours were approximately 4 mg/liter SCN^-, and < 1 mg/liter SCN^- by 12 hours. The group stressed at 4 hours suffered 60% mortality, and none of the fish died after stress at 48 hours (Table 7).

CONCLUSIONS

Solutions of both ferrocyanide and ferricyanide were more acutely toxic to rainbow trout when tested under light than when tested in total darkness. Further, there was a trend toward greater toxicity of either of these solutions at greater light intensity. Both of these potential toxicants are known to decompose under light to produce free cyanide. Although it was not possible for us to measure free cyanide, the concentration of Method-C CN^- was assumed to approximate the concentration of free cyanide.

If free cyanide alone were the toxic agent, and if Method-C CN^- concentrations approximate free cyanide concentrations, then calculation of LC50 values in terms of Method-C CN^- should have been comparable for all tests regardless of light regime. This was not the case; toxicity of the solutions tested in terms of Method-C CN^-, whether considering the LC50 values for either or both sets of tests, or considering the individual tanks with $\leq$ 10% mortality for both sets of tests combined, revealed a relationship between available light and mortality of fish.

We conclude that Method-C CN^- is not a true (approximate) measure of free cyanide under the conditions of our tests, and/or that free cyanide was not the sole toxic agent in the tests conducted. Additional research will be necessary to quantify better the toxicity of solutions of iron cyanide complexes, and the conditions of their photodegradation. In conducting this additional research, greater care should be exercised to standardize light conditions both among tanks for any given test, and between tests that are to be compared for other variables such as temperature. Further, the procedures for analysis of different forms of cyanide in the test waters should be reviewed to ensure that samples collected have not appreciably altered by the time of analysis.

The results of our tests on thiocyanate demonstrate it to be acutely toxic to trout at concentrations lower than those suggested by previous studies (see Doudoroff 1976). The acute toxicity of thiocyanate to trout, however, would appear to be relatively unpredictable. Exposed fish, which seemed healthy, would suddenly and often for no apparent reason begin to convulse and quickly expire. The signs of SDS in trout (convulsions, loss of equilibrium and buoyancy, extreme rigor, among others) are virtually identical to the characteristics of acute thiocyanate toxicity in mammals, including humans (convulsions, vertigo, coma, hyper-reactivity,

Table 7. Persistence of sudden death syndrome in juvenile rainbow trout[a/] maintained in fresh water for different time periods after 96-hour exposure to SCN^- (Test 726).[b/]

Group No.	Exposure concentration, mg/liter SCN^-	Fish alive after 96h exposure	Hours in replacement water after SCN^- exposure and before 30s stress[c/]	Deaths during 45 min period after stress	Percent mortalities from SDS
1	6.7	8	0	6	75
2	7.3	10	4	6	60
3	6.9	9	12	2	22
4	8.0	9	24	3	33
5	7.7	9	48	0	0

[a/] Ten fish per group, mean size and range 1.03(0.37–2.48) g, 4.57(3.25–6.00) cm.

[b/] A single control group of ten fish was maintained in freshwater for the entire 96-hour exposure and subsequent 48-hour stress periods. This group was stressed each time any of the other groups was stressed. No mortalities occurred in this control group.

[c/] No fish died during these periods.

extensor rigidity) (Garvin 1939, Smith 1973). In mammals, these effects are probably due to the SCN^- ion itself, rather than to its metabolic products, HCN, OCN^-, and NH_3 (Smith 1973); administration of sodium thiosulphate, an antidote for cyanide poisoning, has no effect on thiocyanate toxicity in mammals. Thiocyanate toxicity in mammals would appear to be influenced by neural activity, inasmuch as sympathomimetic stimulants (e.g. amphetamines) increase the toxicity of SCN^-, whereas barbiturate anaesthetics (e.g. phenobarbital) decrease its toxicty (Smith 1973). Similarly, the possible effect of photoperiod on thiocyanate toxicity to trout may be related to the observed increase in spontaneous activity of fish under continuous white light relative to fish under continuous dim red light.

SDS in fish may represent a direct effect of the thiocyanate anion on neuromuscular functioning; SCN^- has been shown to enhance the contractility and electrical conduction of frog muscle fibres (Lubin 1957), and to increase the excitability and electrical transmission of spinal neural pathways and motoneurons (Goto and Esplin 1961). Regardless of the exact mechanism involved in SDS, normal rapid movements of wild fish during feeding and predator avoidance probably would be sufficient to trigger SDS as a consequence of thiocyanate exposure.

Standard acute toxicity tests (96-hour LC50 determinations) are of limited value in predicting the toxicity of thiocyanate because of the unpredictability of SDS. Subsequent to the studies reported here, we determined that the correlation between plasma thiocyanate concentrations and SDS provides a more certain measure of thiocyanate toxicity (Heming et al. 1985). Those results demonstrated that fish readily accumulated SCN^-, and 50% of the fish tested would be at risk of SDS when plasma SCN^- concentrations reached approximately 250 mg/liter. The duration of thiocyanate exposure necessary to attain that plasma concentration depends upon the exposure concentration, fish size, water temperature, and ambient water quality. It is possible that, under conditions when uptake of SCN^- is extremely slow, excretion of SCN^- would be able to keep pace with SCN^- uptake and plasma concentrations of thiocyanate would remain low. During long term exposures, however, fish probably would exhibit the chronic effects of thiocyanate.

ACKNOWLEDGMENTS

Elizabeth L. Meyn, Donald R. Skaar, and Richard K. Zajdel were principally responsible for performing the acute toxicity tests, and Ms. Meyn and Terry L. Mudder (Homestake Mining Company) for the water chemistry analyses. This research was funded by the U.S. Environmental Protection Agency, Environmental Research Laboratory, Duluth, Minnesota, Research Grant CR807240, and by the Homestake Mining Company, Lead, South Dakota.

REFERENCES

APHA (American Public Health Association), American Water Works Association, and Water Pollution Control Federation. 1980. Standard methods for the examination of water and wastewater. 15th ed. American Public Health Association, Washington, D.C.

ASTM (American Society for Testing and Materials). 1981. Proposed revision of standard methods of test for cyanide in water, Standard D-2036-81. American Society for Testing and Materials, Philadelphia, Pennsylvania.

ASTM (American Society for Testing and Materials). 1982. Designation D-2036. Annual book of standards. American Society for Testing and Materials, Philadelphia, Pennsylvania.

Barnett, H.J.M., M.V. Jackson, and W.B. Spaulding. 1951. Thiocyanate psychosis. J. Am. Med. Assoc. 147: 1554-1558.

Benoit, D.A., V.R. Mattson, and D.L. Olson. 1982. A continuous-flow mini-diluter system for toxicity testing. Water Res. 16: 457-464.

Boxer, G.E., and J.C. Rickards. 1952a. Determination of traces of hydrogen cyanide in respiratory air. Archs. Biochem. Biophys. 39: 287-291.

Boxer, G.E., and J.C. Rickards. 1952b. Determination of thiocyanate in body fluids. Archs. Biochem. Biophys. 39: 292-300.

Broderius, S.J., and L.L. Smith. 1980. Final Report. Grant No. R805291. U.S. Environmental Protection Agency, Duluth, Minnesota.

Caruso, S.C. 1975. The chemistry of cyanide compounds and their behaviour in the aquatic environment. Carnegie-Mellon Institute of Research, Mellon Institute.

Davenport, H.W. 1940. The inhibition of carbonic anhydrase and of gastric secretion by thiocyanate. Am. J. Physiol. 129: 505-514.

Davies, R.E. 1951. The mechanism of hydrochloric acid production by the stomach. Biol. Rev. 26: 87-120.

Devuyst, E.A., B.R. Conard, and V.A. Ettel. 1982. Pilot plant operation of the Inco SO_2/air cyanide removal process. Can. Mining J. August 1982: 27-30.

Doudoroff, P. 1976. Toxicity to fish of cyanides and related compounds. A review. EPA-600/3-76-038. U.S. Environmental Protection Agency, Duluth, Minnesota.

Epstein, F.H., J. Maetz, and G. de Renzis. 1973. Active transport of chloride by the teleost gill: inhibition by thiocyanate. Am. J. Physiol. 224: 1295-1299.

Epstein, F.H., P. Silva, J.N. Forrest, and R.J. Solomon. 1975. Chloride transport and its inhibition by thiocyanate in gills of seawater teleosts. Comp. Biochem. Physiol. 52A: 681-683.

Garvin, C.F. 1939. The fatal toxic manifestations of the thiocyanates. J. Am. Med. Assoc. 112: 1125-1127.

Goldstein, F., and F. Reiders. 1951. Formation of cyanide in dog and man following administration of thiocyanate. Am. J. Physiol. 167: 47-51.

Goldstein, F., and F. Reiders. 1953. Conversion of thiocyanate to cyanide by an erythrocytic enzyme. Am. J. Physiol. 173: 287-290.

Goodman, L., and A. Gilman. 1970. The pharmacological basis of therapeutics. 4th ed. The Macmillan Co., London, England.

Goto, K., and D.W. Esplin. 1961. Excitatory effects of thiocyanate on spinal cord. J. Pharmacol. Exp. Ther. 133: 129-136.

Habig, W.H., J.H. Keen, and W.B. Jakoby. 1975. Glutathion S-transferase in the formation of cyanide from organic thiocyanates and as an organic nitrate reductase. Biochem. Biophys. Res. Commun. 64: 501-506.

Hamilton, M.A., R.C. Russo, and R.V. Thurston. 1977. Trimmed Spearman-Karber method for estimating median lethal concentrations in toxicity bioassays. Environ. Sci. Technol. 11: 714-719. Correction -- Environ. Sci. Technol. (1978) 12: 417.

Heming, T.A., R.V. Thurston, E.L. Meyn, and R.K. Zajdel. 1985. Acute toxicity of thiocyanate to trout. Trans. Am. Fish. Soc. (In press).

Huiatt, J.L., J.E. Kerrigan, F.A. Olson, and G.L. Potter. 1983. Workshop -- Cyanide from Mineral Processing. Utah Mining and Mineral Resources Research Institute, Salt Lake City, Utah.

Izatt, R.M., J.J. Christensen, R.T. Pack, and R. Bench. 1962. Thermodynamics of metal-cyanide coordination. I. pK, $\triangle H°$, and $\triangle S°$ values as a function of temperature for hydrocyanic acid dissociation in aqueous solution. Inorg. Chem. 3: 828-831.

Katz, A.I., and F.H. Epstein. 1971. Effect of anions on adenosine triphosphatase of kidney tissue. Enzymes 12: 499-507.

Kimball, G.L., L.L. Smith, Jr., and S.J. Broderius. 1978. Chronic toxicity of hydrogen cyanide to the bluegill. Trans. Am. Fish. Soc. 107: 341-345.

Lubin, M. 1957. The effect of iodide and thiocyanate ions on the mechanical and electrical properties of frog muscle. J. Cell. Comp. Physiol. 49: 335-349.

Meyn, E.L., R.K. Zajdel, and R.V. Thurston. 1984. Acute toxicity of ferrocyanide and ferricyanide to rainbow trout (Salmo gairdneri). Technical Report No. 84-1, Fisheries Bioassay Laboratory, Montana State University, Bozeman, Montana.

Mount, D.I., and W.A. Brungs. 1967. A simplified dosing apparatus for fish toxicology studies. Water Res. 1: 21-29.

Pines, K.L., and M.M. Crymble. 1952. In vitro conversion of thiocyanate to cyanide in the presence of erythrocytes. Proc. Soc. Exp. Biol. Med. 81: 160-163.

Smith, R.P. 1973. Cyanate and thiocyanate: acute toxicity. Proc. Soc. Exp. Biol. Med. 142: 1041-1044.

Solomon, R.J., P. Silva, and F.H. Epstein. 1973. Thiocyanate inhibitable ATPase in the gill of Anguilla rostrata. Bull. Mt. Desert Island Biol. Lab. 13: 115-117.

Towill, L.E., J.S. Drury, B.L. Whitfield, E.B. Lewis, E.L. Galyan, and A.S. Hammons. 1978. Reviews of the environmental effects of pollutants: V. Cyanide. EPA-600/1-78-027. U.S. Environmental Protection Agency, Cincinnati, Ohio.

U.S. EPA (U.S. Environmental Protection Agency). 1974. Methods for chemical analysis of water and wastes. EPA-625/6-74-003. U.S. Environmental Protection Agency, Washington, D.C.

U.S. EPA (U.S. Environmental Protection Agency). 1980. Ambient water quality critieria for cyanides. EPA-440/5-80-037. U.S. Environmental Protection Agency, Washington, D.C.

Vennesland, B., E.E. Conn, C.J. Knowles, J. Westley, and F. Wissing. 1981. Cyanides in biology. Academic Press, London, England.

Westley, J. 1973. Rhodanese. Adv. Enzymol. 39: 327-368.

Wolff, J. 1964. Transport of iodide and other anions in the thyroid gland. Physiol. Rev. 44: 45-90.

Wuhrmann, K., and H. Woker. 1948. Beitrage zur Toxicologie der Fische. II. Experimentelle Untersuchungen uber die Ammoniak- und Blausaurevergiftung. Schweiz. Z. Hydrol. 11: 210-244.

Zadunaisky, J.A., M.A. Lande, and J. Hafner. 1971. Further studies on chloride transport in the frog cornea. Am. J. Physiol. 221: 1832-1836.

CONFERENCE ON CYANIDE AND THE ENVIRONMENT
Tucson, Arizona • December 1984
Published by Geotechnical Engineering Program • Colorado State University • Fort Collins, Colorado 80523

THE DETERMINATION OF CYANIDES IN THE HYDROMETALLURGICAL PROCESSING OF GOLD

C. Pohlandt*

The determination of cyanides in cyanidation processes is of considerable importance for several reasons. For example, excessive consumption of the reagent must be prevented for economic reasons; the chemistry of the process must be controlled for efficient operation; and, most important of all, environmental pollution must be avoided. Depending on the pH value of a solution, cyanide can be present as the molecular acid (HCN), as ionic cyanide, or as metal complexes of widely varying stability. Classical methods for the determination of cyanide are invariably tedious and time-consuming, and are rarely suitable for the rapid analysis of large numbers of samples.

Ion chromatography has gained increasing acceptance in the determination of a large variety of anions and, with an amperometric instead of a conductivity detector, it is eminently suitable for the determination of cyanides(1). For the determination of 'free' or 'available' cyanide, the sample simply needs to be diluted and to be injected into the chromatographic system. With a weakly alkaline mobile phase containing ethylene diamine, excellent separation of the cyanide from most other anions, including common interferents such as sulfide and thiocyanide, is obtained. The method is fast, precise, and reasonably accurate, and as little as 50 μg of cyanide ion per litre can be reliably determined. Weak metal cyanide complexes, for example those of cadmium, zinc, and nickel, are decomposed in the alkaline environment of the chromatographic system, whereas strong cyanide complexes, for example those of iron, gold, and cobalt, remain intact and are retained on the anion-exchange separator.

'Total Cyanide'

The determination of 'total' cyanide requires the decomposition of strong metal cyanide complexes. Classical methods of determination require boiling under reflux with acids, usually followed by a distillation step. At the Council for Mintek Technology (Mintek) it was considered that an attractive alternative approach would be to combine ultraviolet irradiation, which results in the photo-ionization of

---

* Analytical Chemist, Mintek, Randburg, South Africa

strong cyanide complexes, with the ion-chromatographic procedure. It was established that, in 3 per cent hypophosphorous acid (50 per cent), all the metal cyanide complexes except that of cobalt decompose competely if they are irradiated for 2 to 3 minutes. Various mercury lamps were tested as irradiation sources. Those with a maximum radiation output at wavelengths longer than 300 nm were preferred because thiocyanate was not decomposed, whereas the recovery of cyanide from the hexacyano cobaltate complex improved. It was established also that a more powerful lamp, i.e. a 400 W instead of the 100 W mercury lamp originally used, further improved the decomposition of the cobalt complex (i.e. 50 per cent), and 96 to 100 per cent of the cyanide present was reproducibly recovered from a mixture of stable complexes. Photoionization is complex, and the oxidation-reduction reactions involved need to be carefully controlled if reliable analytical results are to be obtained. For example, the irradiation of an aqueous solution of ionic canide in the absence of reducing agents results in the quantitative formation of harmless cyanate within 3 minutes. Metal complexes, on the other hand, decompose slowly with the simultaneous appearance of cyanide and cyanate ions. Therefore, pollution of the environment with so-called 'stable' cyanide complexes must be avoided, since irradiation by sunlight would result in the continuous production of small amounts of cyanide over long periods of time, which could be harmful to marine life.

Individual Cyanide Complexes

Recently the Dionex Corporation, U.S.A., issued a series of application notes describing the separation of the complexes of cobalt from gold (I) and gold (III), and also the separation of iron (II) from ion (III) by mobile-phase ion chromatography (MPIC)(2). This procedure utilizes the principles of ion-pair chromatography, and uses a suppressor device to reduce the conductivity of the mobile phase prior to conductimetric detection.

Metallurgical processes that involve the use of resins or carbons frequently suffer from the 'poisoning' of such materials by, for example, metal cyanide species that cannot be eluted under normal stripping conditions. It follows that a knowledge of the kind of complexes present in the system is of considerable importance.

A method based on the information issued by Dionex has been developed that enables the cyanide complexes of copper, nickel, cobalt, iron (III) or iron (II), and gold to be separated (Figure 1). The determination of the copper complex that, due to decomposition in the suppressor, could not be detected conductimetrically, was achieved by simultaneous photometric detection at 240 nm. Calibration graphs for the various complexes were found to be linear over the concentration ranges 0.2 to 10 mg/l; the gold (I) complex was the least sensitive. The separation of the two iron complexes, as claimed by the Dionex Corporation, could not be verified under any experimental conditions. Iron (II) and iron (III) cyanides were found to decompose rapidly when exposed to daylight, and additional peaks due to decomposition products were observed in the chromatogram. Daylight also had a pronounced effect on the hexacyano cobaltate (III) complex, resulting in the formation of the aquo-pentacyano cobaltate (III) complex. Since it is the latter complex that was previously identified as causing resin poisoning, it is of significance that the proposed procedure is able to distinguish between the two cobalt complexes(3).

References

1. R.D. Rocklin and E.L. Johnson, Anal. Chem., vol. 55. 1983. p. 4.

2. DIONEX CORPORATION, Application Notes 40 and 40R and Technical Note 12. DIONEX CORPORATION, Sunnyvale, Ca. 94086.

3. C.A. Fleming and R.D. Hancock, J.S. Afr. Inst. Min. Metall. vol. 79. 1979. p. 334.

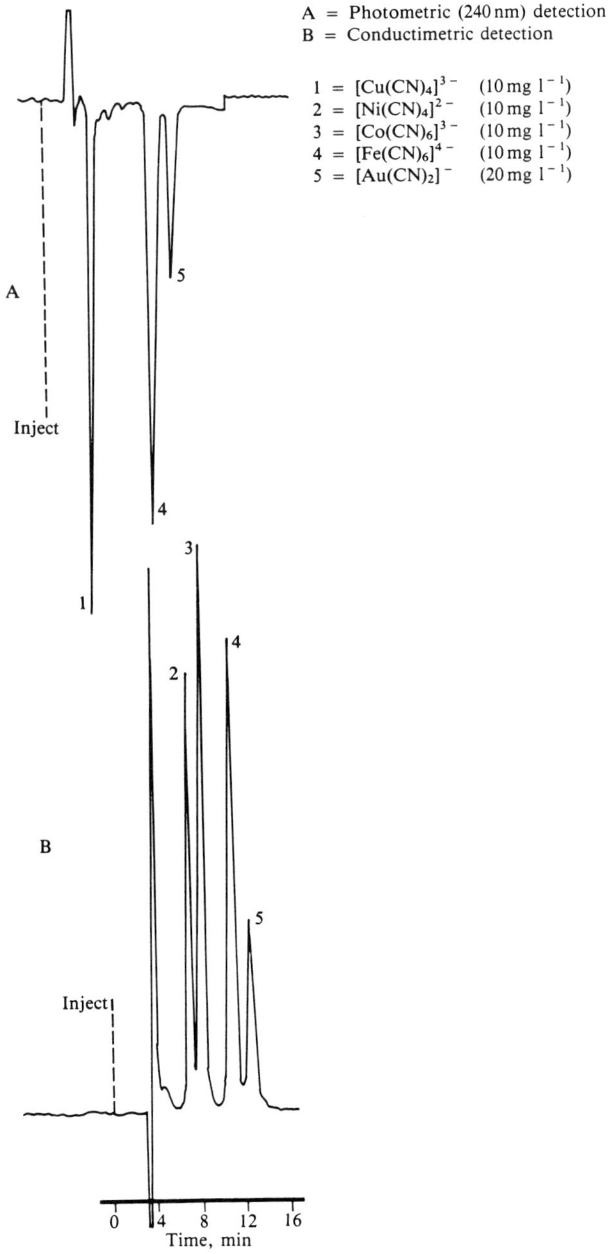

FIGURE 1. The separation of five individual metal cyanide complexes

CONFERENCE ON CYANIDE AND THE ENVIRONMENT
Tucson, Arizona . December 1984
Published by Geotechnical Engineering Program • Colorado State University • Fort Collins, Colorado 80523

DEVELOPMENT OF SITE SPECIFIC DISCHARGE CRITERIA THROUGH TOXICOLOGICAL TESTING

by
Terry Mudder[1], Fred Fox[2], Jim Whitlock[3], and Steve Marshall[4]

ABSTRACT

Employment of aquatic toxicological testing for the selection of viable wastewater treatment alternatives and the development of site specific water quality criteria is increasing. The increase in its usage is due to recognition that such testing is cost effective in solving environmental problems and its use should no longer be considered merely an elaborate research tool. There is a growing spirit of compromise and cooperation surfacing between industry and the regulatory agencies in an attempt to, through rational and practical approaches, solve long standing environmental problems. This paper deals with an approach undertaken at the Homestake Mine in Lead, South Dakota. The approach followed flexible guidelines recently proposed in a new water quality criteria development document published by the EPA. The problem dealt with development of an acceptable wastewater treatment alternative that would provide an effluent compatible with the designated use classifications of Whitewood Creek, the receiving stream.

INTRODUCTION

The use of aquatic toxicological testing in selecting environmentally acceptable wastewater treatment alternatives and establishing site specific water quality criteria is increasing rapidly, due to many factors. Regulatory agencies (state and federal) have recognized that previously calculated water quality and waste load allocation criteria are in certain instances unnecessarily stringent and unwarranted. Enforcement of these criteria may be impractical, leading to public outcry when violations remain unenforced. Both industry and regulatory agencies recognize that construction of tertiary or advanced wastewater treatment facilities in certain instances may result in effluents exhibiting adverse aquatic life effects. These toxicological effects are often attributable to chemical and/or physical factors in the treated effluent which result from a toxic component previously unidentified through chemical analysis. This situation often arises when treatment plant process alternatives are evaluated on a numerical basis only. The reluctance of industry to invest millions of dollars in research, development, and construction of "state of the art" treatment

[1] Terry Mudder, Ph.D., Chief Environmental Engineer, [2] Fred Fox, Environmental Director, [3] Jim Whitlock, Chief Chemist, and [4] Steve Marshall, Bioassay Technician, Homestake Mine, Lead, South Dakota

facilities in an attempt to meet criteria which are technically unachievable or unnecessarily stringent. Finally, there is a spirit of compromise and cooperation developing between industry and regulatory agencies to attempt rational and practical approaches in establishing site specific criteria which will assure protection of beneficial use classifications.[1]

This paper deals with the employment of an aquatic toxicological testing program currently in progress at the Homestake Mine in Lead, South Dakota. The purpose of the program is to establish site specific water quality criteria and waste load allocations to assure protection of the beneficial uses of the receiving stream, Whitewood Creek, a cold water marginal trout fishery. Development of a treatment facility and subsequent development of water quality criteria relied significantly upon the use of toxicological testing and the guidelines proposed in the recent draft of the EPA aquatic life protection and criteria development document.[2]

HISTORICAL PERSPECTIVE

On September 3, 1976, the United States Environmental Protection Agency (EPA), issued to the Homestake Mine in Lead, South Dakota, National Pollutant Discharge Elimination System (NPDES) Permit No. SD-0000043. The permit contained discharge effluent limitations derived from Best Practicable Control Technology requirements under the Clean Water Act and South Dakota water quality standards applicable to Whitewood Creek, the receiving stream. Effective July 1, 1977, the NPDES permit required Homestake to meet very low effluent limitations principally designed to attain and maintain the existing beneficial use classifications of Whitewood Creek below the mine's discharge.

On July 1, 1978 the mine was not in compliance with the permit limitations, despite its attempt to implement Best Practicable Control Technology for the destruction of cyanides and heavy metals in the discharge. At this time, it became clear that accurate and precise laboratory analysis to measure the very low levels in the permit was also a problem.

Numerous treatment technologies representing the Best Available Technology were tested at the mine prior to the selection of a biological treatment process. Construction of a treatment facility was initiated during March of 1983 and completed and placed into continuous operation by August 15, 1984.

If the treated effluent discharged by the mine will not interfere with the attainment and maintenance of the existing designated beneficial uses of Whitewood Creek under South Dakota water quality standards, the State will initiate a proceeding to consider modification of its water quality criteria for Whitewood Creek.[3]

In order to assure attainment and maintenance of the designate uses for the receiving stream and to be certain that the mine can properly analyze for and meet future permit limits, an aquatic toxicological testing program was integrated into the treatment selection program during the spring of 1980.

The program consisted of 1) conducting a bioassessment of the receiving waters, 2) cooperating with State and Federal agencies in modifying South Dakota's surface water quality standards to reflect laboratory testing procedures developed at the mine and allow for development of site-specific criteria for water quality standards and 3) constructing and utilizing an on-site aquatic toxicological testing facility.

BIOASSESSMENT

The first step toward development of site specific water quality criteria and waste load allocations is to establish the beneficial use classification of the discharger's receiving system. In the case of the Homestake Mine, the receiving system is a small cool water stream, Whitewood Creek. A bioassessment was completed in accordance with proposed EPA guidelines and protocol[4] at a cost of approximately $300,000. The actual thirteen month study (March 1981-March 1982) was conducted and designed by a team of university professors, experts in their respective fields, in cooperation with the South Dakota Department of Water and Natural Resources (DWNR) and EPA Region VIII. The study was conducted along Whitewood Creek and two reference streams, Spearfish Creek and Sand Creek. The study assessed the physical, chemical, and biological characteristics of the receiving stream, defining the stream's existing environmental conditions and potential future beneficial uses.

The physical characteristics investigated included surficial geology, stream discharge, stream morphometry, and sediment size classifications and quantification. In addition, chemical analyses were conducted on samples collected from surface waters, sediments and the biota. The biological investigations included a survey of riparian vegetation (including percent cover), qualitative and quantitative macrobenthos, algae, diatoms, and existing fisheries. The detailed study fulfilled the requirements of a water body survey and formed the basis for a petition to request a modification of the beneficial use classification of Whitewood Creek from a "cold water permanent fishlife propagation" classification to "cold water marginal fishlife propogation". The latter classification, which was granted, protects for stockings of catchable size trout, but does not provide protection for reproduction. The results of the study concluded the habitat was limited due to low hydraulic flows and excessive summer water temperatures. In addition to the petition for reclassification of Whitewood Creek, Homestake initiated further specific changes to the South Dakota water quality regulations to upgrade them technically and to make them consistent with current scientific thinking.[5] The changes required modification of the surface water quality regulations through public hearing and final approval by the South Dakota board of water management. They included allowances for toxicological testing and its use in setting site specific water quality criteria. Advances in analytical techniques, specifically the methodology for analysis of weak acid dissociable cyanides, (considered by Homestake an important potential form of toxicologically significant cyanides), were also accepted by the water management board and are presently incorporated into South Dakota law.[6,7]

TOXICOLOGICAL TESTING FACILITY

In conjunction with the water body assessment and the upgrading of the surface water quality regulations, Homestake constructed a toxicological testing facility located adjacent to the site of the new biological wastewater treatment facility. The primary test organisms include Daphnia, macroinvertebrates (stoneflies and caddisflies), and trout (rainbow and brown). Dilution water is pumped continually through the bioassay facility from a pumping station located along Whitewood Creek approximately one mile above Homestake's discharge. The dilution water provides flowing fresh water for the stock fish population and for test purposes. A bioassay facilities manual details the specific protocol employed in the laboratory and is utilized as an educational tool to train bioassay technicians.[8] The basic toxicological testing procedures are in accordance with procedures specified by ASTM[9], Standard Methods[10], and the EPA[11].

The toxicological testing facility was built with a two-fold purpose in mind. First, to evaluate and compare the toxicological effects of various treatment process alternatives. Secondly, to utilize the toxicity data from the process selected for eventual development of site specific water quality criteria and waste load allocations.

Alternative Treatment Selection

The first use of the facility is of particular importance, as emphasis on specific parameter removal through routine numerical evaluations could result in "treated effluents" that meet numerical limits, but still exhibit considerable toxicity. The toxicological characteristics are due to pollutants associated with or produced through breakdown of target parameters not analyzed for and/or removed through further treatment. The employment of whole effluent testing aids in minimizing these possible oversights. One example involved numerical and toxicological comparisons of the copper catalyzed hydrogen peroxide process and the biological process as alternatives for the treatment of Homestake's waste waters. In terms of specific parameter removal, the two treatment alternatives were comparable, based solely upon numerical evaluations of the treated effluents (such as copper and total cyanide removal). However, toxicological evaluations of the effluents indicated the chemical treatment effluent to be quite toxic as compared to the effluent from the biological treatment pilot plants. Further chemical analyses indicated the chemically treated effluent contained significant concentrations of ammonia, not found in the biologically treated wastewater. The ammonia constituted a parameter which would require further treatment to remove if the chemical treatment alternative was to be employed. As a result of comparative numerical and toxicological evaluations, the biological treatment alternative was found feasible and environmentally acceptable at a considerable cost savings over other process alternatives. Design of the biological treatment facility was completed and a full scale treatment plant was constructed and placed into continuous operation on August 13, 1984. A comparison of the various treatment plant alternatives tested can be found in a recent paper presented at the AIME conference is Los Angeles.[12]

The use of toxicological testing aided significantly in the development and selection of a "state of the art" innovative treatment process. The reduced capital and operational costs could save millions of dollars over the design life of the facility, while providing an environmentally acceptable effluent compatible with the designated beneficial use of the receiving stream.

Site Specific Water Quality Criteria Development

With the completion of the bioassessment, modification of the existing water quality regulations, and the construction of the treatment facility, the final step is to establish discharge criteria which are consistent with existing water quality criteria. The criteria development as generally outlined in the proposed EPA guidelines, involves three phases: selection of parameters of concern, recalculation of water quality criteria on a site specific basis, and a toxicological testing program to establish the final permit values for the parameters of interest. The process requires frequent meetings between key technical personnel from industry and the regulatory agencies with emphasis on flexibility, cooperation, and practicality. Due to the beneficial use classification of Whitewood Creek as a "cold water marginal" trout fishery, the approach to developing adequate criteria and the degree and type of toxicity testing is quite novel. With input from all parties, it was agreed that the first step of the process would require the establishment of a list of potential parameters which are of a concern from a water quality and beneficial use aspect. The second phase of the process involves recalculating the site specific water quality criteria for these parameters using existing ambient water quality criteria documents for each parameter.[13]

Based upon the recalculated water quality criteria and comparison of these values with historical background and untreated discharge water quality analyses, the list may be narrowed to those parameters of primary concern. These parameters form the basis for the third phase of the process, the toxicological testing program, which itself involves three modes: 48 hour range finding toxicity tests, 96 hour flow through tests to establish acute toxicities, and 45 day long term tests to establish chronic toxicities and long term effects.

The first mode of testing involves conducting a series of 48 hour static range finding toxicity tests using the primary organism of interest (most sensitive species, trout) to establish an approximate range of lethal concentrations (LC50's) for each of the parameters of interest. The choice of test concentrations is made on the basis of past testing and available literature centered on the organisms and parameters of interest. The results of this and other range finding tests produce toxicity information which is utilized to select a range of parameter concentrations to use in the second mode of testing, the 96 hour flow through toxicity tests.

In meetings prior to the initiation of the toxicity testing program it was mutually agreed that the results of the 96 hour tests would be used to derive instantaneous not-to-exceed in-stream water quality criteria, based upon an acceptable percent death. This approach was in agreement with the degree of protection to be afforded to the stocked fish population to maintain the beneficial use classification.

In order for this data, as well as subsequent long term test data to be utilized in developing waste load allocations for Homestake, a low flow value for Whitewood Creek had to be established. The 7Q25 value selected was 4.5 cfs (2000 gpm) and was derived by extrapolation of low flow conditions from adjacent water shed basins and through examination of existing flow records maintained by Homestake and the USGS. Using the design dry weather flow for the treatment plant of 2600 gpm (3.75 MGD), the resulting critical effluent dilution was 56%. It was decided to operate the flow through tests (both acute and long term) at this effluent/dilution water ratio in all aquaria, except the control. Using this fixed effluent concentration as the base ratio, concentrated solutions of the various test parameters are spiked into the aquaria with the use of a multichannel metering pump to create a series of test concentrations from which a 96 hour acute LC50 value could be obtained. This procedure allows one to study the effects of an individual parameter with the background matrix of the whole effluent present during the test.

No provision for control of water temperature is provided as the wastewater and dilution water temperatures fluctuate considerably during the course of a year. Control of the water temperatures would not reflect actual stream conditions and may lead to difficulties when attempting to extrapolate such information to real situations. As a result, it was decided the testing program would encompass the two most critical temperature periods, that of winter and late summer, both of which correspond to minimum flow conditions.

Following establishment of the maximum in stream values through the 96 hour test program, the final mode of toxicity testing involves conducting a series of long term, or chronic, tests to establish a 30' day average discharge value and subsequent waste load allocation. Since the beneficial use classification focuses upon maintenance of a stocked fish population and not reproduction, the purpose of these tests involving spiked effluent is to gather data on general external appearance, internal organ appearance, bioaccumulation, and of course, death. Based upon surveys and information obtained from local game, fish, and parks personnel, approximately 95% of the stocked fish are removed from a stocked stream section within 45-90 days. As a result, the long term tests will be conducted for 45 days to simulate a protection period. Again, a base effluent concentration of 56% is used into which concentrated solutions of each test parameter are spiked to produce a series of test concentrations. These concentrations are selected through examination of the test results from the previous 96 hour flow through tests. Organisms are fed throughout the long term test, which constitutes the only major difference in test protocol between the two tests. In addition to the testing of fish, indigenous macroinvertebrates which serve as food source organisms for the fish will also be included in the toxicity testing program. The insects tested include primarily stoneflies and caddisflies, as these species were the predominant organisms found in the receiving stream during the water body assessment.

CAPITAL AND OPERATING COSTS OF THE TOXICITY FACILITY

Table 1 presents itemized costs of construction of the bioassay facility and the associated dilution water pumping station. Capital costs will vary considerably from site to site. These costs represent an upper value, with considerable cost savings possible in both construction of the facility and the dilution water feed system. An approximate cost of operation is presented in Table 2, for the various test modes. Neither of these costs reflect the capital cost expended previously for the new Homestake Analytical Chemistry Laboratory.

CONCLUSION

The use of toxicological testing as an aid in selection of wastewater treatment alternatives and in the establishment of site specific water quality criteria is increasing rapidly. The implementation of such testing in an environmental program is cost effective and its use should no longer be considered merely an elaborate research tool, but rather a practical and sound approach to solving environmental problems. The capital expenditures by Homestake are far outweighed by considerable cost savings in developing an innovative wastewater treatment alternative, while providing a treated effluent which is environmentally compatible with the beneficial use classifications of its receiving stream. Also, the Homestake example has shown that industry and regulatory agencies can work together effectively to solve complicated environmental problems.

References

1. Edelman, L.H., Walline, R.E., "Developing a Cooperative Approach to Environmental Regulation"., National Resources Lawyer., Volume XVI, No. 3 pg. 489.

2. Water Quality Standards Handbook., United States Environmental Protection Agency, Office of Water Regulations and Standards, Washington, D.C., December 1983.

3. Consent Decree, Civil No. 78-5094 United States of America, State of South Dakota vs. Homestake Mining Company, February 1980.

4. Herricks, E.E., "Bioassessment of Whitewood Creek, Lawrence and Meade Counties, South Dakota"., 1982. Prepared for Homestake Mining Company, Lead, S.D.

5. Proposed modifications to amend Surface Water Quality Standards, ARSD Chapter 74:03:02., April 1984., Homestake Mining Company, Lead, S.D.

6. Mudder, T.I., Whitlock, J.L., Sharp, C., "Summary of the Toxicological Significance and Analytical Methodology for Free and Complexed Cyanides"., December 1, 1981.

7. "Workshop, Cyanide From Mineral Processing"., Chapter 5, Utah Mining and Mineral Resources Research Institute., February 2-3, 1982, Salt Lake City, Utah.

8. "Facilities and Operational Manual for the Homestake Mining Company Aquatic Toxicological Testing Facility", the Homestake Mine, Lead, S.D., First Edition, July 1981.

9. Proposed Standard Practice for Conducting Acute Toxicity Tests on Aqueous Effluents with Fishes, Macroinvertebrates and Amphibians, Draft 3, June 1, 1983. (T.A. Abrahamsen, Tech Bldg 311, Kingsport, Tenn. 37662, E-47.01)

10. Standard Methods for the Examination of Water and Wastewater, 15th Edition, 1980., pp. 615-743.

11. Methods for Measuring the Acute Toxicity of Effluents to Aquatic Organisms, 3rd Edition, EPA-600/4-82-000, November 1982.

12. Mudder, T.I., Whitlock, J.L., "Biological Treatment of Cyanidation Waste Waters"., presented at the annual AIME conference in Los Angeles, CA., February 1984.

13. "Ambient Water Quality Criteria ....", U.S. Environmental Protection Agency., National Technical Information Service., October 1980.

TABLE 1

CAPITAL COSTS OF CONSTRUCTION OF THE TOXICOLOGICAL TESTING FACILITY

EXPENDITURE PURPOSE	COST($)
Building	30,000.00
Internal piping	15,000.00
Aquaria	3,200.00
Pumps, dilutor system, metering system, tubing, glassware, etc.	6,000.00
Dilution water pumping system	
Pump house/pump	3,500.00
Stream modification for water source	5,000.00
4" buried water supply line to bioassay facility	12,000.00
TOTAL	74,700.00

TABLE 2

OPERATING COSTS OF THE BIOASSAY FACILITY

EXPENDITURE PURPOSE	TEST TYPE		
	48 HOUR STATIC	96 HOUR FLOW THROUGH	45 DAY FLOW THROUGH
Bioassay technician time ($11.50/hr)	$ 92.00	$ 276.00	$ 2,162.00
Chemical analysis ($5.00/analysis) (in house)	$390.00	$1,170.00	$ 8,190.00
Outside Chemical* Analyses	-----	-----	$ 1,500.00
Supervision ($20/hr)	$ 100.00	$ 100.00	$ 500.00
TOTALS	$ 582.00	$1,546.00	$12,352.00

*Outside chemical analysis of whole fish tissue for determination of bioaccumulation

CONFERENCE ON CYANIDE AND THE ENVIRONMENT
Tucson, Arizona . December 1984
Published by Geotechnical Engineering Program • Colorado State University • Fort Collins, Colorado 80523

CYANIDE-THIOCYANATE SPECIATION AND REMOVAL OF THIOCYANATE AND OTHER INTERFERENCES IN AUTOMATED SYSTEMS

by

Nabih P. Kelada[1], Cecil Lue-Hing[2] and John A. Chavich[3]

ABSTRACT

A fully automated system has been developed to measure the different cyanide species as well as thiocyanate in a variety of environmental samples. The system can analyze for three parameters simultaneously at the rate of 20 samples/hour. The system includes automated modules for UV irradiation and thin film distillation as well as direct color development. The different cyanide species and thiocyanate can thus be determined, namely UV total CN, total CN, acid dissociable CN, complex CN and SCN. Explanation of these terms and definitions are presented. The effects of basic factors (pH, temperature, time, and ionic strength) on the measurements are elucidated, thus the analytical behavior of the different species is understood.

Interferences are also discussed and proper treatments are given for turbidity, oxidants, metal cations, sulfides, nitrate-nitrite, aldehydes, carbonate-bicarbonate, fatty acids, and cyanide forming substances. Thiocyanate is determined by the automated system and subtracted from the UV total CN to obtain the true total CN.

INTRODUCTION

Cyanides are known to be toxic to different forms of life, to man and more so to aquatic life at low concentrations. The chemistry of cyanides in the environment is complex and the uncertainty of the proper identification of toxic cyanide species and their concentration levels is complicated by the fact that the analytical methodology needs some improvement. More sensitive, accurate and reproducible methods are needed to furnish proper information about the behavior of the different cyanide species in the receiving environment. This information should be helpful to the concerned authorities in the assessment of the cyanide limits for effluents, stream quality, and land disposal of cyanide bearing wastes.

Cyanides are compounds characterized by having the chemical group -C≡N. Ideally, cyanides can be classified according to their physicochemical properties as free, simple, complex or organic cyanides. In addition, other terms such as total cyanides, oxidizable cyanides, and

----

1. Nabih P. Kelada, Ph.D., Head of Methodology & Toxic Substances
2. Cecil Lue-Hing, D.Sc., P.E., Director of Research & Development Department
3. John A. Chavich, B.S., Sanitary Chemist
The Metropolitan Sanitary District of Greater Chicago

cyanides amenable to chlorination are frequently used. In fact, they reflect the corresponding methods of treatment and analysis.

Current cyanide analytical procedures involve three steps: Separation, absorption and measurement.[1] Separation of cyanides from the sample is a prerequisite step to eliminate several types of interference.[2] Separation usually follows acidification and some form of volatilization to break down the complex cyanides to the free form.[3] Several separation techniques are known, such as distillation at atmospheric pressure[4-6] or under reduced pressure[7] and separation by aeration.[4] Automated methods utilize modified techniques such as flash distillation[8] or thin-film distillation.[9] Absorption of the evolved HCN in an alkaline solution such as sodium hydroxide,[4-5] or sodium acetate[9] is the next step. Spiral flow gas washers[3] and recirculation[9] techniques are used in manual methods, whereas fractionating columns,[8] absorption columns,[9] and coils are used in automated methods. Measurement of the recovered cyanides can be volumetric, e.g., by titrating the absorbed cyanide with silver nitrate using rhodamine indicator,[10] or colorimetric, using color reagents such as benzidine[10], pyrazolone[12], or barbituric acid[13] in pyridine solution. Generally, the colorimetric measurement is for low cyanide levels and is applicable to automation. The type of cyanide determined by the different methods is controlled through selective decomposition and distillation.

One of the main objectives of this study was to develop an automated system to distinguish between different cyanide species at the low levels found in municipal treatment plant effluents and other environmental samples. It was also desirable to develop a reliable method for determination of thiocyanate, CNS^-, in the presence of different cyanide species. Identifying the interferences in the developed automated methods was also a major undertaking as well as establishing effective methods of treatment.

EXPERIMENTAL & DISCUSSION

Reagents:

Acid digestion mixture: 1 L contains 200 mL of (85%) orthophosphoric acid, 40 mL of (50%) hypophosphorous acid, and 2 g of sulfamic acid.

Sodium hydroxide: 0.02 M is used for HCN absorption and preparation of the cyanide working standards.

Phosphate buffer: (resultant pH 6) 1 L contains 83 g of sodium phosphate monobasic.

Acetate buffer: (resultant pH 4) 1 L contains 243 g sodium acetate-trihydrate and 480 g (458 ml) glacial acetic acid.

Chloramine-T: 5% stock solution prepare weekly, and 0.4% daily.

Pyridine-barbituric acid color reagent: 15 g barbituric acid in 1 L flask, and wet with water. Add 75 mL of pyridine and mix to dissolution, then add 15 mL of HCl (specific gravity 1.19). Mix and let cool then complete to volume. Keep in brown bottle and store in dark (stable for 3 months).

Cyanide and thiocyanate standards: Prepare alkaline stock solutions, 1 g/L (as CN), and standardize weekly or monthly. Prepare daily working solutions (1-100 μg/L CN) by dilution with 0.02 M NaOH.

Apparatus & Equipment

Some continuous flow Technicon Auto-Analyzer modules are used, namely sampler, pump, colorimeter, recorder and printer. This is in addition to the newly developed on-line thin film distillation[14] and ultraviolet irradiation.[15] A one channel or three channel system could be made. A schematic flow diagram of the automated system is shown in Figure 1. The rate is 20 samples per hour (1:1 cam), a 15 mm flow cell and a 580 nm colorimeter filter.

The thin film distillation unit is made of borosilicate glass and a schematic is shown in Figure 2. The horizontal tube accommodates the continuous flow of the acidified sample and is connected to the vertical tube to carry the HCN gas evolved to the absorption coil. The nondistilled portion flows to the waste trap. The aluminum bar is heated with a 150-W cartridge and temperature is controlled with a Variac and monitored with a thermometer.

Absorption of HCN gas is achieved by forcing the gas mixture and 0.02 M NaOH solution through a glass coil, 2.4 mm ID and 28 turns (Figure 2). The absorption coil should be placed horizontally or sloped downwards at any desirable angle.

The UV irradiator utilizes a mercury lamp (type A 673-A-36, 550 W Conrad Precision Industries), and a quartz sample coil 3 mm ID tubing, 11 cm coil diameter and 30 turns (Figure 3).

Methodology Concepts

Separation of cyanides from the samples is controlled by three factors: a) acidification, b) air stripping, and c) thin film distillation. The classic use of condensers[9] in automated distillation units was found to be disadvantageous and has been eliminated. Considerable amounts of the liberated HCN gas are refluxed back with the condensed water and thus not recovered. Acidification is made to pH < 1, however, the sample exposure to the heat treatment in the continuous thin film distillation is very short (few seconds). Thus the liberation of HCN is only from the free cyanides and the weak cyanide complexes; i.e., the acid dissociable cyanides, and not from the strong complexes. For total cyanides the breakdown of the strong cyanide complexes, prior to the thin film distillation is achieved by ultraviolet irradiation. The liberated HCN gas is recovered in the absorption coil. Then the color development is made with pyridine-barbituric acid and is measured at 578 nm.

Procedure

The system is set into operation and the temperature of the heating aluminum bar is adjusted so that the distillation ratio equals 17-20%.

MANIFOLD FOR AUTOMATED CYANIDE SYSTEM

Figure 1

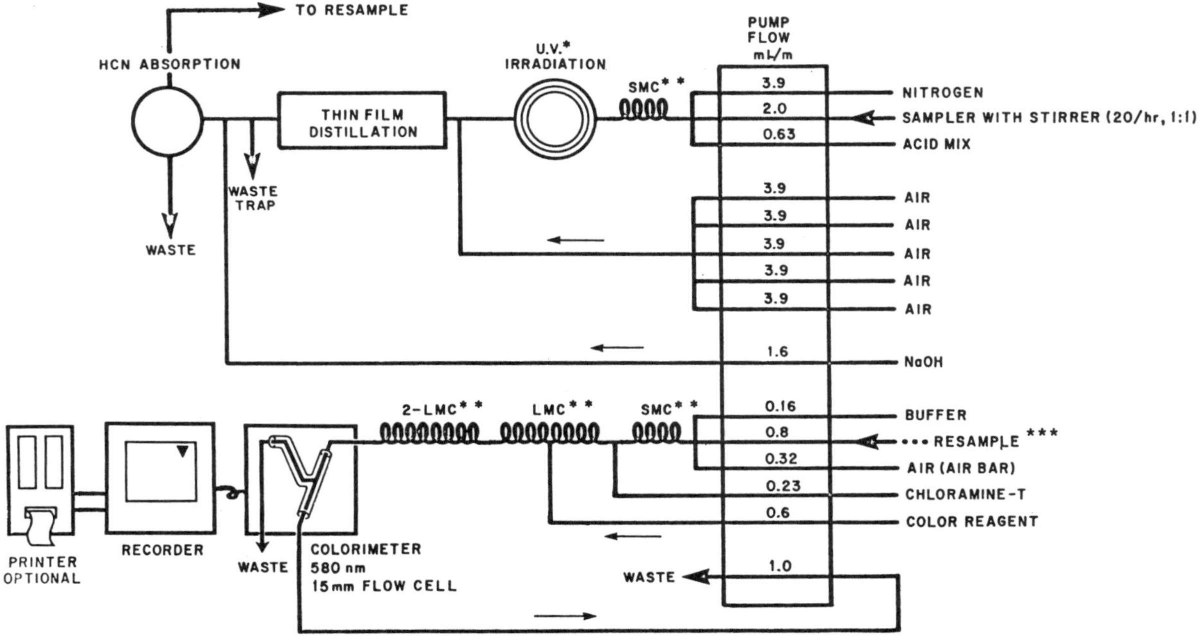

* U.V. IRRADIATION ON LINE FOR TOTAL CYANIDE AND BYPASSED FOR SIMPLE CYANIDE

** SMC and LMC: SHORT AND LONG MIXING COILS

*** FOR DIRECT COLOR, SAMPLE DIRECTLY INTO RESAMPLE LINE

CONTINUOUS THIN FILM DISTILLATION UNIT

FIGURE 2

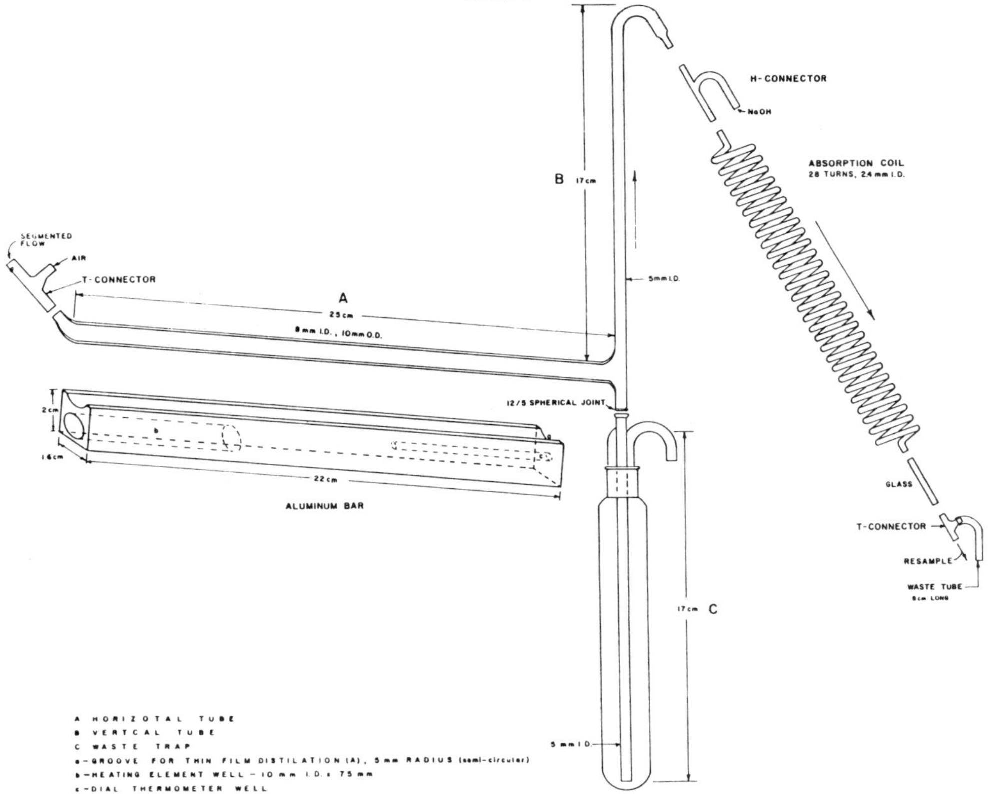

A HORIZOTAL TUBE
B VERTCAL TUBE
C WASTE TRAP
a–GROOVE FOR THIN FILM DISTILATION (A), 5 mm RADIUS (semi-circular)
b–HEATING ELEMENT WELL – 10 mm I.D. x 75 mm
c–DIAL THERMOMETER WELL

ULTRAVIOLET IRRADIATION UNIT (LAMP, COIL & HOUSING)

FIGURE 3

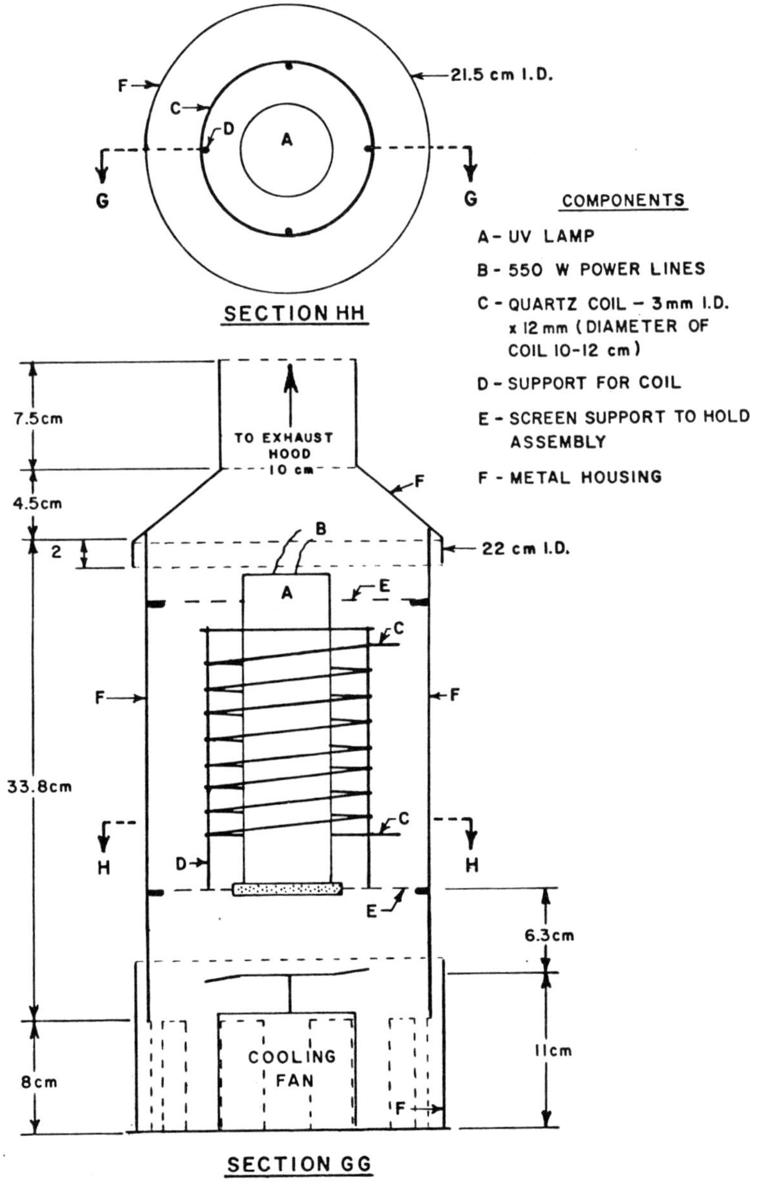

$$\text{Distillation Ratio, \%} = \frac{\text{Volume of Vaporized Portion of Sample}}{\text{Total Volume of Acidified Sample}} \times 100$$

The UV irradiation is required for total cyanide measurement. Nitrogen gas is used instead of air to segment the flow to prevent ozone formation and oxidation of cyanide. The UV is bypassed for the acid dissociable cyanide. For the direct color determination the thin film distillation is also bypassed and samples (at pH $\sim$12) are fed directly into the colorimetric part of the manifold.

Calibration procedures, using 1 to 100 µg/L CN (or up to 500) are made separately for each of the direct color, acid dissociable and total cyanide trains.

Samples should be treated from interferences and preserved at pH > 12 and 4°C, and should be analyzed as soon as possible.

Sediment samples can be mixed thoroughly and homogenized in a heavy duty blender. A suitable weight of sample (1-5 g/L) is transferred to a volumetric flask and volume adjusted with 0.02 M NaOH. The sample is kept in suspension by the use of an ultrasonic disrupter (W 350 sonifier), then fed into the system.

For the direct color determination sediment samples should be leached according to recognized acceptable procedures and the leachate can then be fed into the colorimetric system.

Analytical Behavior of Cyanide and Thiocyanate

The behavior of some inorganic metal-cyano-complexes and their analytical response to the developed automated system were evaluated and found to be largely dependent on the pH and their stability constants (Table 1). Representative data are shown in Table 2, and accordingly, the metal-cyano-complexes can be classified as very strong, strong, and weak complexes.

Very strong metal cyanide complexes such as those of cobalt, platinum and cobalt are difficult to dissociate and are not oxidized to cyanate by agents such as chlorine or ozone. Cobalt (III) complex does not break down by any of the known distillation procedures and, as expected, there was no cyanide detected by either the direct color or thin film distillation. However, the UV irradiation (for total cyanides) was effective in the breakdown of cobalt complex, and good recovery was achieved (Table 2).

Strong iron complexes include ferricyanide and ferrocyanide. All of the cyanide was recovered from these complexes by the UV total cyanide system. On the other hand, both direct color and thin film distillation showed about the same small recovery of 3.6%. This indicates that the thin film distillation does not break down iron complexes, and what was measured probably was due to some decomposition by aging and photoillumination.[17,19]

TABLE 1. SOME METAL-CYANO-COMPLEX IONS AND THEIR STABILITY CONSTANTS

Metal	Complex Ion		Stability Constant at 25°C	Reference
Cobalt(III)	hexacyanocobaltate	$[Co(CN)_6]^{3-}$	1×10^{64}	16
Iron(III)	ferricyanide	$[Fe(CN)_6]^{3-}$	1×10^{52}	17
Iron(II)	ferrocyanide	$[Fe(CN)_6]4-$	1×10^{47}	17
Nickel(II)	tetracyanonickelate	$[Ni(CN)_4]^{2-}$	1×10^{22}	18
Cadmium(II)	tetracyanocadmiate	$[Cd(CN)_4]^{2-}$	7.1×10^{16}	18
Manganese(III)	hexacyanomanganate	$[Mn(CN)_6]^{3-}$	5×10^{9}	16

TABLE 2. ANALYTICAL BEHAVIOR OF CYANIDE COMPOUNDS

Compounds	CN Preparation µg/L	CN Measured (µg/L) Direct Color	Thin Film Distill	UV Irrad.
Metal-Cyano-Complex				
Hexacyanocolbatate	100	ND	ND	97.0
Ferricyanide	100	3.6	3.4	98.5
Ferrocyanide	100	3.5	3.6	97.0
Tetracyanonickelate	100	19.7	98.8	100.2
Tetracyanocadmiate	100	101.5	98.6	98.5
Hexacyanomanganate	100	101.5	98.5	101.2
Organic Cyanides				
Acetonecyanohydrin	100	98.0	103.0	101.0
Acetonitrile	1,000	ND	ND	ND
Acrylonitrile	100	ND	ND	15.0
Adiponitrile	1,000	ND	ND	ND
Cyanate	1,000	ND	ND	ND
Thiocyanate	100	100.5	ND	98.6

ND = Not Detected

Nickel (II) complex showed complete recoveries with both thin film distillation and UV irradiation, whereas the direct color measurement showed significantly lower values. It was also noticed that the percent cyanide measured is affected by pH and inversely proportional to the original concentration. At pH 6 the measured values were 35% at 10 μg/L and 14% at 100 μg/L and at pH 4 the values were 50% and 20%, respectively. Therefore the nickel complex should be treated as an individual case.

Weaker complexes are formed with cadmium (II) and manganese (III); Table 2 shows that all the cyanides were recovered with the direct color, thin film distillation and UV irradiation. It should be noted that the direct color measurement was made at pH 4-6.

Organic cyanides have one or more cyanide groups attached to organic radicals and include the cyanohydrins and nitriles. Acetonecyanohydrin, $(CH_3)_2C(OH)CN$, dissociates completely in solution yielding its cyanide content as evidenced from the direct color measurement. On the other hand, the nitriles generally do not break down to release cyanides. Acetonitrile, CH_3CN, and adiponitrile, $NC(CH_2)_4CN$, did not show any significant values by any measurement. However, acrylonitrile, $CH_2{=}CHCN$ released only about 15% of its cyanide content after UV irradiation. These differences between the cyanohydrins and nitriles should be considered carefully for evaluation of environmental aspects.

Cyanate ion was found to be very stable and did not show any positive results. Other potential cyanide-forming compounds; namely, urea, glycine, cysteine and nitrobenzine, were also examined and no significant values were obtained.

Thiocyanate is a different case, though with the thin film distillation it is not measured at all, it was completely recovered by the UV total cyanide and the direct color determination. Apparently, thiocyanate breaks down by the UV irradiation and gives cyanide values on an equimolar basis. With regard to the colorimetric development with pyridine-barbituric acid reagents, the initial oxidation step with chloramine-T leads to the formation of cyanogen chloride. This is true whether the reacting ion is cyanide or thiocyanate, as shown by the following equations:[20]

$$CH_3C_6H_4SO_2NClNa + CN^- + 2H_2O \longrightarrow CNCl + CH_3C_6H_4SO_2NH_2 + Na^+ + 2OH^-$$

$$4CH_3C_6H_4SO_2NClNa + SCN^- + 4H_2O \longrightarrow CNCl + 4CH_3C_6H_4SO_2NH_2 + 4Na^+ + SO_4^{-2} + 3Cl^-$$

Thus thiocyanate is completely included in both measurements, the UV total cyanide and the direct colorimetry.

Analytical Definitions of Cyanide and Thiocyanate Measurements

It may be beneficial at this point to redefine the types of cyanide-thiocyanate determinations and indicate what they actually measure.

1. Acid Dissociable Cyanide: Utilization of the Thin Film Distillation technique allows for the breakdown of the weak cyanide complexes and measures also all the free cyanide, CN^- and HCN. Iron complexes are not included.

2. Direct Color Determination: This measures the free cyanide, and the dissociated weak cyano-complexes, depending on the pH. It also includes all the thiocyanate.

   Therefore,

   Thiocyanate = Direct color - Acid Dissociable CN

3. UV Total Cyanide: Utilization of UV irradiation breaks down all the strong cyanide complexes, including those of cobalt and iron. Therefore, this measurement will determine all free, simple, complex cyanides, and also all the thiocyanate. Thus, the total cyanide, without thiocyanate, can be obtained by subtraction.

   Total CN = UV Total CN - Thiocyanate

4. Complex Cyanide: This term is meant only for the strong complexes and can be determined as follows:

   Complex CN = Total CN - Acid Dissociable CN

   or

   = UV Total CN - Direct Color

Optimization of Direct Color Development

As mentioned earlier both ions, CN^- and SCN^- react with Chloramine-T giving CNCl. Then CNCl reacts with pyridine-barbituric acid giving the colored compound which absorbs at 578 nm. It was important to find out the conditions at which CN^- and SCN^- react with the same degree to give the same color intensity, so that addition or subtraction can be done with satisfactory reliability.

Two factors were evaluated extensively, that is the pH and ionic strength. Figure 4 shows these effects on CN^- and SCN^- measurements, as represented by the peak heights. As was hoped both react similarly and give comparable peak heights. It is interesting to notice also that, at low ionic strength when no salt (NaCl) was added, the optimum pH range for measurements was wide, from 3 to 6. As the ionic strength was

FIGURE 4. PH AND IONIC STRENGTH EFFECTS ON COLOR DEVELOPMENT

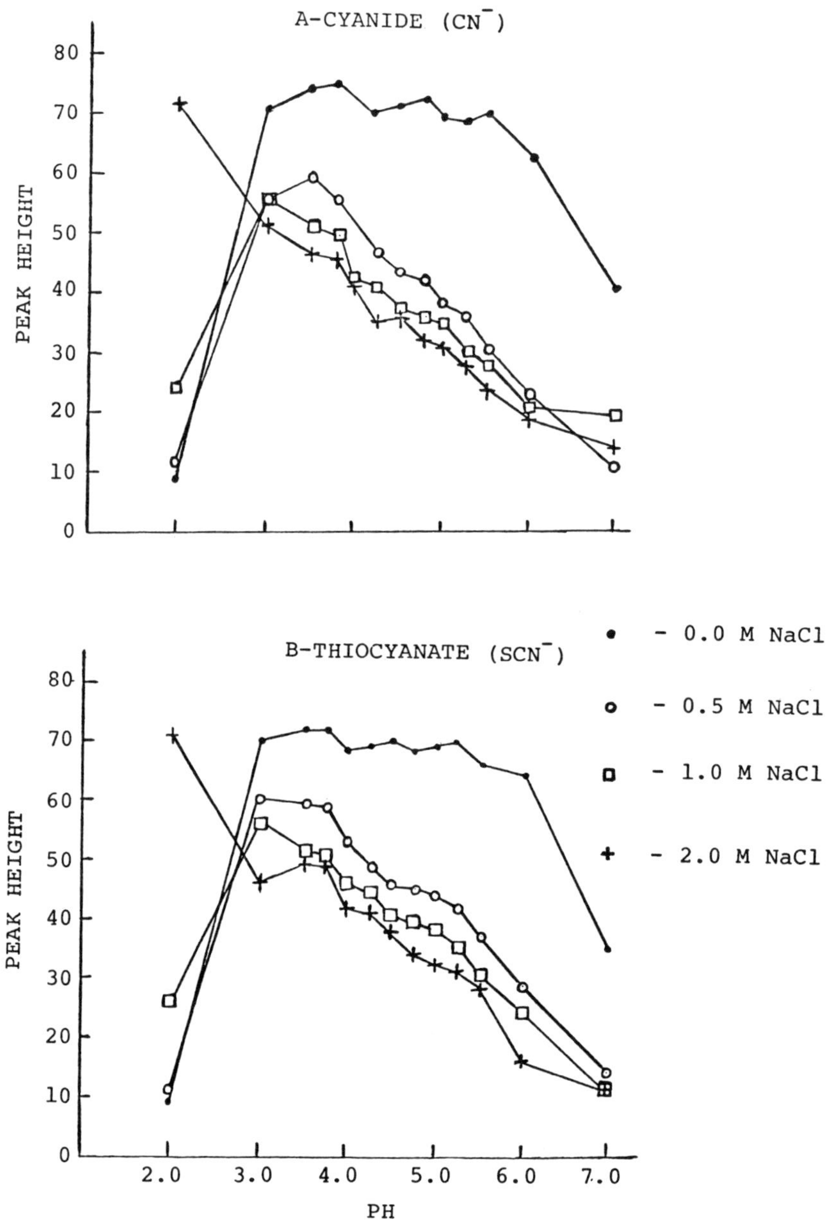

increased the pH range narrowed to about 3-4. With UV irradiation and thin film distillation the ionic strength is fixed by the absorbing solution, 0.02 M NaOH. Whereas in the direct color development there may be wide variability due to the nature of the samples themselves. Therefore, it was advisable to use a buffering system with a high ionic strength and which adjusts the pH to 3.5 or 4. Though at low ionic strength the sensitivity of the color development is higher, and the phosphate buffer (0.6 M, resultant pH 6) was used, yet with the introduction of the direct color development for the thiocyanate determination the acetate buffer ($\sim$ 10 M, resultant pH 4) is now in use. Compensation for the decrease in sensitivity was easily made electronically. Table 3 shows some results for thiocyanate determinations in synthetic mixtures and field samples using both buffers. Good recoveries were obtained with synthetic solutions by both buffers, but with field samples the phosphate buffer gave unsatisfactory results, whereas with the acetate buffer almost complete recoveries were achieved, ranging from 97% to 100%.

Table 3 also shows the thiocyanate results obtained by the Ferric Nitrate Method.[4-5] The method measures the colored compound formed by the reaction of Fe^{3+} and SCN^-, (buffered at pH 5.5-6). The method rendered itself easily to automation, and similar results were obtained by the manual and automated techniques. The results obtained were satisfactory with synthetic preparations. However, with field samples the situation was different and the results were generally much higher than with the presented direct color technique. The spike recovery was somewhat higher than expected (111% and 114% for the two effluent samples shown in Table 3). But more important is that the initial sample result is much higher, not only than the presented direct color method, but also higher than the UV total cyanide, which includes all the thiocyanate in the measurement. Raw sewage samples 1 and 2 contained 21 and 49 μg/L for UV total cyanide and the ferric nitrate method gave 51 and 90 μg/L for thiocyanate alone. The direct color method gave 10 and 48 μg/L, respectively. These latter values are in line with both UV total cyanide and thin film distillation acid dissociable cyanide.

System Performance Characteristics

Recovery evaluation was made with a variety of water and wastewater samples; namely, distilled water, tap water, river water, raw sewage, treated effluents and industrial waste, with a wide range of cyanide and thiocyanate content. The samples were spiked with different levels (up to 100 μg/L) of simple and complex cyanides as well as thiocyanate, then analyzed again to determine the efficiency of recovery. The acid dissociable cyanide recoveries were complete from distilled, tap, and river waters. However, with the raw sewage, effluents, and some industrial waste, losses up to 25% were observed. It appears that such samples contained sequestering components which complex some cyanides, making them not available for determination by the thin film distillation. The total cyanide and thiocyanate determinations showed practically complete recoveries, more than a hundred total cyanide determinations averaged 97%.

TABLE 3. COMPARISON WITH FERRIC NITRATE THIOCYANATE METHOD

Sample and Spike	Cyanide µg/L		Thiocyanate Determination µg/L as CN		
	Acid Dissoc.	UV Total	Ferric Nitrate	Direct Color: Phosphate* Buffer	Direct Color: Acetate* Buffer
Synthetic Mixture**	39.9	113.7 (97%)	41.2	40.2	39.9 (100%)
Final Effluent - 1					
As is	0.9	26.0	27.0	3.5	3.7
+ 50 SCN	1.8	75.2 (98%)	76.8	41.2	52.6 (98%)
Final Effluent - 2					
As is	3.3	14.0	23.6	5.4	3.3
+ 50 SCN	4.2	63.2 (98%)	78.2	39.3	51.6 (97%)
Raw Sewage - 1	4.5	20.6	51.0	8.2	9.5
Raw Sewage - 2	0.0	48.8	89.5	26.8	48.0

*Phosphate Buffer: 0.64 M (lower ionic strength), resultant pH 6

Acetate Buffer: 10 M (high ionic strength), resultant pH 4

**Synthetic Mixture: 40 µg/L (as CN) of CN^-, SCN^- & $[CO(CN)_6]^{3-}$

Reproducibility studies were run in the range 1-100 μg/L using CN^-, $[Co(CN)_6]^{3-}$ and SCN^-, as well as the above variety of field samples. Ten to twelve replicates were used in succession for each case (Figure 5). There was no apparent dependence of reproducibility on the nature of samples. The coefficients of variation were less than 3%, 6%, and 8% for the acid dissociable cyanide, total cyanide, thiocyanate respectively.

The system can analyze up to 20 samples per hour. Calibration is linear in the working range of 0-100 μg/L and up to 500 μg/L (Figure 5). The lower limit of detection is 0.025 μg/L, i.e., less than 1 ng absolute.

The system can distinguish between small differences in cyanide concentration, such as between 1 and 2 μg/L, or between 25 and 26 μg/L (Figure 5). Statistical analysis showed that, for ten replicates each, the confidence level is higher than 99.9% ($P < 0.001$).

INTERFERENCES

Several interferences are encountered with cyanide analysis and have been reported. Many of these interferences could be treated, however, care should be taken to reduce the time of handling and minimize exposure to UV light.

1. Turbidity and Color Contributing Substances

   These may interfere with color measurement. Most of these substances are removed during the thin film distillation. For direct color development a filtration step may be necessary.

2. Sulfide

   Sulfides may cause direct and/or indirect interferences. The direct interference is caused by competition of sulfide with cyanide in the color reactions. This depends on the concentration of $S^=$, CN^- and color reagents. Under the prescribed conditions the automated system tolerates up to 15-20 mg/L $S^=$ without significant interference. (In case $S^=$ is present in high concentration sample dilution may be helpful.)

   The indirect sulfide interference is due to the interaction with cyanide to form thiocyanate, especially at the high pH of preservation. Thus, unless the sample could be analyzed rapidly, sulphide treatment should be made before storage. Treatment with cadmium or lead carbonate is recommended until the lead acetate paper test shows negative results.

3. Oxidizing Materials

   Oxygen, ozone, chlorine and others may oxidize the cyanide and some weak complexes as well as thiocyanate to cyanate and result in lower values. Treatment is to prevent further oxidation but cannot recover what has been oxidized. Ascorbic acid, $C_6H_6O_6$, sodium

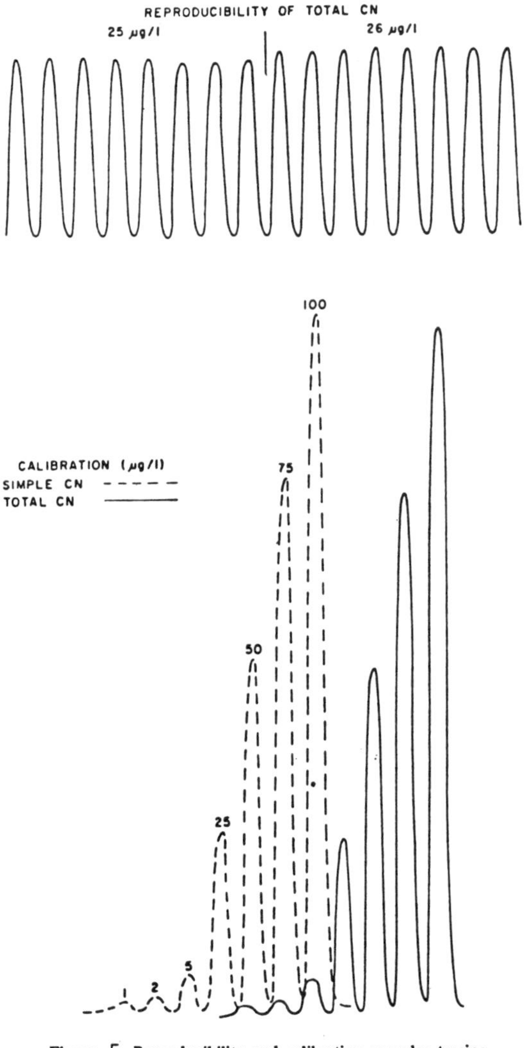

Figure 5 Reproducibility and calibration recorder tracing.

hydrogen sulfite, $NaHSO_3$, Stannous Chloride, $SnCl_2$, and hypophosphorous acid, H_3PO_3, were evaluated and found not satisfactory. They either caused interference themselves or did not demonstrate efficient reduction.

Sodium arsenite, Na_2AsO_3, was found to be very efficient. Only 0.1 g/L can reduce 50 mg/L chlorine. However, in several cases with field samples, containing nitrate and nitrite, arsenite caused high erroneous results.

Oxalic acid, $C_2O_4H_2$, about 2 g/L can reduce up to 50 mg/L chlorine. The reaction is satisfactory, though slower than with arsenite, and requires acidic or neutral pH. Therefore, when treating with oxalic acid, close the sample container, wait 15 minutes, then preserve with NaOH.

4. Nitrate-Nitrite Interference

Nitrate and nitrite do not interfere with thin film distillation or with direct color significantly, contrary to the UV total cyanide measurement where significant positive interferences were observed. The UV irradiation conditions may cause nitrite to react with other sample components. Nitrate may also be reduced to nitrite in presence of the hypophosphorous acid. The interference is much higher with most field samples than with synthetic preparations, and is more pronounced in presence of arsenite.

Sulfamic acid and urea react with nitrous acid or nitrite[21] as represented by the following equations,

$$H^+ + NO_2 + O^{\cdot}SO_2NH_2 \longrightarrow N_2 + HSO_4^- + H_2O$$

$$2H^+ + 2NO_2 + CO(NH_2)_2 \longrightarrow 2N_2 + CO_2 + 3H_2O$$

Sulfamic acid was found to be more effective in removal of the interference. Addition of 2 g sulfamic acid per liter of digestive acid mixture readily removes the nitrate or nitrite interference, up to 100 mg/L (Table 4). It was interesting to notice that the original total cyanide results of field samples frequently decreased after the addition of sulfamic acid. A direct correlation was found between the decrease of the total cyanide value and the nitrate and/or nitrite content in those samples.

5. Carbonate-Bicarbonate

Carbonate and bicarbonate release carbon dioxide upon acidification and may affect the flow pattern and escape with HCN through the waste trap of the thin film distillation. Samples with high carbonate or bicarbonate content, such as coal gasification wastes, or atmospheric emission scrub waters may be stabilized by addition of lime instead of sodium hydroxide.

Table 4. NITRATE INTERFERENCE WITH TOTAL CYANIDE MEASUREMENT AND REMOVAL BY SULFAMIC ACID

Waste Treatment Plant Sample	Nitrate Spike, mg/L				
	0	10	50	100	200
	(Total CN Result, ug/l)				
Plant I					
Raw Sewage	59	65	100	off scale	off scale
Raw Sewage + Sulfamic	50	50	54	57	63
Effluent	57	59	82	95	109
Effluent + Sulfamic	23	23	28	33	33
Plant II					
Raw Sewage	54	57	96	off scale	off scale
Raw Sewage + Sulfamic	52	52	54	58	62
Effluent	41	41	62	84	116
Effluent + Sulfamic	43	42	44	49	69
Plant III					
Raw Sewage	76	85	115	off scale	off scale
Raw Sewage + Sulfamic	71	72	76	81	87
Effluent	27	32	52	69	103
Effluent + Sulfamic	16	16	18	20	25

6. Metal Cations

Metal cations do not interfere with total cyanide measurement, because UV irradiation breaks down all the cyanide complexes. Formation of metal cyanide complexes in field samples is not considered a source of interference to the acid dissociable cyanide or direct color determinations, since the objective is to measure the available species and not the strong complexes.

On the other hand addition of some metallic catalytic compounds during the analytical procedure is not desirable. Dramatic inhibition occurs with mercuric chloride and, to a lesser extent, cuprous chloride when added as catalysts. Due to its high volatility mercury (> 1 mg/L) distills over causing negative interference.

7. Aldehydes

Aldehydes cause negative interference (probably due to formation of nitriles). This interference is noticeable at a formaldehyde concentration > 0.5 mg/L. Treatment with silver nitrate[4] gave erratic results, whereas, ethylenediamine was found to be reasonably effective. Addition of 2 mL of 5% ethylenediamine solution per 100 mL sample gave complete recovery of total cyanide in presence of up to 50 mg/L formaldehyde. Recoveries with thin film distillation and direct color determinations were not complete. Some analytical data are shown in Table 5.

8. Fatty Acids

Mineral oils do not cause interferences. Fatty acids up to 100 mg/L are tolerated by the automated system. Higher concentrations interfere mechanically with the thin film distillation technique and may cause escape of gases through the waste trap. Also fatty acids may distill over and form soap with the NaOH absorbing solution and disturb the flow patterns and the colorimetric distillation.

Excessive amounts of fatty acids can be removed by liquid-liquid extraction. Extraction at pH 6-7 as previously suggested[4] caused significant cyanide losses. In this study extraction at pH 12 with freon, hexane, or isooctane was adequate. One or two extractions with a solvent volume 1/5 of the sample reduced the fatty acids below the interfering level and the cyanide losses were insignificant. Salting out effect by addition of NaCl, 10 g/L sample, enhances the extraction and separation.

9. Potential Cyanide Forming Materials

Several substances; namely, cyanates, nitrobenzine, urea, thiourea, glycine and cysteine, were investigated to find out if they hydrolyze or break down under the analytical conditions and may cause some interference. None of those materials gave any interference with the thin film distillation or the direct color determinations.

TABLE 5. RECOVERY OF CYANIDE FROM ALDEHYDE INTERFERENCE USING ETHYLENEDIAMINE

	mL of 3.5 Ethylenediamine per 100 mL Test Solution													
	0		1		2		4		6		8		10	
	AD	Tot.	AD	Tot.	AD	Tot.	AD	Tot.	AD	Tot.	AD	Tot.	AD	Tot.
Ethylenediamine (alone)					0	0	0	0	0	2	1	2	1	3
KCN, 100 µg/L	100	100			106	102	103	101			111	110		
+Formald.5 mg/L	46	60	72	92	75	99	76	100	83	113	85	112		
+Formald.10 mg/L	31	48	70	110	70	112	70	113	70	112	69	118	68	117
+Formald.25 mg/L	10	26	43	100	42	104	44	111	39	103	38	100	42	112
+Formald.50 mg/L	5	20	22	88	39	106	27	103	28	109	17	102	30	113
+Formald.100 mg/L	1	14	7	51	11	66	12	73	13	83	14	95	15	95

AD = Acid Dissociable Cyanide, µg/L
Tot.= UV Total Cyanide, µg/L

Only the sulfur containing substances gave variable positive interferences with the UV total cyanide. One mg/L thiourea produced a response of about 5 μg/L CN. Cysteine interfered only at very high levels and could be considered negligible up to 100 mg/L. Both thiourea and cysteine are not likely to be found in significant amounts in natural and wastewater.

10. Thiocyanate

As explained earlier in this presentation, all the thiocyanate is completely included in the UV total cyanide measurement. Also it was elucidated how to determine the thiocyanate with the same automated system (direct color). Thus, by simple subtraction the (true) total cyanide is determined.

CYANIDE-THIOCYANATE SPECIES DISTRIBUTION

The developed cyanide-thiocyanate automated system has been utilized to study the distribution of the different cyanide species and thiocyanate in several environmental situations. The automated system also served as a tool to follow up some of the kinetic interactions and transformation of the simple cyanide species to more complex forms and thiocyanate. Special emphasis was made on the waste treatment process and several wastewater, and industrial waste samples were analyzed. Some of the data obtained are presented in Tables 6 and 7 respectively. The species of interest were the acid dissociable cyanide, complex cyanide, total cyanide and thiocyanate. However the UV total cyanide and the direct color are essential measurements and provide some additional information and are also presented in the tables. The waste treatment plants are shown in succession according to their treatment capacity (Table 6). Plant II is in a major industrial area, Plants I and III serve both domestic and industrial area, and Plant IV is in a basically residential community. The industrial influence is shown by the raw sewage of Plant II, about 370 μg/L for the UV total cyanide. The effectiveness of treatment is shown by the low value of the corresponding effluent, 30 μg/L. The thiocyanate and total cyanide were major components in most of the raw sewage samples. It is interesting to notice that in those effluent samples there were no acid dissociable cyanide. Probably the simple cyanide and weak complexes have been oxidized, or complexed by sequestering agents in the sewage, or also transformed to thiocyanate in presence of the sulphide commonly found in sewage.

On the other hand the industrial discharges grab sample shown in Table 7 are generally higher than the treatment plants in the cyanide content, in the mg/L range. In many of these samples the high values were due to the presence of thiocyanate. However, in the Road Salt Dock sample there was no thiocyanate and most of the cyanide found (26 mg/L) was in the complex form. Cyanide is commonly used as anticaking agent for road salt.

TABLE 6. CYANIDE AND THIOCYANATE SPECIES (μg/L)
IN SOME WASTE TREATMENT PLANT SAMPLES

Grab Sample	UV Total CN	Direct Color	Acid Dissoc. CN	Thio SCN	Total CN	Complex CN
Plant I						
Raw Sewage	40.0	31.0	8.0	23.0	17.0	9.0
Effluent	12.0	4.0	0.0	4.0	8.0	8.0
Plant II						
Raw Sewage	369.0	264.7	50.3	213.4	155.6	105.3
Effluent	30.0	10.0	0.0	10.0	20.0	20.0
Plant III						
Raw Sewage	49.0	47.0	23.0	24.0	25.0	2.0
Effluent	14.0	2.0	0.0	2.0	12.0	12.0
Plant IV						
Raw Sewage	30.0	16.0	0.0	16.0	14.0	14.0
Effluent	19.0	2.0	0.0	2.0	17.0	17.0

TABLE 7. CYANIDE AND THIOCYANATE SPECIES (mg/L) IN SOME INDUSTRIAL WASTE SAMPLES

Grab Sample	UV Total CN	Direct Color	Acid Dissoc. CN	Thio SCN	Total CN	Complex CN
Chemical Industry 1	50.90	50.50	0.00	50.50	0.40	0.40
Chemical Industry 2	10.40	10.60	0.03	10.57	0.00	0.00
Coking Operation	25.70	24.90	1.30	23.60	2.10	0.80
Oil Refinery	2.25	2.24	0.00	2.24	0.01	0.01
Plating Company 1	0.27	0.09	0.07	0.02	0.25	0.18
Plating Company 2	0.03	0.02	0.03	0.00	0.03	0.01
Road Salt Dock	25.66	2.52	2.90	0.00	25.66	23.14

It is beyond this presentation to elaborate deeper on the details of the cyanide distribution in the environment. Hopefully the cyanide-thiocyanate automated system presented proves to be a useful analytical tool for further investigations.

REFERENCES

1. Kelada, N. P., D. T. Lordi, and C. Lue-Hing. Cyanide Species Methodology in Water, Wastewater, and Sediments. The Metropolitan Sanitary District of Greater Chicago, R & D Dept., Report No. 77-5, 1977.
2. Hewitt, P. J., and H. B. Austin. Water Poll. Control 381, 1972.
3. Chamberlin, N. S., and H. B. Snyder, Jr., Proc. Purdue Ind. Waste Conf. 10-277, 1955.
4. Standard Methods for the Examination of Water and Wastewaters, 13th ed., Washington, D.C., American Public Health Association, 1971.
5. American Society for Testing and Material. Annual Book of ASTM Standards, Part 23, Designation D2036-72, 1972.
6. "Methods for Chemical Analysis of Water and Wastes," USEPA Water Quality Office, Cincinnati, Ohio, 1971.
7. Robert, R. F., and B. Jackson. Analyst 96-209, 1971.
8. Conetta, A., J. Jansen and J. Salpeter. Pollution Engineering, p. 36, January 1973.
9. Goulden, P. D., B. K. Afghan and P. Brooksbank. Anal. Chem. 44:1845, 1972.
10. Ryan, A. J., and G. W. Culshaw. Analyst, 69:370, 1944.
11. Aldridge, W. N. Analyst, 69:262, 1944.
12. Epstein, J. Anal. Chem., 19:272, 1947.
13. Asmus, E., and H. Garschagen. Z. Anal. Chem., 138:414, 1953.
14. Kelada at al. In Line Continuous Thin Film Distillation System U.S. Patent No. 961-162, 1972.
15. Afghan, B. K., P. E. Goulden and J. F. Ryan. Advances in Automated Analysis, Vol. II, p. 241, Thurman Associates, Miami, Florida.
16. Sillen, L. G., and A. E. Martell. Stability Constants of Metal Ion Complexes, Special Publication 17, p. 107, Chemical Society, Burlington House, London, 1964.
17. Broderius, S. J. Ph.D. Thesis; Oregon State University, 1973.
18. Mirsch, E. Fortschr-Wasserchem, 1:120, 1964.
19. Henrickson, T. N., and L. G. Daignault. "Treatment of Complex Cyanide Compounds for Reuse or Disposal," Report No. EPA-R2-73-269, 1973.
20. Nagashima, S. Anal. Chem., 55:2086, 1983.
21. Vogel, A. I. "A text Book of Quantitative Inorganic Analysis," 3rd Ed., Longmans, Green and Co., London, 1961.

CONFERENCE ON CYANIDE AND THE ENVIRONMENT
Tucson, Arizona • December 1984
Published by Geotechnical Engineering Program • Colorado State University • Fort Collins, Colorado 80523

CYANIDE/THIOCYANATE REACTIONS IN TAILINGS

by
Sandra L. McGill,* James L. Hendrix**
and John H. Nelson***

ABSTRACT

Conditions and rates of reactions for the formation of thiocyanate from various sulfur species were investigated by the Generic Waste Treatment and Recovery Center. Constant stirred, constant temperature reactors were used to react several individual sulfur species as well as some complex gold ores with pH buffered cyanide solutions. Cyanide distillation and the ferric nitrate thiocyanate determination methods were employed as analytical procedures. The effects of concentration of reactants and temperature are presented.

INTRODUCTION

The form that cyanide takes in cyanidation tailings is not well known, and is dependent on the type of ore being processed and the specific operation. Each form of cyanide presents a different environmental impact and therefore the treatment methods have to differ. The type of compounds formed need to be determined so that adequate treatment methods can be applied. The most common commercial practice is by oxidation of cyanide with chlorine, ozone or hydrogen peroxide. Other processes include bacterial action, ion exchange, electrolysis and several others. This study has concentrated on the formation of thiocyanate from cyanide and sulfur species in aqueous solutions which may be present in gold mill tailings.

Thiocyanate (SCN^-) is a common cyanide reaction product found in mill effluents where cyanide is used. A relatively non-toxic compound, thiocyanate, has been shown to be an intermediate which is produced during the biodegradation and detoxification of free cyanide in living systems[1]. Small amounts of free cyanide released

* Sandra L. McGill, Research Associate, University of Nevada, Reno, Reno, Nevada 89557
** James L. Hendrix, Professor of Chemical Engineering, University of Nevada, Reno, Reno, Nevada 89557
*** John H. Nelson, Professor of Chemistry, University of Nevada, Reno, Reno, Nevada 89557.

into the environment can react with various forms of sulfur to form thiocyanate. The reaction of polysulfides and thiosulfate to form thiocyanates has been studied by Luthy and Bruce (1979).[2]

$$S_x^{2-} + CN^- \longrightarrow S_{(x-1)}^{2-} + SCN^- \quad (1)$$

$$S_2O_3^{2-} + CN^- \longrightarrow SO_3^{2-} + SCN^- \quad (2)$$

For our study, several complex sulfide ores were obtained from Duval Corporation and analyzed for major sulfur species. Individual sulfur species were then reacted with varying concentrations of cyanide and varying temperatures, at a pH of 10 to obtain kinetic data for the formation of thiocyanate. A pH of 10 was selected since most gold cyanidation mills maintain this pH. The complex sulfide ores were also studied in the same manner. Solutions were analyzed for SCN^-, free CN^- and total CN^-.

The sulfur species studied and their stoichiometries when reacted with CN^- are shown below:

$$FeS_2 + 8CN^- \longrightarrow Fe(CN)_6^{4-} + 2SCN^- + 2e^- \quad (3)$$

$$FeS + 7CN^- \longrightarrow Fe(CN)_6^{4-} + SCN^- + 2e^- \quad (4)$$

$$CuFeS_2 + 10CN^- \longrightarrow Fe(CN)_6^{4-} + Cu(CN)^-_2 + 2SCN^- + 3e^- \quad (5)$$

$$Cu_2S + 5CN^- \longrightarrow 2Cu(CN)^-_2 + SCN^- + 2e^- \quad (6)$$

$$ZnS + 3CN^- \longrightarrow Zn(CN)_2 + SCN^- + 2e^- \quad (7)$$

$$S^o + CN^- \longrightarrow SCN^- \quad (8)$$

All sulfur species studied reacted with cyanide to form thiocyanate. The highest conversion of sulfur to thiocyanate was that associated with chalcopyrite ($CuFeS_2$). Sulfur associated with chalcocite (Cu_2S) formed a minimal amount of SCN^- but consumed the most CN^-.

MATERIALS AND METHODS

Materials:

All sulfur species were studied at -200 mesh. $CuFeS_2$, Cu_2S, ZnS, FeS, FeS_2 and S^o were high grade minerals obtained from Wards Natural Science Establishment, Inc., and the ferrous sulfide was reagent grade, chemically prepared.

Cyanide solutions were made with reagent grade KCN in a pH 10 buffer made with 4.2 g/l $NaHCO_3$ and 5.3 g/l Na_2CO_3. The strengths of the CN^- solutions were based on the stoichiometries according to equations 3 through 8. 1:1 NaOH and 6M HCl were used when necessary to adjust the initial pH of the buffer to 10. Cyanide solutions were used immediately after preparation.

Methods

One gram samples of the individual sulfur species were placed in stoppered 250 ml erlenmeyer flasks with 200 ml of the CN^- buffer solutions, and were placed in shaker water baths. Periodic samples were taken with syringe pipets to remove 15 ml homogenous samples (mixtures of solid and solution) to maintain a constant concentration ratio. The samples were filtered and the solutions were analyzed for SCN^- according to the ferric nitrate procedure[3] (see Analytical Procedures section). When the runs were terminated, the solutions were also analyzed for free and total CN^- according to the suggested procedures in ASTM[4] (see Analytical Procedures section). Some final solids were analyzed for cyanide by the ASTM procedure to test for metal cyanide precipitates.

ANALYTICAL PROCEDURES

The complex sulfide samples were analyzed by ICP, fire assay, SEM and X-ray diffraction. The individual mineral samples obtained from Wards and the chemically prepared ferrous sulfide sample were analyzed by X-ray diffraction.

Thiocyanate determinations were made using the ferric nitrate colorimetric procedure from Standard Methods for the Examination of Water and Wastewater. The following modifications were made. The ferric nitrate solution was prepared by dissolving 50 g $Fe(NO_3)_2$ in 500 ml of 10% HNO_3 solution. A Beckman ACTA MVII Spectrophotometer was used to measure the absorbance of the ferric thiocyanate complex. Concentration of thiocyanate was determined by a calibration curve of absorbance vs. ppm SCN^- which was constructed from standard solutions. Before analyzing the solutions, an excess of $ZnSO_4$ was added to precipitate any iron (an interference in this procedure) present in the solution.

Free CN^- was measured according to the $AgNO_3$ titrimetric procedure.[3] Total CN^- was detected by distillation and a subsequent colorimetric determination as was suggested in ASTM . The only modification to this procedure was the addition of 20 ml of $HgCl_2$ to assist in the decomposition of the metal cyanide complexes. CN^- in the residues was measured using the method for cyanide in solid waste in ASTM .

To increase our confidence level in the distillation procedure two initial tests were run using the distillation procedure. A known amount of potassium ferrocyanide was introduced to the distillation flask. It was found that 100% of the complexed cyanide was collected by the distillation and colorimetric procedure. Another test was for the detection of SCN^- in the distillation procedure. When a known amount of potassium thiocyanate was added to the distillation flask none of it was distilled and therefore it was not considered an interference. Ammonia was detected with a specific ion electrode.

RESULTS

Table 1 shows the composition of the Duval complex sulfide samples as detected by ICP, X-ray diffraction and fire assay.

The maximum % S converted to SCN^- was that associated with $CuFeS_2$ at all temperatures studied (see Figures 1, 2 and 3).

The effect of temperature on the four sulfur species whose % S converted to SCN^- which were the highest of those studied are presented in Figures 4, 5, 6 and 7.

Table 2 shows both maximum % S converted to SCN^- and % of the original CN^- remaining as free, complexed, and that which was not detected for all sulfur species studied using 1 x stoichiometry of CN^-.

Table 3 shows the effect of the stoichiometry of CN^- on the % S converted to SCN^- for all sulfur species studied.

Table 4 shows the maximum % S converted to SCN^- and % of the original CN^- remaining as free, complexed, and that which was not detected for the complex sulfide samples.

After 10 days, a blank which was run at 45° with 20 g/l KCN in a pH 10 buffer with no sulfur species added had 86% of the original CN^- remaining as free CN^-. 1.9% of the original CN^- was detected as complexed CN^-, and 12.1% of the original CN^- was not detected.

Table 1 Composition of Complex Sulfide Samples

Element	North	South	East
Cu	0.18%	700 ppm	540 ppm
Ni	90 ppm	120 ppm	30 ppm
Pb	240 ppm	140 ppm	56 ppm
Zn	0.27%	0.12%	410 ppm
Au	0.02 oz/ton	0.02 oz/ton	0.03 oz/ton
Ag	0.1 oz/ton	0.1 oz/ton	0.1 oz ton
Al	3.98%	4.29%	3.39%
Ca	0.65%	2.63%	0.33%
Fe	10.84%	7.62%	7.69%
Mg	1.38%	2.82%	0.90%
SiO_2	65.9%	54.9%	74.9%
S_T	8.16%	5.71%	4.70%
S^o	0.05%	0.04%	0.02%
S^{2-}	7.72%	5.03%	4.12%
SO_4^{2-}	1.18%	1.93%	1.69%

Major species in all samples were quartz, pyrite, and feldspar as detected by X-ray diffraction.

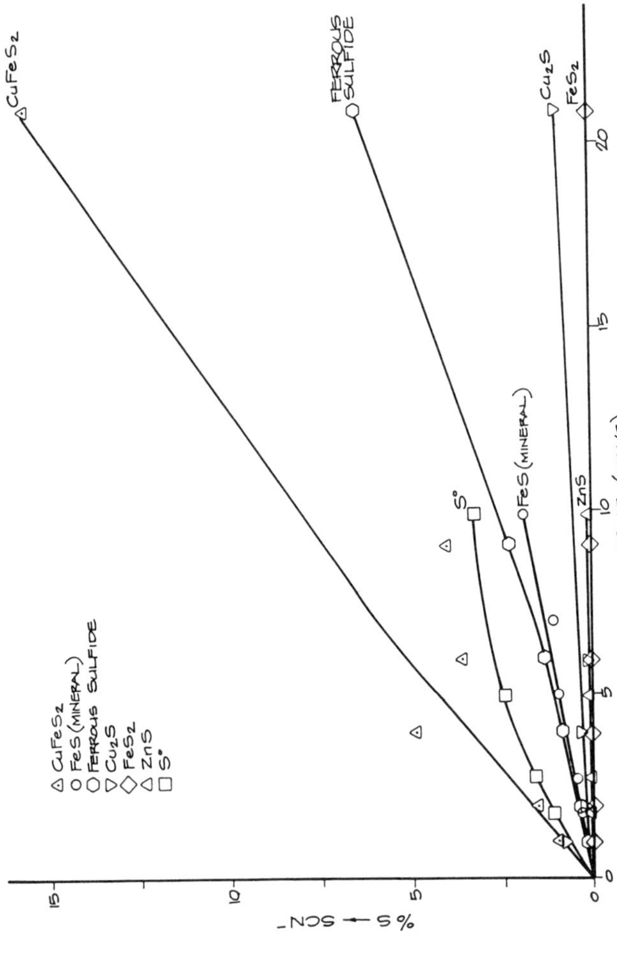

FIG. 1 %S converted to SCN^- vs. Time at 25°C, pH 10, and 1 x stoich. of CN^-

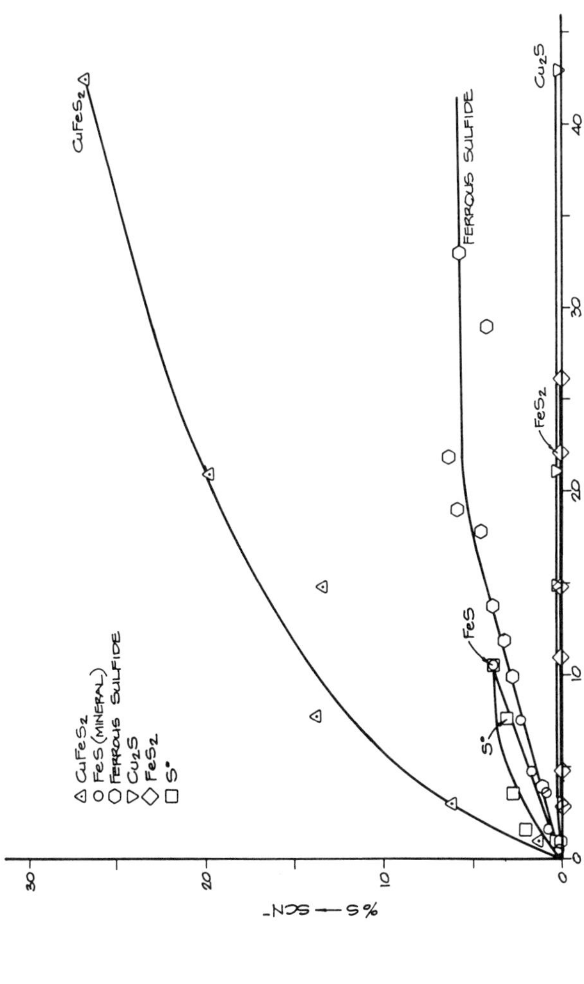

FIG. 2 %S converted to SCN^- vs. Time at 35°C, pH 10, and 1 x stoich. of CN^-

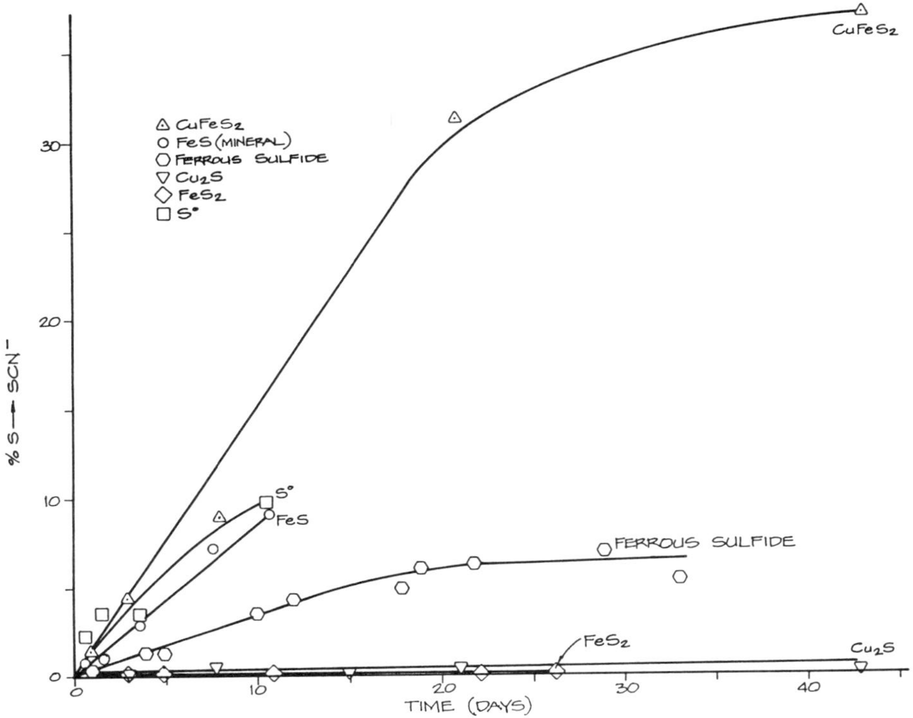

FIG. 3 %S converted to SCN^- vs. Time at 45°C, pH 10, and 1 x stoich. of CN^-

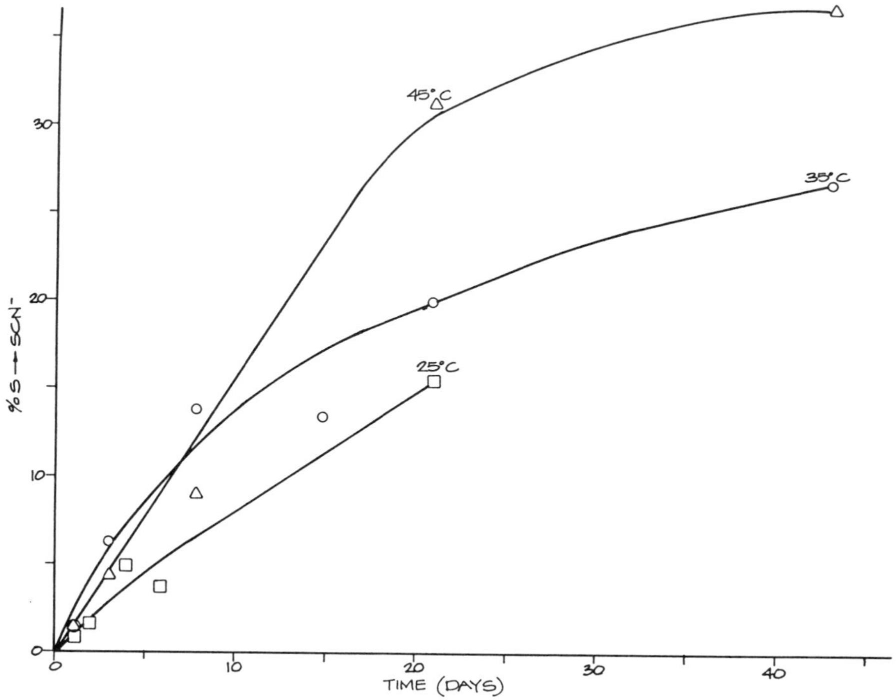

%S converted to SCN^- vs. Time for CuFeS at pH 10, and 1 x stoich. of CN^- at 25°C, 35°C, and 45°C

FIG. 4

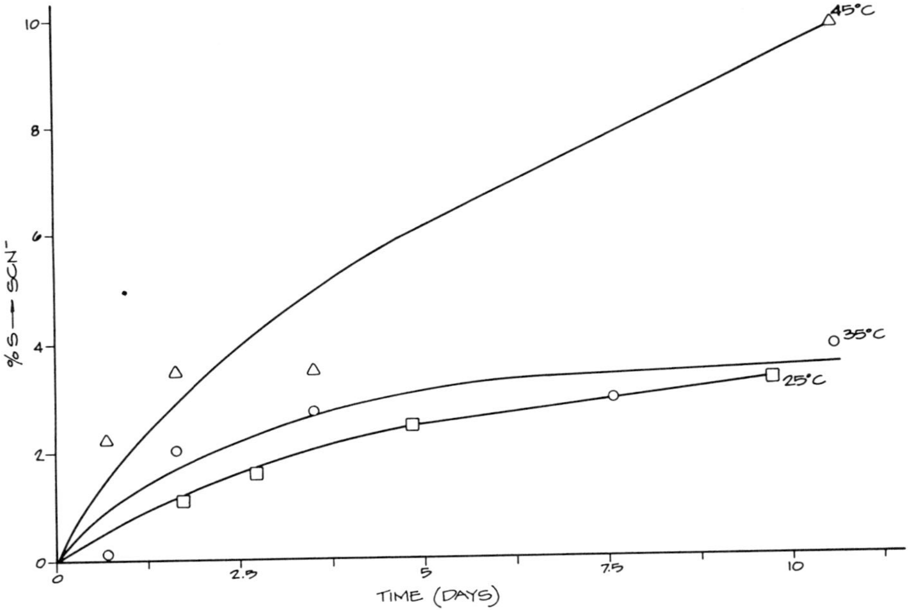

FIG. 5 %S converted to SCN^- vs. Time for S° at pH 10, and 1 x stoich. of CN^- at 25°C, 35°C, and 45°C

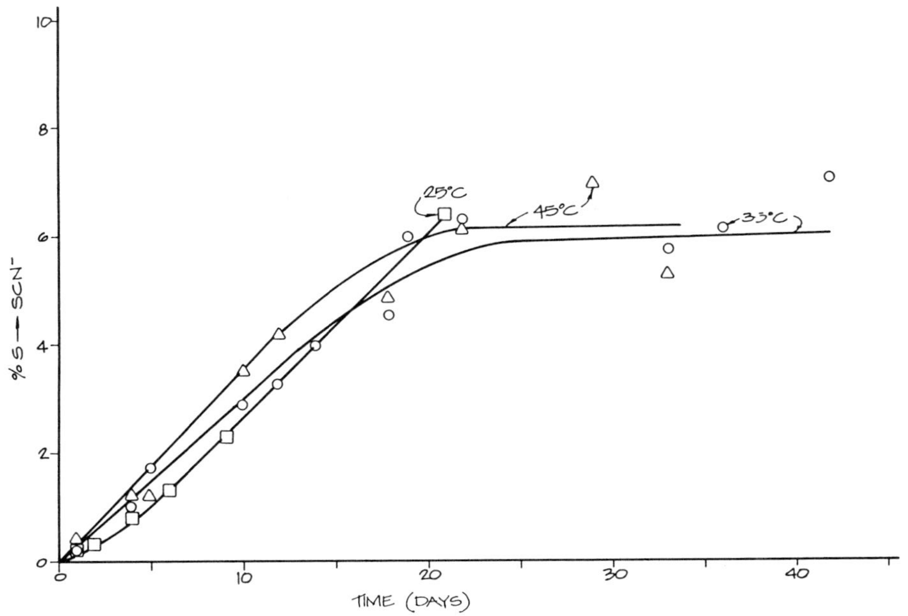

%S converted to SCN^- vs. Time for Ferrous sulfide at pH 10, and 1 x stoich. of CN^- at 25°C, 35°C, and 45°C

FIG. 6

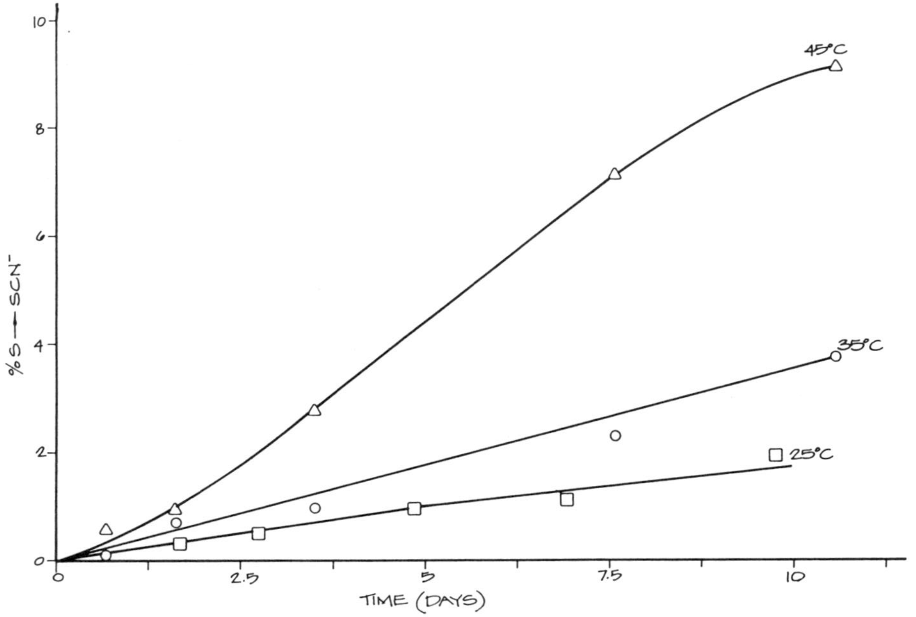

%S converted to SCN^- vs. Time for FeS (Pyrrhotite) at pH 10, and 1 x stoich. of CN^- at 25°C, 35°C, and 45°C

FIG. 7

Table 2. Conversion of S ⟶ SCN^- and CN^- Analyses of Solutions

Species/ Temp. °C		Maximum % S → SCN^- 10 days	20 days	40 days	Elasped days for CN^- Analyses	% of Original CN^- remaining as free CN^-	% of Original CN^- converted to complexed CN^-	% of Original CN^- not detected[1]
$CuFeS_2$	25°	5	15	---[2]	21 days	46	35	19
	35°	14	20	26	43 days	26	44	30
	45°	16	30	38	43 days	8	49	43
Ferrous Sulfide	25°	2.5	5.7	---	21 days	55	22	23
	35°	3.0	5.5	6.0	43 days	45	21	34
Pyrrho-tite (FeS)	25°	1.9	---	---	10 days	87	13	0
	35°	3.6	---	---	10 days	72	3	25
	45°	8.8	---	---	10 days	54	21	25
S^0	25°	3.2	---	---	10 days	77	9	14
	35°	3.5	---	---	10 days	55	0	45
	45°	9.5	---	---	10 days	45	0	55
Cu_2S	25°	0.5	0.5	---	21 days	4	66	30
	35°	0.4	0.4	0.4	43 days	6	23	71
	45°	0.4	0.4	0.4	43 days	6	18	76
ZnS	25°	0.1	---	---	10 days	88	12	0
FeS_2	25°	0.05	0.05	---	21 days	90	8	2
	45°	0.10	0.10	---	26 days	100	0	0

1) CN^- lost to precipitate and decomposition which was confirmed by presence of ammonia.

2) Test wasn't run this long.

Table 3. Effect of Stoichiometry of CN^- on the %S Converted to SCN^- for all Sulfur Species Studied at 25°, 35° and 45°.

Species/Stoich.	CN^-	Maximum % S ⟶ SCN within 1st 10 days 25°	35°	45°
S^0	1x	3.2	3.5	9.5
	2x	4.5	---(1)	---
FeS Pyrrhotite mineral	1x	1.9	3.6	8.8
	2x	1.2	---	---
FeS Ferrous sulfide	0.5X	---	2.5	2.5
	1x	2.5	3.0	3.6
	2x	---	5.0	3.4
	5x	---	4.7	2.8
$CuFeS_2$	1x	8.3	14	16
	1.5x	---	16	---
	2x	14	---	---
	3x	---	14	---
Cu_2S	1x	0.5	0.4	0.4
	2x	9.0	2.0	10
ZnS(2)	1x	0.1	---	---
FeS_2(2)	1x	0.05	0.10	0.10

(1) No test run.
(2) Stoichiometries weren't varied since SCN^- was so low at 1x stoich.

Table 4 Conversion of $S \rightarrow SCN^-$ and CN^- Analyses of Solutions for Complex Sulfide Ore Samples after 10 Days.

Sample Desc.	Temp ^oC	Original CN^- conc. g/l	$\%S \rightarrow SCN^-$	% of original CN^- remaining as free CN^-	% of original CN^- converted to complexed CN^-	% of original CN^- not detected
North	25°	14.2	0.65*	82	0	18
North	25°	20.8	0.56	87	0	13
North	35°	10.4	0.85	81	0	19
North	45°	10.4	0.68	81	0	19
South	25°	20.8	0.69*	87	1	12
South	35°	10.4	1.34	81	0	19
South	45°	10.4	0.94	80	0	20
East	25°	14.2	1.31	92	0	8
East	25°	20.8	0.95	86	0	14
East	35°	10.4	1.61	81	0	19
East	45°	10.4	1.21	80	0	20

* These SCN^- and CN^- solution analyses reported after 20 days elapsed time.

DISCUSSION

The reaction of CN^- with the various sulfur species studied to form SCN^- was relatively slow. Of the compounds studied, chalcopyrite formed the most SCN^- relative to its initial sulfur content, but even so, after 8 days only ten percent of its sulfur had been converted to SCN^-. All species studied had an increase in SCN^- formation with temperature with the exception of Cu_2S. However, the formation of SCN^- from Cu_2S was so low that the decrease of SCN^- with temperature was within experimental errors and is probably not significant in this case. It may be possible that at low temperatures the reaction to form SCN^- is a heterogeneous reaction but at higher temperatures when solubilities of the compounds are higher it becomes more of a homogeneous reaction. Corresponding with higher temperatures and higher solubilities of compounds is an increase in the number of metal ions in solution which compete with the sulfur for the CN^-. It might be that for $CuFeS_2$ which has a low solubility, a surface reaction is more responsible for the SCN^- formation, and for Cu_2S a homogeneous reaction is dominating. In the latter case the presence of more Cu^{+2} in solution to compete for the CN^- might account for the low SCN^- formation.

However, the hypothesis doesn't hold well in the case of FeS_2 and FeS. FeS is more soluble than FeS_2 and also forms more SCN^-. There is more iron cyanide formed from the FeS than the FeS_2 which would support the hypotheses, but there is a definite increase in SCN^- with FeS than with FeS_2.

Copper in an ore is a signal for high cyanide consumption, and so it was not surprising to see the highest complexed cyanide percentages associated with Cu_2S and $CuFeS_2$.

In general, an increase in stoichiometry of CN^- led to an increase in SCN^- formation at all temperatures studied except for ferrous sulfide at 45^oC and five times the stoichiometry of CN^- and a slight decrease was shown for pyrrhotite at 25^oC and two times the stoichiometry of CN^-.

The complex ore samples reacted much in the same way as pyrite. Their reaction to form SCN^- was slow and to a small extent and the cyanide was not complexed with metal ions.

CONCLUSIONS

Cyanide reacts with the sulfur species to form SCN^-. The percent S converted to SCN^- is dependant on the mineral that the sulfur is associated with. Percent S converted to SCN^- increased with temperature and with increasing CN^- stoichiometry. Of the sulfur compounds studied, chalcopyrite produced the most SCN^- relative to its initial sulfur content. Percent S converted to SCN^- for the complex ore samples studied resembled that for pyrite.

ACKNOWLEDGEMENTS

The authors are grateful to the USBM for funding this project through the Generic Waste Treatment and Recovery Center at the University of Nevada, Reno. We are also grateful to Duval Corporation for supplying the samples, and to the USBM Reno Research Center for their assistance with equipment and expertise for a portion of the analytical measurements.

LITERATURE CITED

1. Huiatt, J.L., J.E. Kerrigan, F.A. Olson, G.A. Potter. Workshop-Cyanide from Mineral Processing. Utah Mining and Mineral Resources Research Institute. (1979)

2. Luthy, R.G. and S.G. Bruce, Jr. "Kinetics of Reaction of Cyanide and Reduced Sulfur Species in Aqueous Solutions." American Chem. Soc., Vol. 13, No. 12; Dec., 1979.

3. American Public Health Association, American Water Works Association and Water Pollution Control Federation. Standard Methods for the Examination of Water and Wastewater, 14th edition. 1976.

4. American Society for Testing and Materials. ASTM Designation: D 2036-81. Standatd Test Methods for Cyanides in Water. Reprinted from the Annual Book of ASTM Standards, Copyright ASTM. March, 1981.

CONFERENCE ON CYANIDE AND THE ENVIRONMENT
Tucson, Arizona • December 1984
Published by Geotechnical Engineering Program • Colorado State University • Fort Collins, Colorado 80523

ANALYSIS OF CYANIDE DATA ON THE RED RIVER, NEW MEXICO

by
Herbert S. Garn[1], Bruce M. Thomson[2]

ABSTRACT

One of the world's largest molybdenum mine and mill complexes discharges treated mill process effluent to the Red River, a tributary of the Rio Grande in northern New Mexico. The lower 4 miles of the Red River as well as 48 miles of the Rio Grande downstream from the Colorado state line are included in the National Wild and Scenic Rivers System. Molybdenite (MoS_2) is recovered from the ore by a flotation process. Sodium cyanide is used as a depressant in the process, principally to prevent contamination of the product by iron species.

Cyanide may reach the river as a trace contaminant in the mill's permitted discharge or as a result of accidental spills and pipeline breaks. The discharge has a sufficiently high cyanide limit (25 ug/L) that, under low flow conditions, the cyanide concentration in the river may exceed the EPA criterion for protection of aquatic life (3.5 ug/L).

The toxicity of cyanide to aquatic life is strongly dependent on the chemical speciation; uncomplexed or free cyanides being more toxic than complexed cyanides. Furthermore, analytical procedures for measuring free cyanide as opposed to total cyanide concentrations have only recently been developed and are not widely used. Numerical calculations have been performed to determine the distribution of cyanide species in the system and evaluate their toxicity. In the system described in this paper, the principal cyanide species are found to be copper and iron complexes as well as free cyanide. The most important parameter affecting this distribution is pH, although the total concentration of each element has some effect.

INTRODUCTION

The lower 4 miles (6.4 km) of the Red River in New Mexico as well as 48 miles (77.3 km) of the Rio Grande downstream from the Colorado State line were designated as one of the "instant" components of the National Wild and Scenic Rivers System by the Wild and Scenic Rivers Act of 1968. One of the world's largest molybdenum mine and mill complexes is located within the Red River drainage basin and discharges treated mill process effluent to the river immediately upstream from the wild and scenic river reach.

Under the Wild and Scenic Rivers Act, the Bureau of Land Management (BLM) is directed to administer a component of the national wild and scenic rivers system to protect and enhance the values which caused it to be

[1]Herbert S. Garn, Bureau of Land Management, Santa Fe, NM.
[2]Bruce M. Thomson, Department of Civil Engineering, University of New Mexico, Albuquerque, NM

included in the system. However, almost no water quality data existed at the time this river was included in the system to define base-line water quality conditions.

PROBLEM AND OBJECTIVES

The Red River drainage, containing prospects for gold, copper, lead, silver, zinc and molybdenum, has been a center of mining activity since 1895 (Schilling, 1960). Molybdenum ore was discovered in 1916 and is the only prospect to have seen much commercial success. Production of molybdenum was minimal until the early 1960's. Facilities for expanded mining and milling operations were constructed during 1964-1965, including a change to open-pit mining methods and new tailings disposal facilities. An 8.5 mile (13.7 km) pipeline transports tailings as a slurry containing 38 percent solids by weight along the Red River from the mill to tailings ponds 1 mile (1.6 km) west of the village of Questa. In 1969 the mill was expanded to its present capacity of 15,000 tons of ore per day. The mining and milling of molybdenum results in one of the major impacts to the Red River.

Processing of low-grade molybdenite ore (0.3 percent) consists of crushing, grinding, and multiple stages of froth flotation, followed by dewatering and drying of concentrated molybdenite. Sodium cyanide is used as a depressant in the flotation process to prevent flotation of other minerals that would contaminate the product. Cyanide may reach the Red River as a trace contaminant in the mill's permitted discharge and as a result of past periodic accidental pipeline leaks and breaks that entered the river.

Mining and milling operations were shut down from August 1981 to September 1983 to develop a new underground mine and modify the mill, tailings lines, and tailings disposal facilities. During this time, a wastewater treatment plant was constructed to treat the tailings pond effluent. Tailings decant water now passes through an ion exchange plant which removes residual molybdenum before discharging it into the Red River. The effluent is also treated with hydrogen peroxide, when needed, to reduce cyanide concentrations in the discharge to permitted levels.

Accidental spills resulting in discharge of tailings into the Red River have been common since the beginning of operations. Since 1966, over 80 separate major pipeline breaks have been recorded (NM Environmental Improvement Division, unpublished monitoring reports). The tailings slurry and decant water discharge also contain high concentrations of suspended and dissolved solids, molybdenum and sulfate. High concentrations of other trace elements (cadmium, copper, manganese and zinc) from nonpoint sources may also be a problem in the Red River (Garn, 1984). Water quality impacts in the future should be significantly less than those experienced in the past, because of the new treatment plant and the construction of a new, relocated pipeline which contains a wear-resistant rubber lining.

A water quality monitoring program of the river was initiated by the BLM in October 1978. The objectives of this study were to: 1) characterize existing water quality under natural conditions and at the present level of basin development; 2) monitor changes in water quality resulting from natural and artificial causes; 3) identify and evaluate the nature, importance, and source of existing and potential pollutants; and 4) evaluate water quality in relationship to State and Federal water quality standards and criteria. Cyanide was one of the major toxic elements evaluated. A particular problem which quickly surfaced was comparing cyanide measurements expressed as total recoverable cyanide with the newly-promulgated water quality criteria (Environmental Protection Agency, 1980) expressed as free cyanide (the sum of HCN and CN^-).

STUDY AREA DESCRIPTION

The study area is located in Taos County in north central New Mexico (Figure 1). The Red River is the major perennial tributary to the wild river portion of the Rio Grande and contains both municipal and industrial (mining and milling) discharges to the river. Since the major impact is from the Red River drainage, emphasis was placed on monitoring water quality of this river.

The Red River has its headwaters in the Sangre de Cristo Mountains, containing the highest point in New Mexico at 13,161 feet (4,012 m). The Red River drainage contains a belt of high-angle faults within which rocks were irregularly faulted and brecciated. The more highly brecciated areas served as conduits for hydrothermal solutions which further altered the rocks. The igneous activity and hydrothermal alteration formed the molybdenum ore deposits associated with the stocks and dikes in this area (Schilling, 1956; 1965). These altered, highly weathered and erodable areas are also a natural source of sediment load and dissolved constituents in the Red River.

The pattern of runoff in the Red River is typical of mountainous areas, where snowmelt is the major source of runoff. Streamflows of the lower Red River are maintained by groundwater discharged from springs, which represents a significant contribution, especially during low flows. The total gain in flow from groundwater discharge between the mouth of the Red River and the head of its canyon near Questa averages 35 cfs. The average annual discharge for the Red River at its mouth is 75 cfs. The average discharge below Questa, upstream from the tailings ponds is therefore about 40 cfs.

The Red River component of the wild river is unique in that it is downstream from all developments and effects of man within its drainage basin. Major developments along the Red River, in downstream order, include the town of Red River and a ski area, a molybdenum mine and mill, the town of Questa, molybdenum mill tailings ponds, and a state fish hatchery at the upper end of the wild river segment (Figure 1). The remainder of the basin is undeveloped forest land within the Carson National Forest. The lower Red River and the Rio Grande are renowned for their high-quality rainbow and brown trout fisheries and together represent one of the top trout fishing areas in the State.

METHODS

The location of the sampling stations and water quality consti-

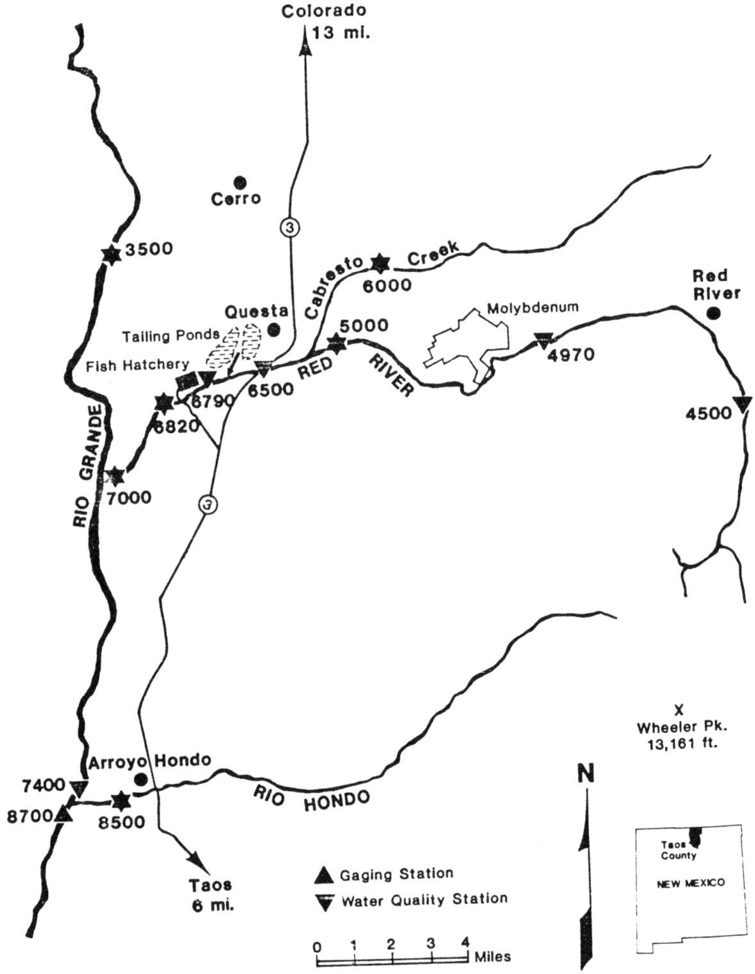

Vicinity map of study area and identification of sampling stations.

Figure 1.

tuents to be measured were tailored to the objectives of the study, environmental conditions, and pollution problems of the area. Sampling stations (see Figure 1) were located upstream and downstream of population and industrial centers, major wastewater outfalls and return flows and natural features that may affect water quality. The frequency of sample collection was about 10 times per year, with emphasis on characterizing seasonal and discharge-related water quality variations. Samples were collected roughly on a monthly basis except during spring snowmelt runoff, when samples were collected near peak flow and during rising and falling stages.

In addition to total recoverable cyanide, samples were analyzed for physical and other chemical characteristics (including common ions, nutrients, and trace elements). Water samples were collected, preserved, and shipped to the U.S. Geological Survey (USGS) Central Laboratory in Denver, Colorado for analysis; standard methods employed by the USGS were used (USGS, 1977; Skougstad, et al., 1979). Time-sensitive constituents such as pH and alkalinity were measured in the field. Each sample was accompanied by a discharge measurement. All data were stored in the USGS WATSTORE computer storage and retrieval system.

CYANIDE SPECIATION CALCULATIONS

Since molecular hydrogen cyanide (HCN) is the species which is most toxic to aquatic life (Thurston, et al., 1979) it is important to determine its concentration in solution. Unfortunately, analytical determination of free cyanide at low concentrations is fairly difficult and therefore not routinely done. An alternative procedure is to assume chemical equilibrium in the solution and to perform speciation calculations of cyanide and related species. This involves solving a series of simultaneous non-linear equations comprised of the equilibrium mass action expressions, a mass balance on each of the dissolved species, calculation of the ionic strength of the solution and appropriate approximations of the single species activity coefficients (Stumm and Morgan, 1981).

A computer model, PHREEQE, developed by the U.S. Geological Survey (Parkhurst et al. 1980) was used in this investigation. It was selected because, in addition to performing simple speciation calculations, it incorporates corrections for non-ideal solutions (i.e. calculation of individual ion activities), and allows variation of oxidation-reduction conditions.

It is important to recognize the fundamental assumptions inherent in speciation calculations when applying them to problems of this nature. The first assumption of chemical equilibrium is that no chemical reactions are occurring and that the free energy of the solution is at a minimum. An assumption of equal importance is the recognition that the model only represents the solution for which data are provided. Chemical speciation calculations require two types of input: thermodynamic equilibrium constants and information about the total concentration of each of the elements or major species in the system. Thermodynamic data for cyanide species and complexes were obtained from the recent compilation by Wagman et al. (1982). The concentration informa-

Table 1
Water quality at Red River at Station 6500 and at tailings outfall

(All units mg/L except as noted)

Parameter	Red River at[1] Station 6500	Tailings[2] Outfall
Cu	.024	.04[3]
CN_{total}	see table 2	.043
Fe	.017	.32
Mn	.293	.44
Mo_{total}	.015	2.92
$Mo_{dissolved}$	.009	
Ni	--	.45[3]
SO_4^{2-}	77.0	1200.
pH	7.0-8.3	6.6-8.3
Avg. Flow (cfs)	40	3.4

[1] USGS water quality monitoring program

[2] USEPA, application for NPDES discharge permit, 1982

[3] Only 1 reported value

tion was based on results of the field sampling program previously described. A summary of the water quality data in the Red River at Station 6500 and in the tailings outfall is presented in Table 1.

RESULTS AND DISCUSSION

A summary of the cyanide concentrations found in the Red River is presented in Table 2. The presence of cyanide in the river at Questa and upstream (Stations 6500 and 5000) is due to acci dental pipeline spills. Cyanide in the Red River below the tailings pond discharge (Stations 6790, 6820 and 7000) is due to a combination of the permitted discharge and accidental spills. Frequency in Table 2 is the number of samples, in percent, that were equal to or greater than 10 ug/L total cyanide.

Table 2
Summary of ambient total cyanide concentrations (ug/L) in the Red River, 1978 - 1983.

	Sample		Statistic		
Station	Size	Minimum	Median	Maximum	Frequency, %
4500	14	0	0	0	0
4970	26	0	0	0	0
5000	32	0	0	10	6
6000	9	0	0	0	0
6500	19	0	0	770	16
6790	22	0	0	110	18
6820	38	0	10	1000	21
7000	12	0	0	60	16

The permitted discharge of tailings pond decant water into the Red River contains a long-term average concentration of 15 ug/L total cyanide, but daily average concentrations have exceeded 40 ug/L, and daily maximums have been as high as 80 ug/L (NMEID, unpublished discharge monitoring reports). The effluent limitations in the permit authorizing the discharge to the Red River are 25 ug/L and 50 ug/L total cyanide for the daily average and daily maximum concentrations, respectively. The average flow of the discharge is about 4 cfs, which varies from no flow to about 7 cfs.

Cyanide data collected during this study were measured as total cyanide because effluent limitations and water quality criteria (EPA, 1977) were expressed in this form. Water samples were analyzed for total recoverable cyanide using the USGS pyridine-barbituric acid method (Skougstad, et al., 1979). Analysis results in the range of 5 - 1000 ug/L were reported to the nearest 10 ug/L. During the course of the study, the total cyanide criterion was criticized (Thurston, et al.,

1979, pp. 106-112) and a new criterion, expressed as free cyanide, was promulgated by the EPA (1980).

The toxicity of cyanides is due primarily to the presence of free cyanide, defined as the sum of HCN and CN^-. Total cyanide could also include stable organic cyanides and metallo-cyanide complexes which do not contribute significantly to toxicity. Therefore, there is a problem of comparing total cyanide data with new water quality criteria and state water quality standards expressed as free cyanide. The EPA water quality criterion to protect freshwater aquatic life is 3.5 ug/L free cyanide as a 24-hour average, and the concentration should not exceed 52 ug/L at any time. The New Mexico water quality standard for hazardous substances states that concentrations should not exceed 5 percent of the 96-hour LC-50 for the form of aquatic life to be preserved (Water Quality Control Commission, 1981). Based on toxicity data from the available literature (Doudoroff, 1976; Koenst, et al., 1977; Kovacs and Leduc, 1979; Smith, et al., 1979), the State standard for cyanide is projected to be 3 ug/L, which is very close to the EPA criterion.

Because of the lack of analytical data on free cyanide concentrations, comparison of the discharge and stream water quality data with the EPA criterion and regulatory standard must depend on the speciation calculations. The values reported in Table 1 were used to determine the distribution of cyanide species concentrations as a function of pH and oxidation-reduction conditions (reported as pe where pe = $-\log\{e^-\}$). Cyanide species which were included in the calculations and their respective formation constants are listed in Table 3.

Table 3
Cyanide species considered and their respective formation constants, calculated from information presented by Wagman et al., 1982.

Species	log (Formation Constant)
HCN	9.23
CuCN	19.47
$Cu(CN)_2^-$	24.00
$Cu(CN)_3^{2-}$	28.63
$Cu(CN)_4^{3-}$	30.31
$Ni(CN)_4^{2-}$	30.12
$HFe(CN)_6^{3-}$	49.81
$Fe(CN)_6^{4-}$	45.63
$Fe(CN)_6^{3-}$	52.62
$CaFe(CN)_6^{2-}$	49.94
$CaFe(CN)_6^-$	55.48

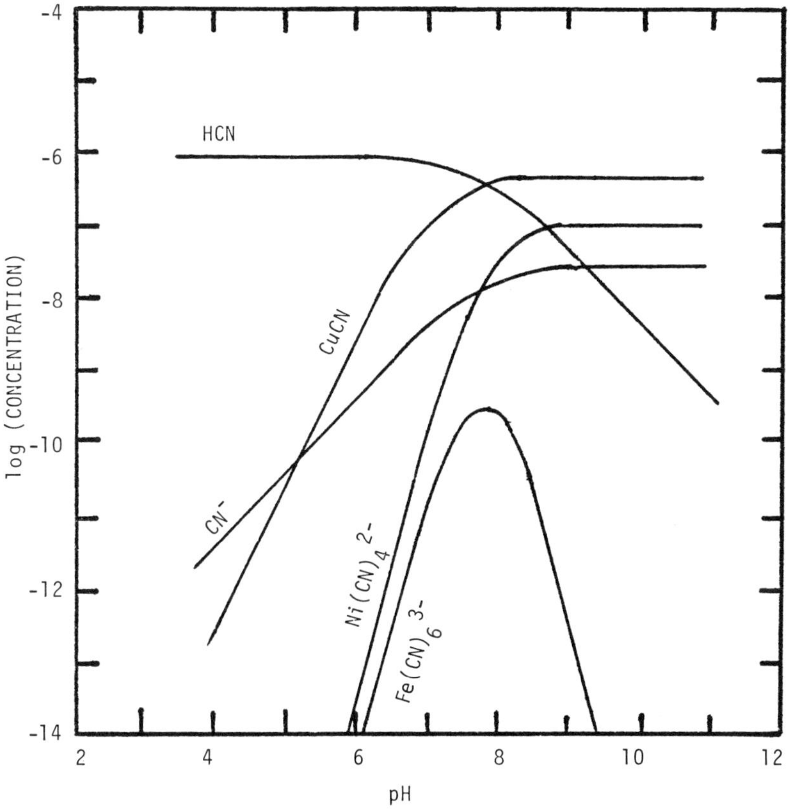

Distribution of major cyanide species. Total concentrations contained in Table 1.

Figure 2.

The dependence of cyanide species on pH under oxidizing conditions is illustrated graphically in Figure 2. The major cyanide species are the free cyanides (HCN and CN^-) and the copper, nickel and iron (Fe(III)) complexes. The one feature of the diagram which is particularly noteworthy is that, above pH 7, there is a significant drop in free cyanide species and a corresponding increase in the complexed species. For the conditions used in these calculations, the free cyanide drops below the 3 ug/L level at a pH of approximately 7.0. This is due to the copper (I) complex and is in marked contrast to the usual assumption that HCN concentrations don't significantly decrease until the pH nears the log of the dissociation constant (pK = 9.23)

The ferrous and ferric iron-cyanide complexes are subject to extensive and rapid photodecomposition by natural light, resulting in the release of HCN (Doudoroff, 1976). Up to one-half or more of the cyanide bound in the complex may be released as free cyanide by this phenomenon. Since the chemical reaction kinetics are little understood and no rate data are available, it was not incorporated into the model and is a source of uncertainty. Complete photo-decomposition may be simulated by omitting the iron complexes from the system. The "real" equilibrium concentrations are expected to be somewhere in between these two extreme cases.

It is worth noting that iron complexes of cyanides are relatively weak in this system although the formation constants are fairly large. The formation constant for the hexacyanoferrate (III) complex (log K = 52.62) is similar to that suggested by Broderius (Doudoroff, 1976). The small concentrations of ferri-cyanide complexes is due to two factors; the higher stability of the copper (I) and nickel (II) complexes, and formation of very stable ferric hydroxide species ($Fe(OH)_3^0$ and $Fe(OH)_4^-$). Figure 3 illustrates speciation calculations performed after omitting ferric hydroxide complexes from the thermodynamic data base. It can be seen that cuprous complexes still dominate. Figure 4 illustrates the effect an absence of copper and nickel complexes has on the system.

The variation of cyanide species with redox conditions has been explored and found not to affect the speciation calculations except under strongly reducing conditions. In such solutions, high concentrations of sulfides are produced due to sulfate reduction and result in metal-sulfide precipitates of most of the transition metals in the solution including Fe, Cu, Mn and Ni.

The toxicity of cyanide solutions to aquatic organisms is almost entirely attributable to molecular HCN (Figures 2 - 4). The CN^- ion is a minor component of free cyanide in most natural waters. Cadmium-cyanide and zinc-cyanide complexes are also of little importance because of their instability and are almost entirely dissociated. Silver-cyanide and copper-cyanide complexes are more stable but do contribute somewhat to toxicity. Ferro-cyanide and ferri-cyanide complexes are highly stable but are subject to photodecomposition by direct sunlight.

A sensitivity analysis of the model, in which the total cyanide and total metal concentrations were varied, indicated that the concentration of free cyanide is relatively insensitive to the metal ion concentrations. Increasing a metal concentration by a factor of 2 decreases the

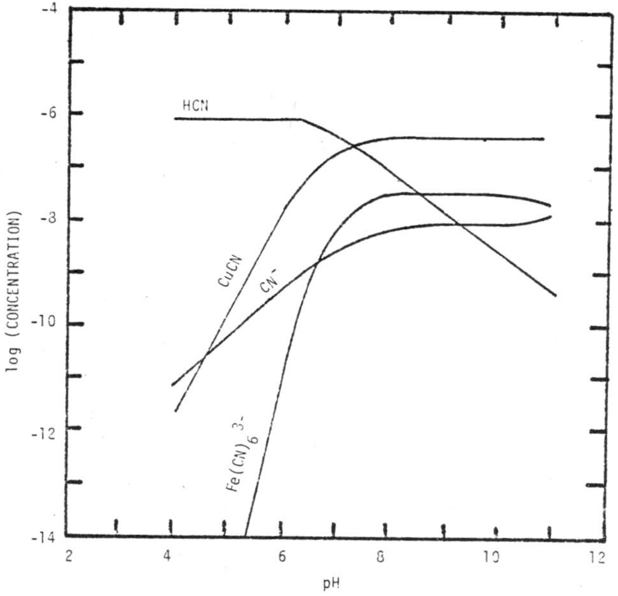

Distribution of major cyanide species.
Iron (III) hydroxide complexes omitted.

Figure 3.

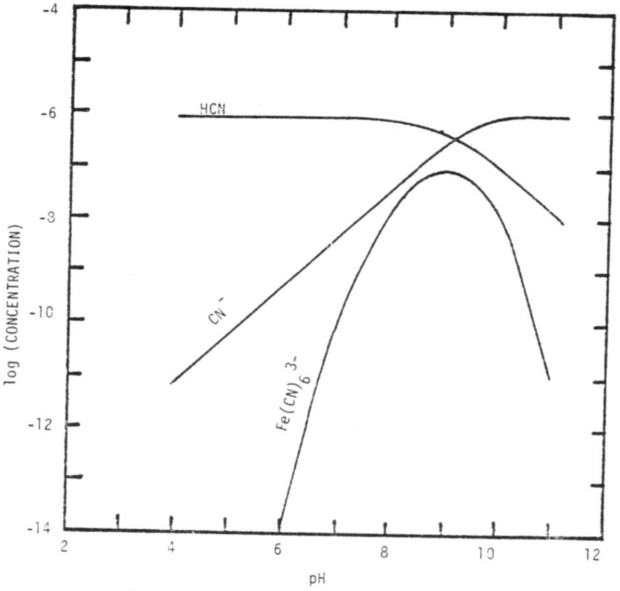

Distribution of major cyanide species. No copper or nickel present.

Figure 4.

HCN concentration by only a few percent of the total. Similarly, increasing the total cyanide concentration maintains the approximate ratio of free to complexed cyanides.

By predicting concentrations of free and complexed cyanide from the cyanide speciation model, one can evaluate the toxicity of total cyanide, as well as more accuratly predict potential impacts. This is based on the premise that free cyanide is a more reliable index of toxicity than total cyanide. The limitations of this approach are primarily the lack of reliable data on metal and complexing anion concentrations and the questionable accuracy of the dissociation constants used in calculating individual species concentrations. These limitations are largely negated by the availability of a comprehensive data base for trace elements and the availability of recently updated thermodynamic data (Wagman, 1982). Although it is more desirable to obtain free cyanide measurements directly, historical data is only available on the total cyanide concentrations. Numerical calculations to determine the free cyanide present in solution is therefore the only current option available when evaluating the impact of cyanide discharges on aquatic life.

Analytical procedures for measuring free cyanide at very low concentrations have only recently been developed (Broderius, 1981; Ingersoll, et al., 1983). These are now capable of measuring free cyanide at a detection limit of 2 ± 1 ug/L.

SUMMARY AND CONCLUSIONS

A computer model of cyanide speciation was applied to estimate solution concentrations of free and complexed cyanides from total cyanide measurements. Such calculations were necessary to evaluate the toxicity of cyanides in a molybdenum mine and mill discharge and to evaluate the impacts to the Red River. Free cyanide was calculated for a variety of conditions using total metal and total cyanide data from the effluent and the receiving stream.

Calculated free cyanide varies greatly with pH. A sensitivity analysis of the model, however, revealed that the ratio of free to complexed cyanides is maintained with changes in metal and total cyanide concentrations. The presence of free cyanide is greatly affected by the degree of complexation with copper and iron and depends upon whether ferric (Fe(III)) or ferrous (Fe(II)) iron is present. The presence of the iron-cyanide complexes may be of limited significance, however, due to their extensive photodecomposition by sunlight. The most probable percentage of free cyanide existing in the effluent is approximately 60 percent of the total cyanide at a pH of 7.5 for the values shown in Table 1.

Predicting concentrations of free cyanide from the speciation model allows for more accurate and meaningful evaluation of the toxicity potential of total cyanide concentrations and the prediction of potential impacts. The permitted discharge and accidental pipeline leaks and breaks that reached the Red River in the past had a sufficiently high cyanide content that the free cyanide concentration in the river may have occasionally exceeded the EPA criterion for the protection of aquatic life. However, impacts in the future should be less than those experienced in the past.

ACKNOWLEDGMENTS

Special gratitude is given to Bruce P. VanHaveren, Bureau of Land Management, Denver Colorado for his constructive review of this paper and to Frances L. Garn for editing.

REFERENCES

Broderius, S.J., 1981. Determination of hydrocyanic acid and free cyanide in aqueous solutions. Analytical Chemistry. 53(9): pp. 1472-1477.

Doudoroff, P, 1976. Toxicity to fish of cyanides and related compounds. A review. EPA 600/3-76-038, Environmental Research Lab. USEPA. Duluth MN. 154 p.

Garn, H.S., 1984. Spatial and temporal variations in water quality of the Rio Grande-Red River Wild and Scenic River, Taos County, New Mexico. In: Selected papers on water quality and pollution in New Mexico. New Mexico Bureau of Mines and Mineral Resources, Socorro, NM; Hydrologic Report No. 7, pp. 49-59.

Ingersol, D., W.R. Harris, D.C. Bomberger and D.M. Coulson, 1983. Development and evaluation of procedures for the analysis of simple cyanides, total cyanide, and thiocyanate in water and wastewater. EPA-600/S4-83-054. U.S. Environmental Protection Agency, Cincinnati, OH.

Koenst, W.M., L.L. Smith, Jr. and S.J. Broderius, 1977. Effect of chronic exposure of brook trout to sublethal concentrations of hydrogen cyanide. Environ. Sci. & Tech. 11(9):883-887.

Kovacs, T.G., and G. Leduc, 1979. Concentration dependence of the acute toxicity of hycrogen cyanide to rainbow trout acclimatized and tested at different temperatures. Proc. Fifth Annual Aquatic Toxicity Workshop, Hamilton, Ontario, Nov. 7-9, 1978, Fish. Mar. Serv. Tech. Rep. 862, 129 p.

Parkhurst, D.L., D.C. Thorstenson and L.N. Plummer, 1980. PHREEQE - A computer program for geochemical calculations. U.S. Geological Survey, Water-Resources Investigations 80-96. Reston, VA. 210 p.

Schilling, J.H., 1956. Geology of the Questa molybdenum mine area, Taos County, New Mexico, NM Bureau of Mines and Mineral Resources, Bulletin 51. Socorro, NM

Schilling, J.H., 1965. Molybdenum resources of New Mexico. New Mexico Bureau of Mines and Mineral Resources, Bulletin 76. Socorro, NM. pp. 26-34.

Smith, L.L., Jr., et al, 1979. Acute and chronic toxicity of HCN to fish and invertebrates. EPA-600/3-79-009. Environmental Research Lab. U.S. Environmental Protection Agency. Duluth, MN. 114 p.

Skougstad, M.W., et al., 1979. Methods for determination of inorganic substances in water and fluvial sediments. Techniques of water resources investigations; Book 5, Chapter A1, U.S. Geological Survey. 626 p.

Stumm, W. and Morgan, J.J., 1981. Aquatic Chemistry, 2nd ed. Wiley-Interscience. New York, NY. pp. 385-399.

Thurston, R.V., et al. (Eds.), 1979. A review of the EPA Red Book: Quality criteria for water. Water quality section, Am. Fish. Soc., Bethesda, MD. 313 p.

U.S. Environmental Protection Agency, 1977. Quality criteria for water. Office of Water and Hazardous Materials, U.S. Environmental Protection Agency, Washington, D.C., 256 p.

U.S. Environmental Protection Agency, 1980. Ambient water quality criteria for cyanides. Document No. EPA 440/5-80-037, Office of Water Regulations and Standards. Washington, D.C.

U.S. Geological Survey, 1977. National handbook of recommended methods for water-data acquisition. U.S. Department of the Interior, Reston, VA.

Wagman, D.D., W.H. Evans, V.B. Parker, R.H. Schumm, I. Halow, S.M. Bailey, K.L. Churney and R.L. Nutall, 1982. "The NBS tables of chemical thermodynamic properties, selected values for inorganic and C_1 and C_2 organic substances in SI units", Journal of Physical and Chemical Reference Data. 11(Suppl. No. 2). 392 p.

Water Quality Control Commission, 1981. Water quality standards for interstate and intrastate streams in New Mexico. Santa Fe, NM.

CONFERENCE ON CYANIDE AND THE ENVIRONMENT
Tucson, Arizona • December 1984
Published by Geotechnical Engineering Program • Colorado State University • Fort Collins, Colorado 80523

THE USE OF RODENTS IN IDENTIFYING AND MONITORING POTENTIAL ENVIRONMENTAL IMPACTS FROM CYANIDE AT A HEAP LEACHING FACILITY IN SOUTH DAKOTA

by
H. Peter Feigley[1], James F. Heisinger[2]
and Richard J. Douglass[3]

ABSTRACT

The South Dakota Department of Game, Fish and Parks required the collection of data from rodent population studies and from monitoring cyanide (CN) levels in rodent tissues to identify and monitor environmental impacts from CN at a heap leaching facility in the Black Hills, SD. Review of appropriate literature and rodent population data collected on site indicate that such studies are probably inadequate.

Rodents are often useful biomonitors because their populations respond quickly to environmental disturbances and their tissues may retain environmental pollutants. However, the use of rodents to identify and monitor impacts from CN is limited due to their ability to metabolize CN, the low toxicity of low CN concentrations, and the lack of bioaccumulation potential of CN. Also, reproductive and dispersal tendencies of rodents as well as instability of rodent populations could mask impacts from CN.

To determine if CN emissions from the heap leaching facility were sufficient to affect rodent populations we examined CN levels in ambient air and maintained caged rodents near the leach pad. Urinary thiocyanate levels in the caged rodents were measured to compare relative levels of exposure to CN at three locations. Preliminary results from these studies failed to demonstrate CN emissions at levels capable of directly affecting rodent populations.

---

[1] H. Peter Feigley, Consulting Biologist, 22 Border Lane #1, Bozeman, Montana 59715.

[2] James F. Heisinger, Professor, Department of Biology, University of South Dakota, Vermillion, South Dakota 57069.

[3] Richard J. Douglass, Professor, Department of Biology, Montana College of Mineral Science and Technology, Butte, Montana 59601.

INTRODUCTION

The heap leaching method of gold ore processing uses dilute cyanide (CN) solution (500 ppm) as the leaching agent. This solution is sprayed onto heaps of crushed ore via a network of small sprinklers. The use of CN in this fashion could result in contamination of the surrounding environment with CN. Contamination could result from either a solution spill or through wind blown aerosols and / or volatilized HCN from the sprinklers and solution containment structures.

At Wharf Resources (USA), Inc.'s Annie Creek gold mine in the northern Black Hills of South Dakota environmental studies were conducted in order to identify CN related problems. These studies included monitoring ground and surface water, ambient air and wildlife. The South Dakota Department of Game, Fish and Parks initially required monthly monitoring of rodent tissues and rodent densities as indicators of CN "build up" and impacts to wildlife. The requirement to analyze rodent tissues for CN was eventually dropped.

Rodents are often useful biomonitors (Douglass 1984 and Skalski 1984). Their generation time is very short and therefore can show population responses to impacts in a convenient time frame. They can occur in numbers (up to 50/ha) suitable for statistical analysis and their movements are confined to small areas (< 5 ha) which minimize confusion with offsite effects. Also, their tissues can serve as indicators of environmental accumulation of toxic substances, such as heavy metals (Johnson et al. 1978, Roberts and Johnson 1978) and organic pollutants (Rowley, et al. 1983).

This paper evaluates the usefulness of monitoring rodents as indicators of terrestrial pollution from CN and presents a more useful method for monitoring relative levels of CN exposure in rodents.

LITERATURE REVIEW

Several aspects of CN affect the usefulness of rodents for monitoring environmental impacts from CN. Although CN can be toxic or lethal, low levels of CN are relatively non-toxic. Rats fed diets containing as much as 300 ppm CN for up to three years showed little chronic effect (Howard and Hanzal 1955). Philbrick et al. (1979) observed neither death nor clinical signs of toxicity in rats fed diets containing 1500 ppm potassium cyanide or 2240 ppm potassium thiocyanate for 11.5 months. Airborne HCN levels greater than 200 ppm are regarded as lethal to mammals while levels of 80 to 160 ppm may cause sublethal toxic effects (Barcroft 1931, Sollmann 1957). Cyanide emissions from heap leaching would have to be quite high (>80 ppm) to potentially affect rodent populations.

In a review of the environmental effects of CN, Towill (1978) indicates that most organisms are able to metabolize and detoxify CN. Mammals (including rodents) convert approximately 80% of ingested CN to thiocyanate which is excreted in the urine (Sollmann 1957, Altman and Dittmer 1964). In addition, CN occurs widely in nature. Numerous plants, bacteria and fungi produce and/ or utilize CN (Goldschmidt et al. 1963, Rangaswami and Balasubramanian 1963, Abrol and Conn 1966, Strobel 1967, Mundy et al. 1973). Free CN also undergoes chemical oxidation in the environment (Ecological Analysts 1979, Rowley and Otto 1980) The natural chemical oxidation and metabolism of CN by organisms tend to remove CN from the environment. Towill (1978) found no evidence that CN either bioaccumulates or biomagnifies in ecosystems.

Since CN is rapidly converted to SCN (relatively non-toxic) and excreted, the analysis of rodent tissues for CN would serve as a poor index of exposure and "build up".

Because CN is relatively non-toxic, readily metabolized and excreted by rodents, we expect impacts upon rodents to be subtle, except in the event of a large CN spill. Since we expect impacts to rodents to be subtle, examination of rodent densities may be insufficient to detect such impacts.

Demographic characteristics of rodent populations could act to obscure subtle effects that CN may have upon rodents. Rodent populations are often unstable and can double in density or become locally extinct in periods as short as two weeks (Krebs and Myers 1974). Even under conditions of stability the reproductive capacity and dispersal tendencies of rodents can replace individuals removed from a population (e.g. by poisoning) in a short time (less than two weeks) (Gaines and McClenaghan 1980). For example, Krebs (1966), in enclosure experiments, was able to remove 30 % of a Microtus californicus population (during the increase phase) every two weeks without causing the density to decrease. Immigration of new individuals into a population could also replace poisoned animals quickly. Gaines and McClenaghan (1980) reviewed several studies examining the recovery rates of rodent populations after being exterminated by trapping. Microtus pennsylvanicus was able to replace 6% of its population in one week (Tamarin 1977)and M. ochrogaster was able to replace 23% of its population in one week (Gaines et al. 1979). Deer mice (Peromyscus maniculatus) have been found to replace 18% and 48% of their populations in one week (Sullivan 1977). This replacement of individuals through reproduction and immigration (recruitment) could confound our ability to detect changes in density caused by low concentrations of CN. Also, by studying only monthly densities, major demographic events (doubling of density or extinction) could be missed or misinterpreted.

If CN were actually affecting rodent populations, examination of densities alone may not be sufficient to identify the impacts. Douglass (1984) demonstrated that even though densities of two populations of deer mice were similar, the recruitment rates and survival rates of the populations were significantly different. Therefore the populations were different. For this reason it is important to examine the survival and recruitment aspects of rodent demography.

To determine if we could detect responses of rodent populations to CN from the leaching process we examined rodent density as well as recruitment and survival. However, it seems appropriate that prior to using intensive rodent population studies for identifying and monitoring impacts from CN, the following question should have been asked: Are CN emissions from the leaching process sufficiently high to potentially affect rodent populations? If not, then studying rodent populations for evidence of impacts from CN would be inappropriate.

In order to evaluate the potential for CN emissions from leaching to affect rodents we measured the concentration of CN in ambient air and measured relative exposure of caged rodents near the leach pad.

METHODS

Rodent populations were sampled by standard live trapping techniques. Four trapping grids (experimental) were constructed near the leaching facility (within 150 meters of the leach pad) and two control grids were located farther away in "unaffected" areas. Each grid contained 100 trap stations in a 10x10 configuration and were spaced at 15 m intervals. Assuming a 7.5 m band (0.5 of the distance between traps) around the periphery of each grid, the area sampled per grid was 2.2 ha. One Sherman live-trap (8x9x23 cm) was placed at each trap station. Traps were covered with 20x30 cm pieces of plywood to protect them from the sun. Peanut butter and oatmeal were used as bait. Synthetic cotton was added to each trap for nesting material. Trapping was conducted for three consecutive days every two weeks, for a total of six sampling periods on each grid. Trapping began in late July so that it would be completed prior to heavy snowfall.

An individually numbered ear tag was placed on each animal that was captured. The following data were recorded: Tag number, species, whether it was new or recaptured, grid location , weight, sex, and breeding condition (testis -- abdominal or scrotal; vagina -- perforate or non-perforate; nipples -- large or small; pubic symphysis -- open or closed; whether it was pregnant).

Because of non-random sampling problems (Krebs 1966) Lincoln index mark-recapture population estimating techniques were not used. Instead the minimum number known to be alive (MNA) (Chitty and Phipps 1966) was used as an estimate of population size during each trapping period. Population variables such as survival rates (SR), recruitment rates (RR), and turnover rates (TR) were calculated from the MNA statistics. Since turnover rates are calculated by dividing the recruitment rate by the survival rate (TR=RR/SR), this statistic can serve to summarize the population data. If CN is affecting rodent populations, we would expect to see a decrease in survival rates which could stimulate an increase in recruitment (immigration) rates. A decrease in survival rates and/ or an increase in recruitment rates would cause an increase in turnover rates. This paper discusses turnover rates as a summary of the population data. Density estimates (MNA, SR and RR) from experimental grid 1A are discussed as an example of the demographic events frequently observed in rodent populations.

Cyanide in ambient air at the leaching facility was measured using the Analytical Method for Cyanide in Air, No. 808 (Katz 1977). Samples were collected for one hour by pumping air (liters/ minute) through a midget impinger containing 0.1 M NaOH. The samples were collected on platforms which were two meters high and located near the leach pad during leaching. The NaOH solution samples were analyzed for total CN at Travis Laboratories, Rapid City, South Dakota.

Caged rodents were used to determine if CN emissions would affect them and potentially affect wild rodent populations. Two cages, each containing five long-tailed voles (Microtus longicaudus), were placed near the leach pad. Each vole was numbered by toe clipping. Voles were fed a diet of oatmeal, carrots and potatoes. Cage A was placed three meters from the N (downwind) corner of the leach pad while cage B was placed 50 m N of the pad. After four weeks cage B was moved to 100 m N. Relative levels of exposure of the voles to CN at these locations were compared by examining urinary thiocyanate (SCN) levels. Paired data were collected at three and 50 m during leaching (29 days of sprinkler operation). The second set of paired data was collected at three and 100 m, after most leaching was completed. However, the ore was releached for five days during the period when the second set of paired data was collected. One vole was removed from each cage (A and B) and placed in a separate metabolic cage for 24 hours, then returned to its appropriate cage. While in the metabolic cages the voles were fed pieces of carrot and potato. After cage B was moved to 100 m from the leach pad, seven days passed before urine collection was resumed. Urine collection tubes on the metabolic cages were immersed in an ice bath to prevent sample evaporation. The volume of each 24 hr urine sample was recorded, placed in a labeled vial, and frozen. Thiocyanate determinations were made using a colorimetric procedure described by Pettigrew and Fell (1972) and performed at the University of South Dakota, Vermillion. Thiocyanate concentrations were expressed as micromoles (uMol) SCN/ 24 hrs. Data pairs (simultaneous samples collected from voles from cages A and B) were compared statistically by a paired sample t-test (Zar 1974).

RESULTS

Rodent Populations

From July 26 to October 9, 1983, 10,800 trap nights were expended on six live trapping grids at the Annie Creek mine area. During that time six species of rodents were captured. Red-backed vole (Clethrionomys gapperi) , long-tailed vole, and least chipmunk (Eutamias minimus) were the only species captured on all six grids. Densities of least chipmunks were low ($\leq$8/grid) on all six grids. Only red-backed voles and long-tailed voles yielded sufficient data to adequately compare experimental and control grids. To summarize the data we discuss turnover rates of red-backed voles and long-tailed voles. The leaching process commenced on September 1, 1984, which was between trapping period 3 and 4.

Average turnover rates of long-tailed voles (Figure 1) on experimental and control grids decreased from period 2 to 3. Turnover rates on experimental grids increased from period 4 to 5 and decreased by period 6. Turnover rates on control grids decreased slightly between period 4 and 5 and increased sharply by period 6. Statistical analysis (ANOV) of these turnover rates showed a significant difference among six grids ($0.01<P<0.025$). However, there were no consistant differences between experimental and control grids (SNK).

Average turnover rates of red-backed voles (Figure 2) on experimental and control grids decreased from period 2 to 4. Turnover rates on experimental grids continued to decrease to period 5 then increased slightly at period 6. Turnover rates on control grids increased sharply between period 4 and 5 and decreased by period 6. Turnover rates of red-backed voles, among the six grids, were not significantly different (ANOV).

Figure 3 demonstrates the demographic events frequently observed in vole populations. Long-tailed vole density, on experimental grid 1A, doubled between period 2 and 3 (a sampling interval of two weeks). The density then decreased by 53% in two weeks (period 4 to 5). The number of survivors followed a similar pattern, but at much lower numbers. The data show that the changes in density of long-tailed voles on grid 1A closely followed the number of recruits. The number of recruits may be related to reproduction and subsequent immigration. On Grid 1A the number of obviously pregnant females captured dropped from three at period 3 to zero at periods 4,5, and 6. Also, at period 2, 88% of the females captured were in breeding condition

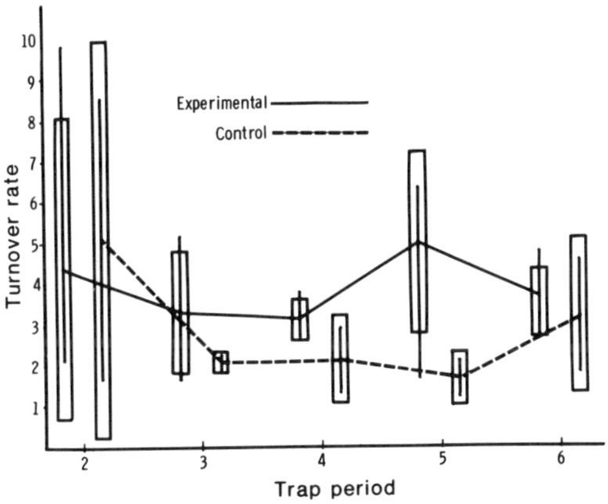

Figure 1. Average turnover rates of long-tailed voles on experimental (N=4) and control (N=2) grids.

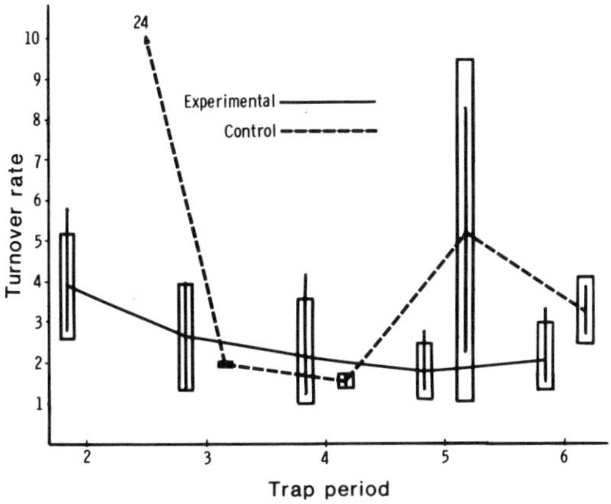

Figure 2. Average turnover rates of red-backed voles on experimental (N=4) and control (N=2) grids.

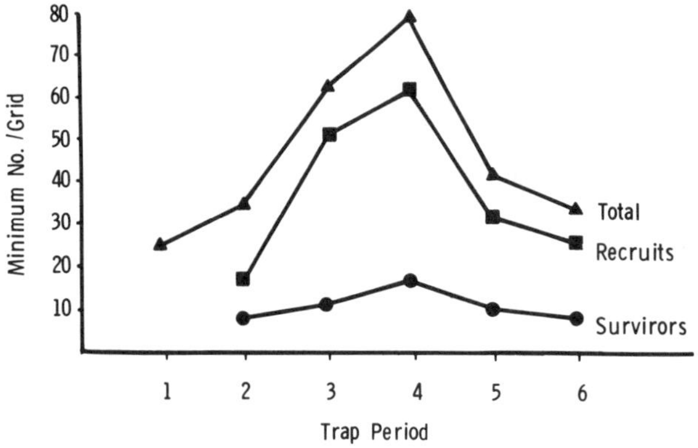

Figure 3. Long-tailed vole densities on experimental grid 1A.

(vaginas perforate). By period 5 all females were non-perforate. These data indicate that the breeding season ended by period 5, which probably accounts for the decrease in recruitment.

Cyanide in Ambient Air

Seven one hour samples of CN in ambient air were collected during 1982 at a test leach facility and seven samples were collected during fall, 1983 at the production leaching facility. The highest level of CN recorded in ambient air was 5.95 ppm at a location two meters from the leach pad during sprinkling of CN solution. Mean CN concentrations in ambient air (Figure 4) were highest close to the leach pad and decreased with distance from the pad, except for one sample collected at 50+ m. Two samples collected at this distance measured 0.29 and 2.88 ppm CN. The sample measuring 2.88 ppm CN was collected downwind from the CN solution containment ponds during winds of 25+ mph.

Urinary Thiocyanate

Of the ten long-tailed voles placed in cages at the leaching facility, two mortalities were observed during the urinary SCN experiment (September 15 to November 1, 1984). One vole from cage B (50 m from the leach pad) died after being returned to the cage, after collection of a urine sample. The carcass showed evidence of fighting (tooth marks in musculature). Another vole died in cage A (three meters from the leach pad). Necropsy of this vole showed no evidence of fighting.

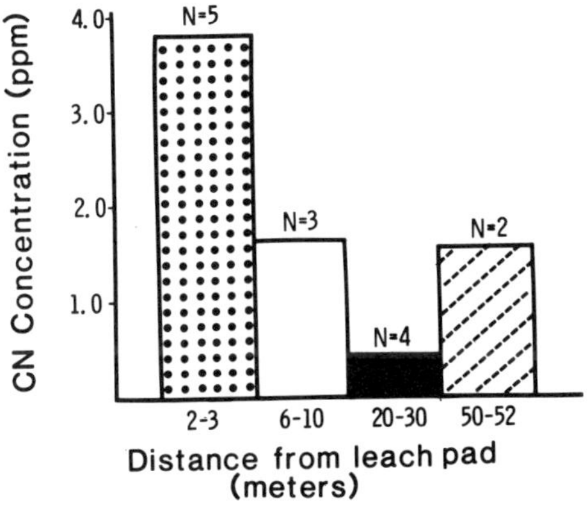

Figure 4. Average cyanide concentration in ambient air.

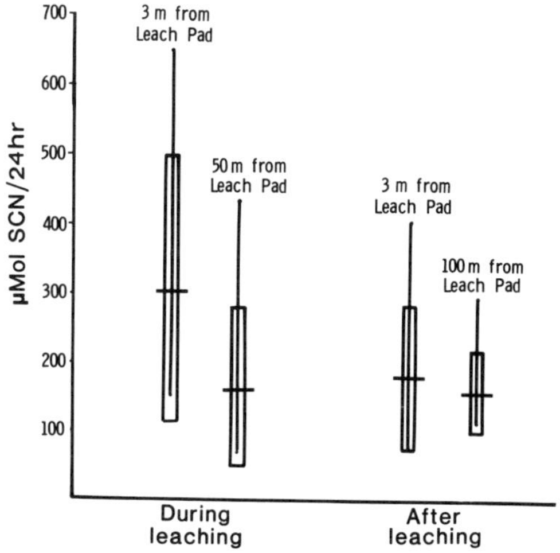

Figure 5. Average urinary thiocyanate levels of caged voles.

Mean urinary SCN levels per 24 hr sample (Figure 5) were higher in those voles located three meters from the leach pad ($\overline{X}$=306.6 uMol SCN, N=7) than in those voles located 50 meters from the leach pad ($\overline{X}$=166 uMol SCN, N=7) during leaching. Mean urinary SCN in voles three meters from the leach pad dropped to $\overline{X}$=181 uMol SCN, N=8 after most leaching was completed. Those voles moved from 50 to 100 m from the leach pad showed little decrease in urinary SCN ($\overline{X}$=161.5 uMol SCN, N=8). Statistical comparison of the data pairs showed that the mean urinary SCN at three meters from the leach pad during leaching was significantly higher than the mean urinary SCN at 50 m during leaching ($0.01<P<0.02$). The sample pairs collected at three and 100 m after most leaching was completed were not significantly different.

DISCUSSION

The rodent population study tested the hypothesis that sprinkling of CN at the leaching facility would not affect populations of rodents. Rejection of the hypothesis could be accomplished in two ways. The first would be if populations on experimental grids in the vicinity of the leach pad were consistantly and statistically different from those on control grids. The second would be if the populations on control and experimental grids fluctuated synchronously (though possibly at different densities) before leaching commenced (before September 1, 1984) and asynchronously after leaching commenced. If rodents were being exposed to levels of CN capable of causing toxic or lethal effects, this should become apparent in the turnover rates of the populations. We expected that toxic or lethal effects of CN upon rodents would cause a decrease in survival rates and, possibly, result in an increase in recruitment rate (replacement by immigration of animals removed from the population). Both decreased survival and increased recruitment would result in an increase in turnover rate.

Turnover rates of long-tailed voles on experimental grids increased after leaching commenced. This suggests that there may have been some effect from CN. However, the SNK test indicated that experimental and control and grids were not consistantly different. There were no significant differences in turnover rates of red-backed voles among the six grids. Based upon this information, the hypothesis that the leaching process (sprinkling of CN) had no effect upon rodent populations must be accepted.

The population data also exemplify demographic characteristics which can confound our ability to identify subtle impacts. As the literature indicated, small mammal populations can be extremely unstable (Gaines and McClenaghan 1980). Long-tailed vole density on grid 1A clearly demonstrated this: density doubled and also decreased by 50% in two week periods. The data showed that the long-tailed vole density followed the recruitment of new individuals into the population. At the end of the breeding season (trap period 4) recruitment , as well as density, began to decrease. The dramatic fluctuations in density demonstrate why monthly monitoring of rodent densities would be inappropriate. If sampling were conducted monthly and designed to monitor only densities, major demographic events could easily be missed or misinterpreted.

Ideally, population studies directed at detecting impacts to rodents should be conducted after the breeding season (mid September). This would alleviate confusion caused by large recruitment rates. At Annie Creek the elevation (6200 ft) and subsequent snow accumulation make live trapping at that time impractical.

Our inability to identify impacts from CN by monitoring rodent populations was not totally unexpected. Literature concerning CN toxicity indicated that rodents would have to be exposed to fairly substantial levels of CN (>80 ppm) in order to be affected. Preliminary data (although limited) examining levels of CN in ambient air at the leaching facility showed CN levels (<6 ppm) to be well below levels capable of causing toxic or lethal effects in rodents. In addition, only one of five voles died in cage A, located three meters from the leach pad. These animals were continuously exposed to the highest concentrations of airborne CN. This also indicates that CN emissions would be insufficient to affect rodent populations. The studies examining CN emissions from the heap leaching process verified conclusions that could have been drawn from the literature. Until the concentrations of CN being emitted from the leaching facility were measured, there was no reason to expect that rodent populations would respond to those emissions. Unless CN emissions are expected to be (or known to be) unusually high, rodent population studies are probably not effective in identifying or monitoring potential impacts from CN. Considering the information presented above, it is necessary for regulators to become familiar with pertinent literature and understand the ecology of the organisms being studied. Failure to do so can result in the improper assessment of environmental problems.

By examining the levels of urinary SCN excreted by caged long-tailed voles at three locations near the leach pad, we were able to demonstrate the relative level of exposure of these animals to CN. During leaching urinary SCN levels of voles three meters from the leach pad were significantly higher than in voles 50 m from the pad. When leaching ceased, urinary SCN levels from the voles located three meters from the leach pad decreased substantially (from 307 to 181 uMol SCN/ 24 hr). Urinary SCN levels from voles that were moved from 50 m (during leaching) to 100 m (after leaching) from the leach pad showed virtually no change. This suggests that if there is an area of concern regarding exposure of organisms to CN, it is probably less than 50 m from the leach pad.

Although rodent populations are probably not good indicators of impacts from low CN concentrations, monitoring urinary or blood SCN levels of native rodents could possibly provide useful information concerning exposure of terrestrial organisms to CN emissions. Such a study would have to take into account naturally occuring CN, which could confound the data.

The data collected at Annie Creek did verify that CN was being emitted from the heap leaching facility at Annie Creek, South Dakota. However, levels of CN in ambient air appear to be well below levels hazardous to terrestrial organisms. There is a possibility that the CN in ambient air could be deposited on the soil near the leaching facility during precipitation. Cyanide in the soil can affect soil microbes positively or negatively (Rangaswami and Balasubramanian 1963). It is not unreasonable that over the operational life of a heap leaching facility (10+ years) prolonged exposure of soil organisms to low levels of CN could have a measurable environmental impact. Positive or negative impacts upon soil microbes could affect soil respiration and microenvironment. Such an impact could eventually affect vegetation and ultimately result in secondary impacts to rodent or other wildlife populations. Further research in this area may be warrented.

LITERATURE CITED

Abrol, Y. P. and E. E. Conn. 1966. Studies on cyanide metabolism in Lotus arabiscus L. and Lotus tenuis L. Phytochem. 5:237-242.

Altman, P. L. and D. S. Dittmer. 1964. Biology data book. Fed. Amer. Soc. Exp. Biol. 194 pp.

Barcroft, J. The toxicity of atmospheres containing hydrocyanic acid. J. Hygiene 31:1-34.

Chitty, D. and E. Phipps. 1966. Seasonal changes in survival in mixed populations of two species of vole. J. Anim. Ecol. 35:313-331.

Douglass, R. J. 1984. The use of rodents in monitoring ecological impacts of oil shale development in the Piceance Basin, Colorado. Thorne Ecol. Inst. Tech. Publ. 14:70-75.

Ecological Analysts, Inc. 1979. Cyanide: An overview and analysis of the literature of chemistry, fate, toxicity and detection in surface waters. Prepared for the Inter-Industry Cyanide Group, June, 1979. Towson, Maryland.

Gaines, M. S. , A. M. Vivas and C. L. Baker. 1979. An experimental analysis of dispersal in fluctuating vole populations: demographic parameters. Ecology 60:814-828.

Gaines, M. S. and L. R. McClenaghan, Jr. 1980. Dispersal in small mammals. Ann. Rev. Ecol. and Syst. 11:163-196.

Goldschmidt, S. B., G. W. Butler, and E. E. Conn. 1963. Incorporation of hydrocyanic acid labelled with carbon-14 into asparagine in seedlings. Nature 197:718-719.

Howard, J. W. and R. F. Hanzal. 1955. Chronic toxicity for rats of food treated with hydrogen cyanide. Ag. Food Chem. 3:325-329.

Johnson, M. S., R. D. Roberts, M. Hutton, and M. J. Inskip. 1978. Distribution of lead, zinc and cadmium in small mammals from polluted environments. Oikos 30:153-159.

Katz, M. 1977. Methods of sampling and analysis. Method #808. Analytical method for cyanide in air. Am. Pub. Health Assoc. 2nd Ed.

Krebs, C. J. 1966. Demographic changes in fluctuating populations of Microtus californicus. Ecol. Monogr. 36:339-273.

Krebs, C. J. and J. H. Myers. 1974. Population cycles in small mammals. Adv. Ecol. Res. 8:267-399.

Mundy, B. P., F. H. S. Liu, and G. A. Strobel. 1973. Aminobutyronitrile as an intermediate in cyanide fixation by Rhizoctonia solani. Can. J. Biochem. 51:1440-1442.

Pettigrew, A. R. and G. S. Fell. 1972. Simplified colorimetric determination of thiocyanate in biological fluids, and its application to investigation of toxic amblyopias. Clinical Chem. 18(9):996-1000.

Philbrick, D. J., J. b. Hopkins, D. C. Hill, J. C. Alexander, and R. G. Thompson. 1979. Effects of prolonged cyanide and thiocyanate feeding in rats. J. Toxicol. Env. Health 5:579-592.

Rangaswami, G. and A. Balasubramanian. 1963. Release of hydrocyanic acid by sorgum roots and its influence on the rhizosphere microflora and plant pathogenic fungi. Indian J. Exp. Biol. 1:215-217.

Roberts, R. D. and M. S. Johnson. 1978. Dispersal of heavy metals from abandoned mine workings and their transference through terrestrial food chains. Env. Pollut. 166:293-310.

Rowley, M. H., J. J. Christian, D. K. Basu, M. A. Pawlikouski, and B. Paige. 1983. Use of small mammals (voles) to assess a hazardous waste site at Love Canal, Niagra Falls, New York. Arch. Env. Contam. and Toxicol. 12:383-397.

Rowley, W. J. and Otto, F. D. 1980. Ozonation of cyanide with emphasis on gold mill wastewaters. Can. J. Chem. Eng. 58:646-653.

Skakski, J. R. 1984. Towards the use of faunal populations as cost-effective biomonitors. Thorne Ecol. Inst. Tech. Publ. 14:76-83.

Sollmann, T. 1957. A manual of pharmacology. W. B. Saunders Co. Philadelphia, PA. 982-990.

Strobel, G. A. 1967. Cyanide utilization in soil. Soil Sci. 103:299-301.

Sullivan, T. P. 1977. Demography and dispersal in island and mainland populations of the deer mouse, Peromyscus maniculatus. Ecology 58:964-978.

Tamarin, R. H. 1977. Dispersal in island and mainland voles. Ecology 58:1044-54.

Towill, L. E. 1978. Reviews of the environmental effects of pollutants: V. Cyanide. Final report. NTIS PB-289 920/1GA. National Technical Information Service, U.S. Dept. of Comm., Springfield, VA.

Zar. J. H. 1974. Biostatistical analysis. Prentice-Hall, Inc. Englewood Cliffs, NJ. 620 pp.

CONFERENCE ON CYANIDE AND THE ENVIRONMENT
Tucson, Arizona . December 1984
Published by Geotechnical Engineering Program • Colorado State University • Fort Collins, Colorado 80523

MODIFIED FREE CYANIDE - FIELD TEST ELECTRODE METHOD WITHOUT DISTILLATION

by

F. W. De VRIES AND O. B. MATHRE

Abstract

Gold and silver milling process streams generally contain complex iron cyanides, free sodium cyanide and a number of metal cyanide complexes that is measured as weak acid dissociable (WAD) cyanide by generally accepted methodology. The cyanide is released from the WAD complexes in the milling stream samples by reaction with zinc dust in the presence of ammonia and sodium hydroxide. Sulfide, a common interference in the determination of cyanide in milling process solutions and waste water is removed by reaction with lead carbonate to form lead sulfide which is filtered off. There is also some evidence that some of the thiocyanate may be removed with the sulfide. The cyanide is finally measured with an ion specific electrode.

Introduction

There has been a need for a rapid method to determine WAD cyanide in gold and silver milling process and waste streams and could be useful in field applications away from conventional laboratory facilities. The generally accepted methodology requires facilities normally found only in a laboratory and needs more than one hour to complete. By use of chemistry closely related to that used in old gold and silver milling technology a method for release of the cyanide from the common WAD complexes has been evolved so that the cyanide in the sample can be determined by well established electrode technology.

This method has been applied to the determination of cyanide in mill process solutions. The electrode method is particularly useful for analysis of samples containing less than 20, preferably 0.4 - 10 mg WAD cyanide per liter. It is preferable to titrate the cyanide with silver nitrate using potassium iodide as an indicator when the cyanide concentration in the sample is above 10 - 20 mg/L.

Chemistry

It is well established that zinc dust will remove silver and gold from alkaline cyanide solutions as the metals thus releasing the cyanide complexed with them. In addition it was shown that copper is also completely removed as metal when ammonia is present in the solution. However, the zinc dust will not release the cyanide complexed by the iron. Equations 1 - 5 represent at least part of the chemistry that is involved in the sample preparation.

$$2\ Ag(CN)_2^- + Zn = 2\ Ag + Zn^{+2} + 4\ CN^- \quad (1)$$
$$2\ Au(CN)_2^- + Zn = 2\ Au + Zn^{+2} + 4\ CN^- \quad (2)$$
$$2\ Cu(CN)_2^- + Zn = 2\ Cu(I) + Zn^{+2} + 4\ CN^- \quad (3)$$
$$Cu(I) + SCN^- = CuSCN\ (solid) \quad (4)$$
$$Cu(I) + (0) = Cu(II) \quad (5)$$

It is necessary to remove the zinc dust from the sample solution before determination of the free* cyanide by titration. It has not been determined if this is necessary for the electrode method but has been done to avoid any possibility of interference.

Sulfide interferes with both the titration of cyanide with silver nitrate solution using potassium iodide as an indicator and with the measurement of cyanide with an electrode. This occurs because the silver sulfide is much more stable than soluble silver cyanide complexes. The sulfide gives a "false" reading with an electrode and obscures the titration end point. It also deactivates the surface of a cyanide electrode so that it will not sense cyanide until the sulfide layer has been removed by polishing. It is removed from solution in the conventional manner by reaction with lead carbonate to form lead sulfide which is removed by filtration before analysis by either titration of electrode measurement.

The direct colorimetric test for cyanide in waste water is used as a rapid test for process waste stream samples in the electroplating industry. This method is described in ASTM Standard 2036-82 D. It is generally not useful for gold and silver mill effluents because thiocyanate in large amounts interfere with the determination of small amounts of WAD cyanide. When the weight ratio of thiocyanate to cyanide exceeds about 10 the accuracy is generally poor. Errors in the determination of cyanide can be greater than 20% of the value in the sample. The uncertainty generally increases as the thiocyanate cyanide ratio increases.

The WAD reflux distillation method described in ASTM Standard 2036-82 C is commonly used to separate cyanide from thiocyanate in the analysis of waste water samples. The determination of the cyanide collected in the absorber can be determined by titration, by electrode or by colorimetry. This method was used to generate reference data in this work. The reproducibility of the distillation data and accuracy of cyanide spike recovery was within the limits described in the precision and accuracy statements in the standard.

The cyanide specific ion electrode contains silver iodide that is slightly soluble in dilute cyanide solutions. The silver iodide also has a very small but measureable solubility in the dilute sodium hydroxide that is necessary to maintain cyanide as the ion in solution so that it can be measured. The addition of other compounds such as ammonia that form complexes with silver increase the solubility of the silver iodide in the solution without cyanide present. This raises the lower level of detection for cyanide in a solution. Since ammonia is required to prepare the sample for analysis it will be present when the cyanide is to be measured by the electrode. Figure 1 shows the effect of the ammonia on the electrode calibration curve in 0.20 M sodium hydroxide. This shows that the cyanide electrode is not very useful to determine cyanide in solutions that contain much less than 5 mg/L.

The silver/sulfide specific ion electrode can be used to measure cyanide in solutions that contain ammonia. The sensing element is much less soluble in solutions so that it can be used to measure cyanide at much lower concentrations than is possible with the standard cyanide electrodes. It measures the concentration of free silver ion in solution at the surface of the electrode. Since there is a 2:1 ratio of cyanide to silver in the complex the electrode response for a 10 fold change in the cyanide concentration is about twice that obtained with the cyanide electrode. However, it is more important to maintain the same stirring rate as is used for the calibration. Figure 2 shows that the electrode response is linear over the range of interest to this work. The broken line shows that ammonia does affect the mV reading but that it does not limit the use of the electrode as was found with the cyanide electrode.

FIGURE 1

CYANIDE ELECTRODE

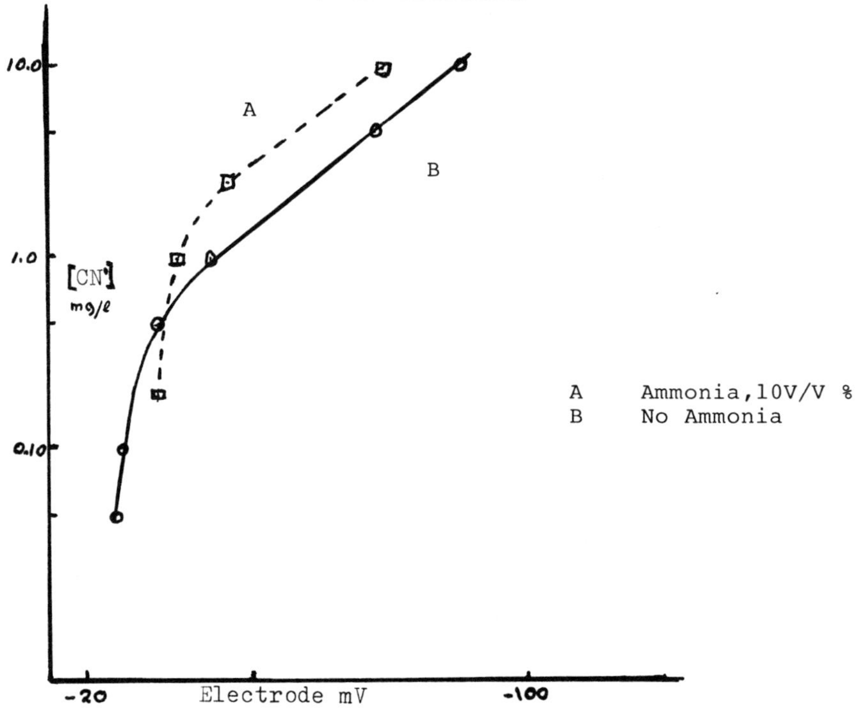

FIGURE 2

SILVER/SULFIDE ELECTRODE

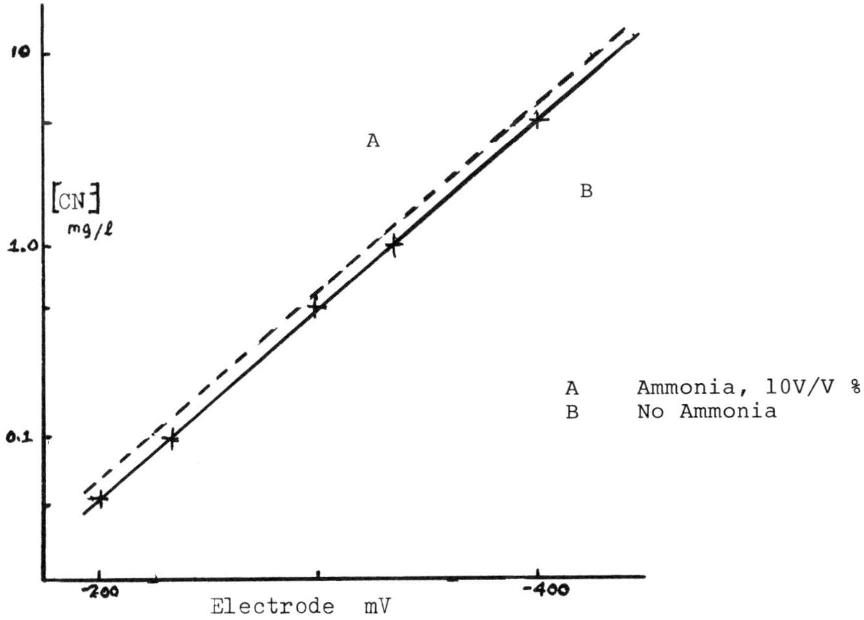

Since the stirring rate should not vary much during the calibration and the analysis the method of standard addition is used to improve the data and to make the analysis easier to run. The calculation can be run easily on a calculator with a log function.

Experimental

Since the titration method is preferred for the determination of cyanide above 10-20 mg/l the chemicals and procedure are included in this paper. If desired the electrode method may be used in preference to the titration method if a small enough sample is taken. Preferably the cyanide concentration during the electrode measurement should be in the range 0.2-5.0 mg/l.

Safety

1. Lead carbonate should be handled according to practices required for protection from acceptable exposure to the dust.

2. Zinc dust wet with alkaline solutions may be pyrophoric. Avoid letting air pass through the filter until it has been washed with water. Do not discard alkaline filter cake in containers or locations that contain combustible materials.

TITRATION PROCEDURE

Apparatus

1. Buret, micrometer syringe type. The Hach Chemical digital titrator with standard solution supplied in plastic syringe cartridges has been used. The Gilmont digital pipet, "Teflon" piston, 2-mL size with a buret tip, has also been used with conventional standard 0.0200 N and 0.100 N silver nitrate solution.

2. Filter paper. Fast filtering paper is generally preferred. Medium speed filter paper should also be available if the fast filter paper does not remove all of the solids in the sulfide filtration.

3. Magnetic stirrer. These units are available from a laboratory supply house and may be powered with a

battery powered tire pump. They will also run with ordinary laboratory air or water supplies.

4. Standard laboratory glassware. Graduated cylinder and pipets to measure samples, Erlenmeyer flasks or bottles to do the reactions and titrations in and a filter system (gravity or syringe operated pressure) for separation of solids (both lead sulfide and zinc are needed).

Reagents

1. Ammonia,ACS reagent.

2. Indicator, Deniges. Dissolve 10.0 potassium iodide in 100-mL reagent ammonia solution. Use 2.0 mL for each 100 mL of solution to be titrated.

3. Lead carbonate, ACS reagent. It has been found that a 10% w/v solution of lead acetate can be used if the sulfide content is not too high. This reduces the possible exposure to dusts of lead salts during analysis. However, the excess reagent must be controlled more carefully.

4. Potassium iodide, ACS reagent. This is needed to make up the indicator solution.

5. Sodium hydroxide, 5 M. Dissolve 200 g sodium hydroxide in about 500 mL water. Dilute to one liter. Store in a plastic bottle.

6. Standard silver nitrate, 0.100 N and 0.0200 N. Prepare with dilute solution by diluting 20.0 mL of 0.100 N solution to 100 mL with deionized water.

   Alternately, the silver nitrate solution may be purchased in cartridges for the Hach digital titrator and used as supplied.

7. Zinc, dust. ACS reagent has been satisfactory. Granular zinc reacts too slowly and does not generally have enough surface area to be satisfactory for this procedure.

Procedure

Sample Preparation

1. Measure 50 mL solution into the reaction bottle or flask.

If the sample is expected to contain less than 5 mg WAD cyanide/L, use 100 mL.

If the sample is expected to contain more than 200 mg WAD cyanide/L, then use 10 mL of sample and add 15 mL deionized water to the reaction bottle.

2. Add about 0.1 g of lead carbonate to the sample and swirl vigorously to react the sulfide with the lead. If the black lead sulfide forms, then add 1 g more and swirl vigorously to react the sulfide. Filter through medium filter paper into another reaction bottle. Wash the filter with about 10 mL of water. This should have removed the sulfide. If there is doubt about it, then the procedure should be repeated.

   If it is known that there is no sulfide in the sample, then this step may be omitted.

3. Add 10 mL ammonia and 3 g zinc dust. Then add quickly 10 mL of 5 M sodium hydroxide.

4. Mix vigorously for 15 minutes. A mechanical stirrer is very helpful for this step. An air powered magnetic stirrer can be used with air, water or a compressed-like carbon dioxide in field use if they can be made available.

5. Filter the solution through a rapid filter paper into a titration bottle or flask. As soon as the solution is through the filter, wash the filter with 50 mL of deionized water.

   NOTE: Remove the filter from the funnel and put into a vented jar containing enough water to cover the filter paper. This will eliminate the chance of spontaneous combustion of the zinc dust.

Titration

6. Add 3 mL (4 mL if 100-mL sample was taken) indicator solution to the titration bottle.

7. Titrate the solution with the standard silver nitrate (0.0200 N) to the first cloud point. If the WAD cyanide content is expected to be above 40 mg/L, then use 0.100 N silver nitrate for the titration.

   The cloud point should be just "off white" in shade and should not be dark. If it is dark brown or black, it is quite likely that the sulfide was not removed completely. The analysis should be repeated. Test the solution after the lead carbonate treatment with lead acetate paper or with a bit of lead carbonate to determine if the sulfide removal is complete.

Calculation

8. CN, mg/L = mL $AgNO_3$ x N x 52/mL sample taken x 0.001

NaCN, mg/L = mL $AgNO_3$ x N x 98/mL sample taken x 0.001

NOTE: If the Hach digital titrator is used, then the cartridge will probably have the factor on it or it will be in the formation supplied by the vendor.

ELECTRODE PROCEDURE

Apparatus

1. Specific Ion Meter or Expanded Scale pH Meter. The instrument must read to 0.1 mV.

2. Electrodes, An Orion model 94-16 Silver/Sulfide electrode used with an Orion model 90-02-00 double junction reference electrode have been used satisfactorily.

3. Pipets, micro, Eppendorf or Oxford disposable tip pipets have been used satisfactorily. The Eppendorf Repeater dispenser is a convenient and excellent substitute.

4. Standard laboratory items as described in the titration procedure.

Reagents

In addition to the reagents available in the titration procedure a standardized cyanide solution is needed:

1. Sodium Cyanide, 1000 mg CN/l. Transfer 0.95 g sodium cyanide to a 500 ml volumetric flash. Add 5 ml of 5 M sodium hydroxide and 100 ml distilled water. Swirl to dissolve, dilute to 500 ml with distilled water, mix and store in a plastic bottle.

Standardize by titration with 0.100 N silver nitrate. Use 5.00 ml sample for titration. Measure it by pipet into a flask. Add 50 ml distilled water, 1 ml Aeniges reagent and titrate to the first cloud point.

$$\text{CN mg/ml} = \frac{\text{ml } AgNO_3 \times \text{N } AgNO_3 \times 52.04}{\text{ml cyanide solution take}}$$

2. Electrode calibration solutions 0.50 mg cyanide/l and 5.00 mg cyanide/l in 0.20 M sodium hydroxide and 10 to V/V ammonia.

   Pipet 0.50 ml standard 1000 mg CN/l solution into one liter volumetric flask. Add 100 ml ammonia solution and 40 ml 5M sodium hydroxide solution. Dilute to one liter, mix and store in a plastic bottle. Label 0.50 mg CN/l.

   Pipet 5.00 ml standard 1000 mg cyanide/l into another one liter volumetric flask. Add 100 ml ammonia solution and 40 ml 5 M sodium hydroxide into the flask. Dilute to one liter with distilled water, mix and store in a plastic bottle. Label 5.00 mg cyanide/l.

Electrode Calibration

1. Pour 100 ml of each standard (0.50 mg/l and 5.00 mg/l) into beakers. Add stirring bars.

2. Place the electrodes in the first solution successively and stir at about 120 rpm. Record the mV (E_1) after about 60 seconds. Repeat with the second solution (E_2).

3. Calculate the difference in mV reading. It is generally 95-115 mV. This is the slope ($S=E_1-E_2$) used in the calculation.

Sample Analysis

1. Prepare the sample in the same way as for the titration method. Choose a sample size that will give a concentration of 0.2-10.0 mg cyanide per liter before electrode analysis.

2. Dilute the sample after filtration to 100-150 ml with distilled water. Immerse the electrodes in the solution, stir and read the mV (E_1 after about one minute).

3. Add stock cyanide solution from a pipet or repeater to give a change in the mV reading of 10-80 mV. Record the mV reading (E_2) and the ml of standard cyanide solution added.

4. Calculation

Calculate $\Delta E = (E_2 - E_1)$ for sample

$$\text{mg CN/l} = \frac{\text{ml cyanide Spike}}{\text{ml sample taken}} \times \left(\frac{1}{10^{\frac{\Delta E}{S}} - 1} \right) \times 1000$$

DISCUSSION AND CONCLUSIONS

The titration and the electrode methods were tested on several gold mill effluents. The results were compared with those obtained by the ASTM WAD reflux distillation method. Since the cyanide concentrations in several of the samples were too high for the electrode the samples were diluted with water before analysis. Typical data is summarized in Table I. Replicates of these samples and synthetic samples used during the initial stages of method development were generally within ± 6 - 10% of the mean. This precision is within the limits commonly expected for the WAD reflux distillation procedure. To date a significant bias has not been observed for the analysis.

TABLE I

RAPID TEST FOR CYANIDE IN GOLD MILL PROCESS SOLUTIONS

CYANIDE (mg/l)

SAMPLE	ELECTRODE	TITRATION	DISTILLATION
I		125,118	122
I (a)	0.17, 0.15		0.14
II	37,41,45		42
II (a)	0.07, 0.08		0.09
III	0.45, 0.50		0.49
IV	0.92, 1.00	0.95,1.1,1.02	0.98

SAMPLE	ELECTRODE	TITRATION	DISTILLATION
V (a)	0.10, 0.13		0.11
VI	2.6, 2.3	2.1,2.2,2.4	2.4

This test appears to be useful for the rapid determination of easily dissociable cyanide in gold and silver mill process streams. The data shows that for these samples the values are essentially equivalent to those obtained by distillation. The results obtained with this method still should be compared with the results obtained by the WAD reflux distillation method to determine if there is any interference problem.

DISCUSSION

Question (F. Clark): Would you explain the silver sulfide electrode? The method I use in the field is simple titration, but I think the silver sulfide electrode would probably be a better method. Could you explain that a little bit, and where do you get them?

Answer (O. Mathre): The silver sulfide electrode can be purchased at any of the chemical supply houses. I got mine from the Fischer Scientific Co. but you could pick any one of them. They run about $250 each. You need a reference electrode with it. The silver sulfide ion-specific electrode, as they call it, is only one-half of the measurement battery or cell. We have been pleased with it. We have used it to follow relative changes in free cyanide concentrations in solution, and the change is 110 mV for each 10-fold change in cyanide concentration.

CONFERENCE ON CYANIDE AND THE ENVIRONMENT
Tucson, Arizona • December 1984
Published by Geotechnical Engineering Program • Colorado State University • Fort Collins, Colorado 80523

A SIMPLE LEACH PROCEDURE FOR DETERMINING THE TOTAL CYANIDE CONTENT OF HEAP LEACH TAILINGS

by
William R. Ray[1]

ABSTRACT

The environmental impact of heap leach tailings depends upon the total amount of cyanide present. The measurement of this impact is hampered by the lack of a suitable method for the determination of total cyanide. Current methods are only suitable for liquid samples and have severe disadvantages when solid samples are analyzed directly. A leach procedure would allow these chemistries to be employed more efficiently and increase the overall reliability of the results. A leach solution also allows the various cyanide species to be identified and enumerated to give a better understanding of the environmental fate of these compounds in the abandoned heap.

INTRODUCTION

Cyanide heap leaching for gold values is a common removal/benefication process used by mining interests in the Desert Southwest. It's large scale and small operating costs make it attractive for many low grade ores. However, the tailings represent a potential and; at present, uncertain environmental problem. Assessment of the environmental impact is hampered by the unavailability of suitable methodology for the analysis of solid samples. Current accepted methodologies are designed for liquid samples, therefore, a leachate procedure that soluablizes all cyanide compounds allows the full use of these methods. In solution, the various cyanide compounds are also ammeanable to any particular chemistry suitable in identifying the individual species present.

Analysis of the solid directly has many drawbacks. The amount of sample analyzed is restricted by the configuration and procedures of the digestion/distillation step. Limiting the sample size necessarily limits the detection levels. For a 0.5 gm sample, as described in Standard Methods; and the pyridine-barbituric acid colorimetric finish the detection limits would be 2 mg/Kg of cyanide. A more important considertaion is the reproducibility of analysis. Heap leach tailings are not homogeneous by nature. Common sample preparation practices used to assure a representative aliquot cannot be performed as cyanide may be lost. Even if sample compositing is practiced, the grainy nature of most tailings does not allow 0.5 gm to be representative.

[1]William R. Ray, State of California Regional Water Quality Control #7, Palm Desert, California.

Three candidate solutions: deionized water, 1 N KNO_3 and 1.25 N NaOH were examined. The three solutions represent three different approaches to cyanide solubilization. Deionized water relies solely on the solubility of the various compounds; 1 N KNO_3 provides a suitable counter-ion in an otherwise neutral solution; while 1.25 N NaOH provides a counter-ion and the presence of a basic medium. An acidic medium is not advisable due to the loss of cyanide ion via HCN volitilization. The solution of 1.25 N NaOH was successful when compared with direct analysis.

REAGENTS AND APPARATUS

Methodology used is found in the USEPA Methods of Chemical Analysis for Water and Wastes. The analytical finish used was the pyridine-barbituric acid colorimetric. The distillation apparatus (see diagram) described in the referenced method was modified to provide better condensation rates. The destruction of complex cyanides and the rate of air stripping depend upon the amount of energy deposited into the reaction flask. The supplied cold finger condenser was not efficient enough except at low energy imputs, especially during summer months in the desert when cooling water was warmer than normal. The changes made in the connecting tubing is to provide greater flexibility when assembling the apparatus. All reagent solutions needed for the distillation and finish methods are prepared with analytical reagent grade chemicals, except where none are available; as with cloramine T and barbituric acid. Cyanide solutions used for preparation of standards were standardized versus a silver nitrate solution freshly standardized against standard sodium chloride.

The methodology followed for the leachate procedureis as follows:

weigh out 20 $\pm$ 1 gm to the nearest 0.01 gm of well mixed sample, as received.

mix by inversion, weighed sample and 100 ml of the candidate leachate solution in a wide mouth plastic container of sufficient size, a 125 ml volume is usually adequate.

allow the sample and leachate solution to set in the dark at room temperature for a least 24 hr.

mix the contents of the container and filter the mixture by gravity through glass fiber filter paper (Whatman GF/C or equivalent) into a 100 ml graduated cylinder.

rinse the filter paper with small amounts of leachate until the volume of leachate collected is 100 ml.

analyze the leachate via the distillation/destruction method and the colorimetric finish compute the concentration of cyanide in the solid via

$$\text{mg/Kg CN} = \frac{\mu\text{g CN in receiving flask} \times 5}{\text{ml leachate distilled}} \times \frac{100}{\text{gm solid}}$$

$$\mu\text{g/gm} = \text{mg/Kg}$$

All reagents used for leachate solutions were analytical reagent grade. The sample was collected from an abandoned tailings site known to be high in cyanide; both simple and complex forms. The sample was well mixed by inversion and rotation but no other preparation steps were taken. The sample was analyzed as received without preliminary drying.

RESULTS AND DISCUSSION

The data for the sample analyzed by the direct method and the three leachate solutions is summerized in Tables 1 through 4. The data from Table 1 averages out to 108 $\pm$ 45.9 mg/Kg. The spread in the data (45.2 low 196 high) is expected as the 0.5 gm aliquots cannot be representative of the sample as a whole.

Data from the leachate replicates clearly indicates that only the 1.25 N NaOH solubilized cyanide at a level similiar to that found for the direct analysis, 108 $\pm$ 45.9 mg/Kg versus 96.2 $\pm$ 34.3 mg/Kg. The fit is even better if the two values 47.9 mg/Kg and 43.2 mg/Kg are eliminated; the average becomes 113 $\pm$ 16.5 mg/Kg. This average points out one of the major advantages of using larger sample sizes; the reproducibility of results is greatly increased. Reproducibility can be increased even further by using larger quantities of the solid sample. Simply increase the amount of leachate solution in proportion at the ratio of ; 5 to 1 liquid to solid.

Table 5 lists some of the subsequent samples analyzed by the above outlined leach procedure using 1.25 N NaOH. In general most heap leach operations found within the boundries of the Regional Board contain relatively small amounts of total cyanide. High values of total cyanide have been noted for operations reporting significant levels of cyanicides such as copper or iron.

The leachate obtained has more uses than simply determing total cyanide. The metal complexes associated with the solid have varying environmental fates. Knowing the types and quantities of each of the various complexes allows them to be monitored over time. The fate of these complexes is, at present, one of the most important unanswered questions of cyanide environmental chemistry. Environmental fates, at present only conjectured, may now be determined and the assumption of environmental inertness of the iron cyanide complexes checked. These complexes in solution allow a wide variety of chemical finishes: i.e. chromatography, or colorimetry to be used. Current projects at the Regional Board include the development of suitable methodologies for complexes.

REFERENCES

1. Standard Methods for the Examination of Water and Wastes, 15th ed. 1980, APHA-AWWA-WPCF, pub by American Public Health Association

2. Methods for Chemical Analysis of Water and Wastes, March 1979, U. S. Environmental Protection Agency EPA-600/4-79-020

3. 1976 Annual Book of ASTM Standards, Part 31 Water, 1976, American Society for Testing and Materials

4. Accuracy and Precision of the EPA Reflux Method for Cyanide in Gold-Processing Waste Streams, Sharp-Beltch, C. and Baker, D. R., February 1981

5. Development and Evaluation of Procedures for the Analysis of Simple Cyanides, Total Cyanide, and Thiocyanate in Water and Wastewater, October 1983, SRI International Menlo Park, Ca, pub by NTIS PB84-112663

TABULATED ANALYTICAL RESULTS

All values are in mg/Kg

Run #	Table 1 Direct	Table 2 DIWater	Table 3 1N KNO_3	Table 4 1.25 N NaOH
1	45.2	0.8	0.6	142
2	125	0.6	0.4	47.9
3	77.5	<0.2	<0.2	43.2
4	57.3	<0.2	<0.2	109
5	179	0.6	<0.2	106
6	114	0.2	0.4	91.9
7	129			116
8	88.1			114
9	98.3			
10	170			
11	196			
12	104			
13	114			
14	59.9			
15	65.1			
Average	108	0.4	0.2	96.2
± 1 S.D.	45.9	0.3	0.3	34.3
			less run # 2 & 3	113 ± 16.5

Table 5

TOTAL CYANIDE VALUES FOR VARIOUS SAMPLES

All values are in mg/Kg

Run #	Results
samples low in iron	
1	0.97
2	0.41
3	0.24
4	0.42
5	0.12
6	0.27
7	1.5
8	0.90
samples high in iron and copper	
9	75
10	34
11	9.0
samples high in iron, mined for silver	
12	17.1
13	5.9
14	11.2
15	105
samples high in copper	
16	41
17	83
18	91
19	5.7
samples low in cyanicides	
20	0.82
21	<0.05
22	<0.05
23	<0.05
24	1.0
25	0.07
26	<0.05
27	0.12
28	0.20
29	<0.05
30	<0.05

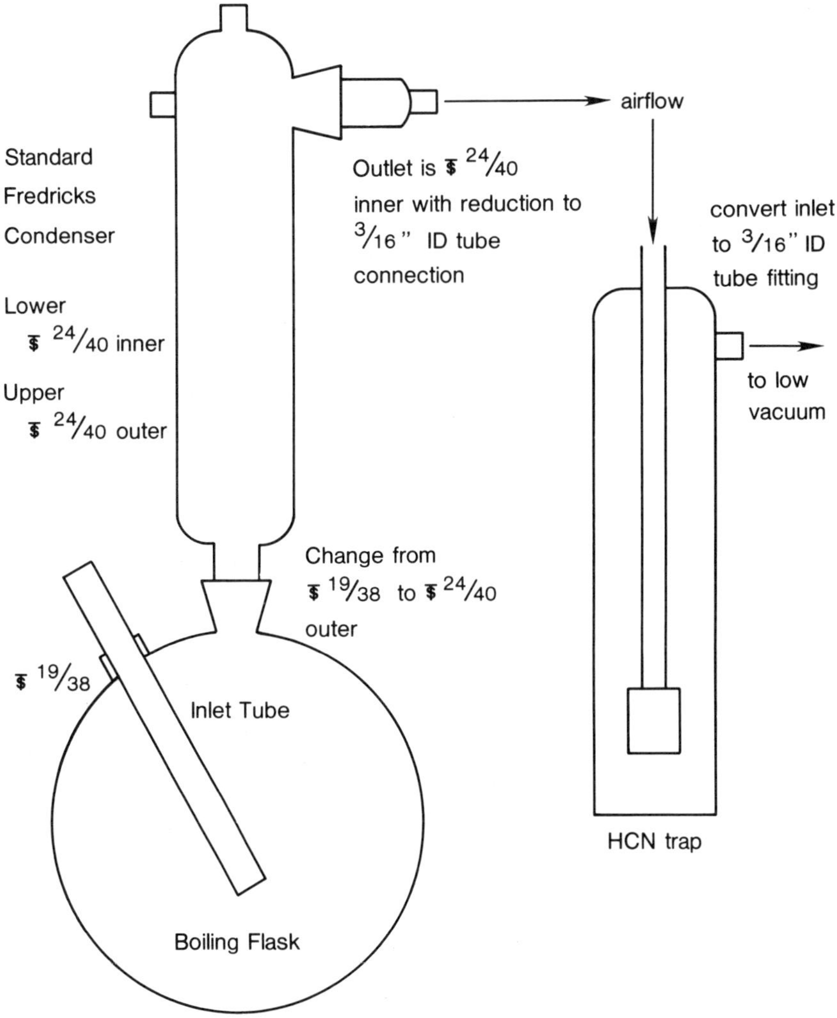

Changes to Standard Cyanide Distillation Configuration
ref 15th ed <u>Standard Methods</u>

DISCUSSION

Questions and Answers during Session

Answer (to inaudible question on sample size) (W. Ray): In the past I used 20 grams, but I have sometimes increased sample size to 100 grams. The important thing is to maintain a solid to liquid ratio of 1 to 5. For a 20 g sample I use 100 ml; for 100 g, 500 ml of leachate. The size of the sample depends on how reproducible it is: if the material is very coarse-textured, you would want a larger sample weight, whereas a smaller sample could be taken in more finely divided or better crushed material. Sample homogeneity dictates the appropriate size of the sample.

Question (F. Clark): Mr. Ray, in order to successfully neutralize a heap leach, what is the acceptable level in parts per million?

Answer (W. Ray): In California, unfortunately, it depends on the Regional Water Quality Control Board. Our Regional Board (Palm Springs) has adopted a new free cyanide level, using a different analytical procedure, of 50 mg/kg. I'd like to point out that when my research started, our level was 1 mg/kg total cyanide, but our current level is 50. In other places I understand the requirements involve not necessarily the solid, but that any leachates or runoff waters are assayed for cyanide. Some Boards don't even have tailings levels.

Comment (F. DeVries): There is every indication that the removal of cyanide from larger particles is diffusion-controlled. It can take weeks for cyanide in crevices, for example, to work its way to the surface. How can we readily analyse these things when, as the rock sits in that solution, the cyanide that has already been removed can react? How do you preserve the cyanide already in solution while you're waiting for the rest of it to come out? Your analysis might very well come out erroneously low. My concern is about setting criteria at low levels of cyanide when there may be more present that is not available to the environment. Then when the technique is perfected, the analytical results will suddenly go up and people will not be able to meet the regulations.

Answer (W. Ray): The method assays total cyanide regardless of environmental availability, that's true. I'll be the first to admit that it's not an actual representation of an environmental model. An exact representation of an environmental model would require monitoring a heap leach tailings pile over time to see what kinds of things come out of it. This method is simply one tool for obtaining some information about that material. As some operators have discovered, cyanide passage through heap leach tailings is not a perfect representation of the cyanide present in the system. Some operators had to re-leach heaps to process more gold out, so environmentally, it's not a model, but is an analytical tool.

Question: I think that's a neat, simple method of analysis, and we should be looking for simple analytical methods such as you've devised for practical applications. However, I really want to stress the futility, in my opinion, of looking for cyanide-- soluble cyanide, say--in that kind of sample. Isn't your region in Southern California in the desert region? Are you advocating taking into account the specific locations of these heaps when you consider a permit?

Answer (W. Ray): The problem we have is that this is an abandonment level, and the operator closing down may be going just down the road to begin another operation, or he may be leaving the state or even the country. In our region, tailings are not dismantled, but left standing in the abandonment procedure.

Comment: May I push for recognition of the fact that perhaps the best place to leave that residual cyanide is right there in the heap. After the first rains it will have been taken care of.

Answer (W.Ray): That is definitely true for the simple cyanides, and we have agreed that the complex cyanides are relatively stable and will not be affected. However, we in the regulatory agencies are constantly bombarded by the hindsight clairvoyants who say: 'Why didn't you think of that 30 years ago?'. So we like to look many years down the road so that if information comes out that, for example iron cyanides, do degrade, we can take that into account later.

Written Questions and Answers

Question (J. Mavis): You commented that because cyanide is present in gold process tailing residues, its concentration needs to be regulated. Since cyanide becomes immobile with time, and since there are no demonstrated effective processess for destroying iron-bound cyanide associated with the solid phase, what constructive purpose is there to regulating immobilized cyanide (since water quality would not be affected)? What control methods would you suggest?

Answer (W. Ray): I believe the problem revolves around the use of the terms 'immobilized' and 'inert' to refer to those cyanides not removable by distilled water leaches. These compounds, under the right conditions, are mobile and do degrade to simple cyanide quite readily. The conditions necessary and their impact on heap leach tailings have not been examined. Regulatory agencies are concerned with the future impact of a waste, as well as the present hazard, and if there is no information of the fate over time then, as a conservative assumption, the 'worst case' is assumed. With a known time-related rate, a more realistic approach may be taken and truly 'inert' and 'immobile' substances may be ignored.

Possible controls for cyanide would depend upon how 'inert' and 'immobile' the metal complexes are. Simple cyanide is easy; the environmental fate and toxicity are known and there are treatment systems available. Limits on the other cyanides would depend upon how readily they convert to simple cyanide. Since accepted treatment systems do not work (I have a thought on a non-standard approach) my approach would depend upon how fast degradation occurred. A slow rate may not require any steps be taken, while a quick rate would call for some means of impoundment for protection. My thoughts do not require that the more stable cyanides be treated directly, but that whatever simple cyanide is formed not be a problem. To restate again, my methodology is not for regulatory purposes, but to provide a means of obtaining those degradation rates that, at present, are not known.

Comment (J. Hendrix): I wish to take this opportunity to commend Mr. Ray's efforts related to the difficult subject of measuring cyanides in ore heaps used in gold processing. His paper is a good beginning to the complex problem. The methods he describes are certainly relatively easy to do and also, I believe the chemistry utilized is proper.

Before this technique comes to be viewed as 'state of the art' for determining the total cyanide content of heap leach tailings, I believe some questions concerning the sampling and analytical methods should be addressed. First, I question the sample size used in the tests. 20 grams of coarse heap material is a very small amount indeed. It must be kept in mind that a heap is heterogeneous in composition. Many of the compounds found in the heaps may be attached to the surfaces of the solids, or they may be adsorbed into the larger particles a small depth. Sample size may explain the high standard deviation found on Table 4 when caustic was used. Before reproducible results can be obtained for total cyanide contained in heaps, the problem of sampling must be overcome. Frankly, I don't have a solution to that problem either. Representative samples would be too large for ordinary laboratory equipment to be utilized. Unfortunately, size reduction of particles also introduces many other potential pitfalls.

The chemistry used by Mr. Ray is generally what we use when we study the total cyanide content found in mill tailings. We also use a caustic leach. Mr. Ray's use of glass fiber filter paper will certainly be adopted by us. Reading through his analytical procedure, I ponder why the sample and leachate solution is allowed to sit in the dark for a minimum of 24 hours. Our laboratory experience has shown that we lose less cyanide if we filter shortly after the dissolution step.

In summation, I think the paper offers a technique for the determination of total cyanide within heaps that should be explored further. The chemistry is sound, but as yet we have no answer to the question of sample size and sample preparation when dealing with coarse materials found in precious metal ore heaps.

Comment (D. Collins, FMC Corp): While the analytical technique Mr. Ray describes appears to be sound and reliable, its accuracy is completely dependent on the quality of the sample being analyzed. A 20-gram sample is not representative of a heap leach pile containing tens or hundreds of thousands of tons of material that could, on any individual rock, range in size up to 3 inches. If the Pierre Gy sampling criterion is used to determine the size of sample that needs to be taken to ensure a sampling error contribution to the standard deviation of 1 on a 100 ppm determination, then a 15-ton sample must be taken if the top size in the heap is 10 inches. This sample would then have to be reduced in size to about 0.1 inch before a 20-gram sample could be taken with the assurance that the sampling error contribution to the standard deviation is 1.

If we reverse the above, and determine the sampling error associated with a 20-gram sample taken from a heap leach dump containing 100 ppm of assayable material, we find that one standard deviation would be about 200: clearly an unacceptable degree of inaccuracy on a 100 ppm determination. This variability can be seen in the results reported by Mr. Ray. His average cyanide value is 108 with a standard deviation of 45.9. I would venture to say that the variability is a direct result of sampling error and not the result of the analytical procedure.

Caution is therefore advised. An analytical procedure to determine the amount of cyanide in heap leach tailings has been described but the results are only as good as the sample on which the analysis is performed. On heap leach piles, unless a very large sample is taken, the sample will be non-representative of the whole.

Regulatory and Environmental Aspects

CONFERENCE ON CYANIDE AND THE ENVIRONMENT
Tucson, Arizona • December 1984
Published by Geotechnical Engineering Program • Colorado State University • Fort Collins, Colorado 80523

Regulatory Aspects

by
Donald R. Baker

In any review of regulatory considerations associated with a mining property, there are a few general factors that are almost always encountered. First, the process of education of the public, and sometimes the regulating community, is almost always necessary. Second, the process will probably be frustrating and time-consuming. Third, the degree of control initially proposed by the regulators will almost always far exceed the degree of hazard. Fourth, and probably the most frustrating factor, is that the permitting process will present a moving target. The proposed constraints on a new operation will vary, not only among various state and federal agencies, but will often show significant variations during the negotiations with a given agency. There can be no question that the scope of regulatory influence has greatly increased during the past ten years. Along with this increased level of control has come a significant elevation in the level of both activity and awareness on the part of the general public. All of this has had the net effect of creating a significant barrier to the development of new mines. While the barrier is significant and one that must be overcome prior to commencing construction, it does not represent an insurmountable obstacle.

It is inappropriate for industrial representatives to believe that permitting will become easier in the future; this is highly unlikely. There are many reasons to believe that there will be an increased level of activity impacting mining operations on both the state and federal level in the coming years. In addition, economic constraints will make it increasingly difficult for a company to agree to questionable constraints on what may already be a marginal property.

An often overlooked impact on potential mining operations is the National Environmental Protection Act (NEPA). Many mining operations have been required to prepare a review of the potential environmental impacts for the proposed project. These reviews are sometimes prepared under the direction of the federal agency or the state agency. While the complexity of the study can vary significantly depending on the project and the lead agency, the general impression prevails that the law regarding NEPA is well established. While there is a large body of well developed law pertaining to the implementation of NEPA, it must be pointed out that recent court decisions have extended the level of preconstruction examination. For example, there is reason for concern that some recent opinions could require that the environmental consequences of a process be proven prior to issuance of a permit. Obviously it is the degree of "proof" that will be of concern.

Another development that appears to be forthcoming would be a permit requirement to conduct studies to demonstrate the continuing level of environmental protection associated with a project. Requirements such as this, while giving an ongoing assurance to the general public, could develop data that would significantly facilitate the permitting of subsequent projects. This could be in industry's best interest, if properly designed. The direction and scope of this type of work must be carefully considered.

The regulation of water associated with a mining operation has been a fact of life for over 10 years under the Federal Clean Water Act. For many types of mineral (Gold & Silver heap leach) processing operations, the regulation under the Federal Clean Water Act is a very straightforward matter. THERE CAN BE NO DISCHARGE. Of course, this can always be complicated by varying definitions of "no discharge". It is possible to have discharges associated with excess precipitation and associated with certain on-site facilities that are not considered to be part of the process. However, these are generally minor exceptions. In many situations the potential impact, or lack thereof, of a discharge on receiving streams becomes a non-issue since the discharge is prohibited. This same relationship exists for permitted discharges when there is a federal technological base.

This is in contrast with most of the rest of the world, Canada in particular presenting the most familiar example. Much work has been conducted in Canada between the mining industry and Environment Canada in a mutual effort to evaluate and develop treatment approaches and to study the potential impact of discharges on receiving streams. Unfortunately much of this work, while of a high scientific caliber, has little or no applicability to the U.S. regulatory scene because of the absolute prohibition. There is a tangential applicability, however, because of the potential for discharge of runoff water from the plant, mine, and disposal areas.

There are several problems that immediately come to mind in such an evaluation. First and foremost is the huge tonnages of all these materials. The second is the extremely complex chemical and physical interaction that can occur. Mining is faced with a unique situation among American industries by being required to manage, in an environmentally and economically sound manner, huge tonnages of material having very low concentrations of contaminants and this is complicated by the fact that most of these contaminants are still in their natural state.

For mining facilities using cyanide, the perception of these problems is magnified considerably because of the large number of possibilities that arise as a result of the interaction of basic cyanide solutions with natural products. This is, of course, complicated by the highly reactive and transient nature of the cyanide ion, as contrasted with most parameters of environmental concern.

Up to this point I have only laid out, in general terms, some of the boundary conditions that must be considered. Let us now turn our attention to a specific example in an effort to demonstrate an approach that has been used.

The best example of which I am aware involves the State of California. California, as I am sure you know, is generally viewed as being a stringent state for environmental permitting, in addition to being on the national forefront on overall standard development. As an example, I would like to point out that in October, 1981, Jerry Brown, Governor of California, issued a proclamation stating that the State of California was going to implement regulations to prohibit the land disposal of certain waste.

One of the wastes that immediately attracted the attention of the gold and silver mining industry was cyanide. The initial statement listing materials to be banned for land disposal included cyanide waste having a total cyanide content of greater than 1,000 mg/kg. After much work on the part of the mining industry, through the good auspices of the California Mining Association, a group working as the CMA Hazardous Waste Subcommittee was able to help direct the final prohibition directed toward free cyanide contained in the free liquid at concentrations greater than 1,000 mg/l. There are several major changes in this. First, the final prohibition addressed only free cyanide. Secondly, it addressed only the component that was mobile; that is, in the free liquid, and third, it expressed the limitation in terms of soluble concentration or mg/l as opposed to mg/kg. The major reason for raising this example is to point out that the final wording of the prohibition regarding cyanide that originally started in California in October of 1981, was passed by Congress as part of the 1984 Reauthorization of RCRA. Thus, what was accomplished in California by involvement in the regulatory process has now come out of the halls of Congress and been signed into federal law. In the environmental area, there are many examples that strongly support industrial involvement in the rule-making process. In my opinion, this ranks high on the list.

During the past three years, there has been a major regulatory approach on the part of the State of California to fine-tune numerous aspects of their waste disposal regulations, while at the same time increasing the level of protection. Part of this has come about as a result of the many investigations around the country regarding Superfund sites. There are two major points that become apparent with most Superfund investigations. These are: first, and foremost, the cost of cleaning up even a small hazardous waste site is very large. A second point that is often overlooked relates to the conditions existing when the site was in operation. In many, if not most of these sites, the disposal was carried out in conformance with the existing regulatory structure and generally using what was viewed to be good engineering practice. Thus, it is not surprising that the regulatory community, both state and federal, has been under considerable public pressure to improve their level of examination and investigation prior to permitting new sites. This also places a large burden on industry to develop improved systems for waste treatment.

One of the first issues that must be addressed in evaluating a potential hazardous waste disposal problem centers around the definition of "hazardous". This is of special interest for cyanide, since most of the approaches currently being employed involve test procedures that are appropriate to metals. Because of large quantities of leached residues, test procedures are very important.

In the late 1970's, considerable work was conducted evaluating many approaches for the generation of a leachate from solid waste. The USEPA adopted the 24-hour acedic acid leach based on modelling of municipal landfills. The applicability of such a procedure to monofill disposal of the type used in the mining industry is, of course, very questionable.

In the recent evaluation by the California Department of Health Services, a procedure utilizing citric acid at a pH of 4.5 was adopted to make a determination regarding the potential environmental availability of a parameter. The citrate ion, being a strong complexing agent, generally results in higher extractive values than does the use of the acetate ion.

An important factor involved in any leaching procedure being applied to a solid waste is the liquid/solid ratio. The USEPA uses a liquid/solid ratio of 20:1, while the California Department of Health Services uses a ratio of 10:1. It is also possible to find state and regional agencies using other ratios. Obviously the total quantity of material dissolved from a solid waste will vary depending on the liquid/solid ratio. The manner in which this variation occurs will be a reflection of the chemical and physical nature of the solid.

Some test procedures require that all solids be finally milled prior to extraction. Some require that the material be extracted as received, while others require that the material be dried and then extracted. To further complicate the matter, USEPA and some state agencies employ a structural integrity test. The potential impact of these varying requirements is a function of the nature of the particular parameter being examined. For example, if the parameter of interest is uniformly distributed in the solid, it is expected that milling will increase the quantity extracted. In contrast, if the parameter under examination is localized on the surface of the particles as would be expected in a treatment process, there is no reason to believe that milling would significantly change the results.

Examination of a parameter that is closely related to the surface area presents an interesting problem. Obviously cyanide would fall into this category since it is added to the system as part of the process and it is reasonable to expect that its presence would be related to surface area. In samples to be tested for surface related parameters, the sampling technique employed becomes a crucial factor. The variation in particle size that can be found in a typical heap leach operation, can contribute a significant variation in the analysis of small portions such as 10 to 100 gram samples. As a general rule, it can be expected that the surface area to weight ratio will be much higher for small sample sizes. Thus, it is anticipated that regulatory agencies will increasingly rely upon requirements for multiple samples using a statistical analysis of the results, as opposed to significant increases in the sample size.

In making a determination regarding the level of a parameter that is viewed as hazardous in an extract, it is not only important to consider the liquid/solid ratio previously discussed, but also to make a determination regarding the environmental attenuation factor that should be applied. The use of an environmental attenuation factor acknowledges that a soluble parameter leaving a landfill will interact with the environment in various manners prior to being consumed by a human being. These interactions can be of a broad scope, i.e.; dilution, complexation, precipitation, oxidation reduction, physical adsorption, volatilization.

Several studies have been conducted in an effort to develop reasonable attentuation factors. USEPA, in the regulations promulgated under RCRA in 1980, adopted an environmental attenuation factor of 100 based upon mathematical modelling. It is interesting to note that this is the same number that has been adopted by the California Department of Health Services, based on experimental work conducted by Battelle. California has gone even further than USEPA in adopting a factor of 1000 for some parameters that are known to interact extensively with the environment. While the California Department of Health Services has not addressed cyanide, it is reasonable to expect that the transient nature of the parameter would result in the adoption of an environmental attenuation factor at least as high as 1000, possibly even higher.

There is a very disturbing trend developing in several states regarding the use of data obtained from leaching tests. This approach involves multiplying the concentration of the parameter found in the leachate by the liquid/solid ratio and expressing the result as mg/kg of the soluble component in the solid waste. It was recently proposed by the California Department of Health Services. However, during the public comment period, many industry groups demonstrated that the limitations and environmental attenuation factors were all developed using the concentration of the parameter in the leachate, not the factor expressed in terms of mg/kg. Expressing the parameter in terms of the soluble quantity per kiligram of waste assumes that all of the soluble material can be dissolved in the first drop of leachate leaving the waste. This is an example of a worst case assumption resulting in a worst case solution. The first drop approach will be applicable only in the situation of a small quantity of a very soluble material in a system having little or no common ion effect. It can be readily demonstrated from thermodynamic calculations that for a system showing the impact of the common ion effect or one containing sparingly soluble materials, this approach overstates the potential hazards associated with the system. Even in systems that exhibit steep elution curves, projections based on this approach are misleading.

There is probably more uncertainty associated with the treatment of cyanide content in residues than any other issue. The uncertainty centers around the methods for evaluation of the cyanide content, the type of cyanide to be considered, and the criteria to be applied. Any of these considerations can easily be the subject of extensive discussions.

It is most important to realize that most of the above points can be very time consuming in negotiations associated with the permitting process, and are almost always of significant potential impact on the operation.

Today the wise path involves becoming involved in regulatory development and interpretation. Proper use of information gained in these efforts can serve to guide efforts regarding the development of technology, which can save cost by reducing the quantity of hazardous waste being sent for disposal. Increasingly companies are becoming aware that proper handling of waste materials can reduce their toxicity, quantity, and the increasingly mounting cost of disposal.

CONFERENCE ON CYANIDE AND THE ENVIRONMENT
Tucson, Arizona . December 1984
Published by Geotechnical Engineering Program • Colorado State University • Fort Collins, Colorado 80523

THE EFFECTS OF CYANIDE-BEARING, GOLD TAILINGS DISPOSAL ON WATER QUALITY IN THE WITWATERSRAND, SOUTH AFRICA

by
Adrian Smith[1], Alison Dehrmann[2] and Rob Pullen[2]

INTRODUCTION

The workshop on "Cyanide in Mineral Processing" held in Salt Lake City in February 1982 identified the following problems with respect to the fate of cyanide in the environment:

> "Limited information is available on the fate of cyanide from leaching and flotation operations in soils, aquifers, and/or old tailings dumps. Temperature, natural oxidants, sunlight, bacteria, organic and inorganic materials, type of soils, water chemistry, mineral constituents of tailings, permeabilities of soils and tailings, type of cyanide compound, concentration of the cyanide compound, rate of migration of cyanides, and materials of construction and design of leach pads and tailings ponds all have an effect on the ultimate fate of cyanide in the environment. Accurate knowledge of the fate of cyanide is necessary if meaningful, practical regulations are to be established for monitoring or controlling mineral process effluents. Nearly all regulations are now handled on a site-specific basis. Any information concerning fate of cyanides and related compounds will be of considerable value to the mine operator and to the monitoring agency."

For the past two years, Steffen Robertson and Kirsten have been cumulating information on the levels of cyanides in tailings, surface waters and near-surface groundwaters associated with cyanide-bearing gold tailings disposal from Witwatersrand, South Africa. In addition, cyanide data has been collated from the drilling and monitoring of tailings impoundments allowing the construction of a cyanide profile through the tailings mass. It is believed that these data will serve as a useful adjunct to data from North American tailings disposal operations.

The collection of data is not complete. This paper represents a presentation of the data available as of November 1984 and may be considered an interim statement of results. Due to the confidential nature of individual data, no specific sources have been identified and remain entirely anonymous. This does not detach from the value of the data which are considered to represent the Witwatersrand area as a whole.

1 Steffen, Robertson & Kirsten (B.C.) Inc., Vancouver, Canada.
2 Steffen, Robertson & Kirsten (Mining) Inc., Johannesburg, South Africa.

BACKGROUND

It is almost one hundred years since the first gold was mined in 1886 on the Witwatersrand, the "ridge of white waters", in the Transvaal Highveld of South Africa. Mining on the Witwatersrand, the principal centre of the South African gold mining industry, has resulted in the accumulation of over 300 tailings impoundments through the area. The majority of the mills producing these tailings used sodium cyanide in the gold extraction process and hence there is normally a residual quantity of unused cyanide reporting to the process tailings.

The combination of geology and climatic regime on the Highveld are such to have produced a groundwater regime over a significant part of the area where two principal aquifers are formed:

- a deep, regional aquifer (in the Transvaal dolomites) bearing good quality groundwater; and

- a near-surface, sometimes non-perennial aquifer, which is normally in hydraulic continuity with the surface waters of the area, when they are present.

The latter aquifer, developed due to the intense weathering of the surficial rocks of the Witwatersrand, is highly permeable and relatively vunerable to surface pollution sources. Slow leakage may or may not occur from this near-surface aquifer to the deeper, regional groundwater. The disposal of cyanide bearing, gold tailings can represent a potential pollution threat to both aquifer regimes by direct runoff, erosion of tailings and seepage from the tailings impoundments themselves.

REGULATORY CONTROL

Discharge of cyanide-bearing effluents or seepage from mining and milling operations is covered by regulations made under the Water Amendments Act 1984 (No. 9330), or, if discharge is made to a potable water resource, in terms of the South African Bureau of Standards (SABS 241-1971) specifications.

Discharge is regulated in terms of total cyanide levels. The general effluent standards specify a total cyanide level of 0.5 mg/L, while the potable water standards are 0.01 mg/L "recommended" limit and 0.2 mg/L "maximum allowable" level. These are broadly similar to both World Health Organization and U.S. Public Health recommendations.

MONITORING PROGRAMS

All the current and past cyanide monitoring has been done as and when time and resources have permitted, in addition to the regular water quality monitoring programs Steffen Robertson and Kirsten undertake. The collection of data has not been as complete as is possible, but efforts have been made to encompass the following variations in good tailings disposal (see overleaf):

- operational, recently-decommissioned and older, abandoned tailings impoundments;
- milling operations which extract uranium in addition to gold, the two elements occurring together in some of the Witwatersrand ore;
- vertical variation within the tailings mass; and
- variation in the interstitial waters in the tailings and in the associated near-surface groundwater adjacent to the tailings impoundment.

The results of the monitoring program are tabulated in the subsequent section. These data are from:

- an operational impoundment, ± 5 years in age;
- an operational impoundment, ± 10 years in age;
- a recently-decommissioned impoundment (within the last 5 years), approximately 20 years in age; and
- an abandoned dam, > 20 years in age.

The cyanide profiles through the deposited tailings are results of drilling two impoundments, both of which have been abandoned in the last ten years.

All data are for total cyanide. They were determined by using prescribed South African Bureau of Standards methods which are essentially the same as those monthly in use in North America.

CYANIDE MONITORING RESULTS

Cyanide monitoring data have been collated in five tables. These are:

- Table 1: total cyanide in the tailings system for a gold/uranium mill;
- Table 2: cyanide profile in interstitial water in a decommissioned tailings impoundment;
- Table 3: chemistry of oxidised, intermediate and reduced zones in tailings impoundments (mean values);
- Table 4: comparison of cyanide (total) in tailings impoundments and near-surface groundwater: (mean and range); and
- Table 5: comparison of total cyanide levels in near-surface groundwater with general groundwater composition.

TABLE 1

TOTAL CYANIDE IN MILLING SYSTEM FOR A GOLD/URANIUM MILL

	RANGE	MEAN	REMARKS
DISCHARGE FROM GOLD PLANT	—	±9	PRIOR TO U PLANT
DISCHARGE AT THICKENERS	0.05–0.08	0.06	MOSTLY PRESENT AS THIOCYANATE
POOL AT TOP OF DAM	—	<0.01	ADJACENT TO DECANT TOWER
SOLUTION TRENCH	—	<0.01	—
RETURN WATER DAM	—	<0.01	USED FOR WATER STORAGE ALSO

1. NEAR-GROUND AND DEEP GROUNDWATER CARRY <0.01 TOTAL CYANIDE ALSO.

TABLE 2

CYANIDE PROFILE IN INTERSTITIAL WATER IN A DECOMMISSIONED TAILINGS IMPOUNDMENT

BOREHOLE	PIEZOMETER NO.	DEPTH m [2]	TOTAL CN mg/l
A	1	11	0.16
	2	17	0.21
	3	25	0.57
B	1	27	1.54
	2	30	0.16
	3	47	<0.01 [4]
C	1	18	0.22
	2	22	2.92
	3	26	0.35
D	1	19	N/S [3]
	2	24	1.09
	3	28	1.86

1. CYANIDE DISCHARGE CONCENTRATION VARIED BETWEEN 8-19 mg/l DURING OPERATION.
2. TOTAL HEIGHT OF TAILINGS IMPOUNDMENT, 32 m (104 ft.).
3. N/S, NO SAMPLE.
4. SAMPLES TAKEN BELOW 32 m ARE IN THE SEDIMENTS BELOW THE IMPOUNDMENT.

TABLE 3

CHEMISTY OF OXIDISED, INTERMEDIATE AND REDUCED ZONES IN TAILINGS IMPOUNDMENTS (MEAN VALUES)

	PH	TDS	SO_4	Fe*	Mn	TOTAL CN
OXIDISED ZONE 0-3m	6.6	3350	1850	47	4	0.6
INTERMEDIATE ZONE 3-15m	6.6	3600	2210	21	11	2.0
REDUCED ZONE 15-35m	6.6	2850	1600	8	20	0.9

1. PH; UNITS OTHEWISE ALL VALUES IN mg/l.
2. TOTAL CYANIDE IN NEAR-SURFACE GROUNDWATER BELOW IMPOUNDMENT WAS 0.08 mg/l (MEAN VALUE).
3. TWO IMPOUNDMENTS ± 20 YEARS OLD.
4. SAMPLE TOTAL = 149

* TOTAL IRON

TABLE 4

COMPARISON OF CYANIDE (TOTAL) IN TAILINGS IMPOUNDMENTS AND NEAR-SURFACE GROUNDWATER (MEAN AND RANGE)

	DECRIPTION OF DAM	TAILINGS		GROUNDWATER	
		RANGE	MEAN	RANGE	MEAN
1	OPERATIONAL DAM ± 5 YEARS AGE	—	0.25	—	<0.01
2	ABANDONED DAM <20 YEARS AGE	—	(0.1?)	0.03-0.04	0.04
3	RECENTLY DECOMMISSIONED DAM ± 20 YEARS AGE	0.6-2.9	1.3	<0.01-0.16	(0.08)
4	OPERATIONAL DAM ± 10 YEARS AGE	—	<0.01	—	<0.01

TABLE 5

COMPARISON OF TOTAL CYANIDE LEVELS WITH GROUNDWATER COMPOSITION

DESCRIPTION OF DAM	TOTAL CN	TDS	SO_4	Fe	Mn	PH
(1) OPERATIONAL DAM ± 5 YEARS AGE	<0.01	712	317	0.1	15	6.8
(2) ABANDONED DAM >20 YEARS AGE	0.04	500	400	34	69	2.9
(3) RECENTLY DECOMMISSIONED DAM ± 20 YEARS OLD	0.08	300	70	4	0.8	5.8
(4) OPERATIONAL DAM ± 10 YEARS	<0.01	500	—	—	—	7.5
(5) "BACKGROUND" WATER QUALITY	<0.01	250	50	0.1	0.1	7.8

1. ALL VALUES IN mg/l, EXCEPT PH; UNITS

ANALYSIS OF MONITORING DATA

The data which follow the progress of cyanides from the gold extraction plant through to the water return facility at a mill with both gold and uranium extraction facilities, given in Table 1 illustrate that disposal of tailings from such mills may not represent a cyanide pollution to water resources. While a typical total cyanide level of 9 mg/L is discharged from the gold plant, the discharge at the thickners after the uranium plant is less than 0.1 mg/L, the bulk of which is believed to be in the form of thiocyanate. The cyanide is apparently either destroyed or otherwise lost in the uranium extraction process, which may involve solvent extraction, ion exchange, precipitation or a combination of these processes. For the remainder of this passage through the disposal facility, the aqeous phase associated with the tailings reports cyanide levels less than detection at < 0.1 mg/L. In addition, there is no remobilization of cyanide, should it report to the solid phase of slurried tailings, as both the near-surface groundwater and the regional aquifer adjacent to this impoundment were found to carry levels of cyanide less than 0.1 mg/L also.

The cyanide profile with respect to interstitial waters in a gold only tailings impoundment is given in Table 2. The interstitial water is taken to be typical of any seepage which may be discharged from the base of the impoundment to the groundwater regime. Given that the cyanide levels in the tailings slurry varied between 8-19 mg/L during operations at the mill, the maximum value in the interstitial water is now less than 3 mg/L. Therefore either the cyanide has decomposed during or after discharge, or it is being held on/in the solid phase of the tailings.

The actual cyanide profile is of interest. The upper portion of the profile to 20 m depth (66') is depleted in cyanide with values less than 0.22 mg/L. Between 20 m and 28 m (92'), the total cyanide levels increase and are in the range of 0.4-3 mg/L CN. These levels may decrease below this depth, although there is only one value of 0.16 mg/L to support such a conclusion. By comparison, the interstitial water in the sediments below this impoundment give cyanide levels less than 0.01 mg/L indicating no cyanide contamination from the impoundment.

In a second tailings impoundment, about 150 samples of interstitial water were taken from three distinct chemical zones within the tailings mass. These chemical zones - oxidised, intermediate and reduced - have been described in detail by Smith et al (1982, 1983). Table 3 illustrates the general chemistry of the three zones together with their respective total cyanide levels. These data are mean values, at least twenty samples being taken from each chemical zone.

In general, there is not a great variation in the major ion chemistry of the waters of the three zones. While the pH values are the same, the TDS and sulphate values are slightly higher in the intermediate zone and lower in the reduced zone as compared with the upper, oxidised zone. There is, however, a very clear increase in manganese levels with depth in the interstitial water coupled with antipathetic behaviour of total iron. Cyanide values then follow the major ion pattern, with highest values occurring in the intermediate zone (average value, 2.0 mg/L).

In addition, it should be noted that while the lower, reduced tailings have an interstitial water cyanide level of 0.9 mg/L, the near-surface groundwater below and adjacent to the impoundment have a mean total cyanide level of only 0.08 mg/L.

The data comparing cyanide in interstitial tailings waters with groundwater (Table 4) and cyanide in groundwater with the general groundwater chemistry (Table 5) can be considered together. Cyanide levels from the tailings examined vary from < 0.01 mg/L to about 3 mg/L with a mean value probably less than 1 mg/L. Known discharge levels for gold only mills are up to 20 mg/L and therefore the cyanide is either being destroyed prior to being held in the interstitial water within the tailings or combined with the tailings itself. Once the interstitial water is lost from the impoundment to the near-surface groundwater, it appears at levels no greater than 0.08 mg/L and, on average, less than 0.03 mg/L. Again, this may be fixation onto a solid phase or decomposition of the cyanide itself, with the addition of dilution by cyanide-free groundwater.

GENERAL DISCUSSION

From the foregoing data analysis, the following observations require some further discussion and possible explanation:

- the relatively low levels of total cyanides in interstitial tailings water, despite significantly higher cyanide discharge levels; and

- the apparent lack of contamination of the groundwater regime, even in close proximity to the impoundments.

It is suggested that there are several possible processes which may be responsible for the breakdown and/or fixation of the cyanide, removing from the aqeous system in the tailings and preventing groundwater contamination. These are:

- the method of tailings disposal: the so-called "semi- dry" or "sub-areal" disposal technique;

- the prevalent climatic conditions;

- the presence of partially or wholly oxidised iron in the tailings; and

- the presence of iron in the highly weathered, semi-lateritic or lateritic near-surface aquifer.

Sub-areal tailings disposal seeks to optimize tailings/water ratios, permitting the impoundment to be constructed by a self-build technique without the requirement of a water-retaining dam, as commonly practiced in North America. Lower water volumes on the impoundment result in smaller seepage volumes and hence limited solute transport. In addition, the presumed free cyanide-bearing tailings liquid is held in a very shallow pool on top of a dam and is readily available for interaction with available oxygen and solar radiation.

The Witwatersrand, at 2000 m (6000 ft.) in the Transvaal Highveld, has an "ideal" climate for maximizing natural cyanide oxidation; a mean yearly temperature of 15°C (60°F), in excess of 290 sunshine days per year - with only 5-10 cold days/nights, moderate but high intensity rainfall and high summer temperatures. The duration of high levels of incoming radiation resulting from the altitude and cold-free days/nights promote conditions for natural oxidation of cyanide, which are maximized by extensive area, shallow depth pool of liquid held on top of the tailings impoundment.

Pyrite, or residual pyrite, which may form between 0.5% and 5% of the tailings is subject to strong oxidation in the tailings, as evidenced by the red-brown iron minerals which form on the surface of the tailings, from the essential grey material which is deposited initially. The evidence for fixation, and hence attenuation, of cyanide by formation of iron species is documented in the literate (see discussion in Chapter 4, Huialt et al, 1983) and an active oxidation system which is in chemical disequilibrium, such as a tailings impoundment, has significant potential for immobilization of free cyanide species from the aqeous phase.

A similar potential which exists to a limited extent is the near-surface aquifer below the tailings impoundment itself. Almost without exception, the mineralogy of this aquifer, derived from quartzitic, dolomite or shale types of strata, compromises some iron minerals. Again, this provides a mechanism for cyanide removal, attenuation and fixation.

SUMMARY

A number of observations on the dearth of cyanide contamination from cyanide bearing, gold tailings disposed on the Witwatersrand, South Africa, can be made: These are:

- despite cyanide discharge levels from gold plants of up to 20 mg/L cyanide (and perhaps significantly more), there is little available total cyanide in interstitial waters in gold tailings impoundment, the general level being about 1 mg/L;

- There is little evidence of cyanide contamination of the groundwater regime below or adjacent to gold tailings disposal facilities, the general total cyanide levels in near-surface groundwater being about 0.03 mg/L; and

- a combination of the sub-areal/semi-dry method of tailings disposal, the climate of the Witwatersrand which greatly facilitates oxidation, ultraviolet radiation involved cyanide decomposition, and the availability of iron species for cyanide complexation may be processes which contribute to cyanide reduction prior to seepage discharge to the groundwater regime.

REFERENCES

Huiatt, J.L., Kerrigan, J.E., Olson, F.A. and Potter, G.L. (1983) - Proceedings of a Workshop on Cyanide From Mineral Processing Sponsored by NSF, Grant PAG 8119007, USBM and Industry.

Smith, Adrian, Dehrmann, A.A. and McPhail, G. (1982 and 1983) - Internal Reports: Steffen, Robertson and Kirsten (Mining) Inc., Johannesburg, South Africa.

DISCUSSION

Question (P. Saletta): Concerning final reclamation at the sites you worked at, were there any requirements for drainage control and top-soiling to minimize infiltration and thereby eliminate some additional hydrologic problems?

Answer (A. Smith): In South Africa there are no specific requirements. By law the mine manager is responsible for ensuring that there is no pollution from any of his facilities, but this responsibility ends when the mine stops operations. The government has agreed to take on the responsibility for any pollution problems generated by tailings impoundments that were built before 1954, I believe. What a mine manager has to do, though, is to get a certificate of safety or clearance of his tailings impoundment before the mine is finally decommisioned, so to that extent the regulators can impose conditions on tailings impoundments. However, the requirements have been minimal in terms of vegetation establishment.

Question (P. Feigley): I have a comment about your comparison of total cyanide levels with the groundwater composition. I think the data very decisively point out attenuation of cyanides over time, but my comment is directed toward possible misuse of terminology. Although your data clearly demonstrate there is no evidence of pollution from cyanide, in order to state that cyanide has no environmental effect, you'd need data examining environmental aspects.

Answer (A. Smith): My apologies; you're quite right. I mean it has no water quality impact.

Question (R. Soniassy): Dr. Smith, you showed some cyanide down in the tailings impoundment close to the bottom that had been sitting there for about 20 years or longer. You said that the total cyanide was 0.04 mg/l, but you showed some extremely low pH values of 2.9. Can you explain these very highly acid pH values?

Answer (A. Smith): In South African tailings impoundments, the gold ore carries both uranium and pyrite. In recent years a lot of the mines have removed the uranium and they're now floating the pyrite since it's used in sulfuric acid manufacturing. But many old mines did not remove the pyrite, and we're seeing quite severe pyrite oxidation. Iron oxidation from divalent to trivalent iron can create acid conditions and that explains the low pH. It's due to acid seepage from the impoundment itself.

CONFERENCE ON CYANIDE AND THE ENVIRONMENT
Tucson, Arizona • December 1984
Published by Geotechnical Engineering Program • Colorado State University • Fort Collins, Colorado 80523

HANDLING CYANIDE AT SUPERIOR MINING COMPANY'S STIBNITE HEAP LEACHING OPERATION

by
William G. Stotts[1]

LOCATION

The Stibnite Project is an open pit/cyanide heap leach gold property located in the Yellow Pine mining district of central Idaho, approximately 95 miles northeast of Boise, in Valley County. The nearest community is Yellow Pine, 14 miles from the project site. Access is either from McCall or Cascade, Idaho, via 80 miles of paved and unpaved roads, or by light aircraft with landing sites near Yellow Pine and Stibnite. (Figure 1)

Topography in the area is typical of central Idaho with narrow, steep sided canyons and swift flowing streams. The regional climate is characterized by short, mild summers and long, cold winters.

The plant and office facilities are located in the Stibnite valley at an elevation of 6,500 feet. The plant facilities are near the conjunction of the East Fork of the South Fork of the Salmon River and Meadow Creek. The plant facilities extend up the canyon floor west of Meadow Creek. All the plant facilities are on national forest land and the boundaries of the River of No Return Wilderness Area lay 3 miles north and 5 miles east of the plant. (Figure 2)

HISTORY

Like many mining districts, Yellow Pine has a long history of production. In the 1920's and 1930's, the district produced gold. In the late 30's, tungsten was discovered in the Yellow Pine mine. The district became the major producer of tungsten during World War II.

The low grade, disseminated gold deposit presently being mined by Superior was discovered by Bradley Mining Company in the early 1940's. In 1973, Twin River Ventures Ltd. of British Columbia leased the property and in 1975 Superior Mining acquired operational control. Twin River Ventures retains a 25% interest in the deposit.

---

[1]William G. Stotts, Mining Engineer, Superior Mining Company, Boise, Idaho.

In early 1978, Superior Mining initiated work on an Environmental Impact Statement for the Stibnite project in conjunction with the U.S.F.S. (Payette National Forest). James M. Montgomery Consulting Engineers, Inc., were retained to conduct the environmental studies and prepare the E.I.S. The E.I.S. was approved in the summer of 1981 and construction of the mine and plant facilities began in July. The project started production in July, 1982.

GENERAL OVERVIEW OF OPERATION

Due to weather conditions and the nature of the operation, both the mine and processing plant operate on a seasonal basis starting in mid-May and ending in mid-November.

The mine produces 400,000 tons to 500,000 tons of ore annually, ranging in grade from .05 oz/ton to .08 oz/ton of gold at a stripping ratio of 2 to 1. Mining is done by using conventional open pit mining methods. The drilling is done with track mounted air drills. The drilling pattern is 10 feet by 10 feet. Holes are drilled to a depth of 24 feet, producing a 20 foot bench. All drill holes are sampled for ore grade control. The ore is loaded out of the pit with hydraulic shovels and hauled from the pit to the crusher in 35 and 40 ton off-highway trucks. The ore is then crushed to 1 1/4" minus material. The crushing equipment, vibrating grizzly jaw crusher, cone crusher, rolls, and vibrating screens are portable, trailer mounted units. For pH control in the leaching process, 1 1/2 to 2 pounds of lime are added per ton of ore in the crushing circuit. The crushed ore is transported in 10 yard trucks to the leaching pads where it is stacked into heaps with a front-end loader.

During the operating season, the plant processes 3,000 tons of ore daily, producing approximately 25,000 to 30,000 ounces of gold annually. The gold recovery plant employs standard cyanide heap leaching techniques. The plant facilities consist of 5 leach pads, a carbon adsorption system, a carbon desorption circuit, and 4 solution ponds. When plus 30,000 tons of crushed ore has been heaped on a pad, a weak solution of sodium cyanide is sprinkled on the heaped ore. The solution percolates through the heap, dissolving the gold. The gold laden (pregnant) solution is then collected and directed into an impervious storage pond, pumped into the plant, and passed through a series of five columns filled with activated carbon. The carbon adsorbs the gold from the pregnant solution. The gold is then desorbed from the carbon in a pressure vessel using a hot solution of concentrated cyanide and caustic soda. The gold is removed from this enriched liquor by electrowinning onto steel wool cathode. The wool cathodes are fluxed with silica and borax, producing a dore bar of 650 fine gold and 350 fine silver. (Figure 3)

CONSTRUCTION

Cyanide was a major concern throughout the E.I.S. studies. Emphasis was put on the safe handling of cyanide while being transported to the millsite and when used in the recovery.

All materials delivered to Stibnite must be transported over 80 miles of narrow, winding mountain roads adjacent to major tributaries of the Salmon River. All chemicals are delivered to the site in enclosed vans preceeded by a pilot car to insure against collision with other vehicles. To maintain better coordination of chemical shipments and to insure a good working relationship with the U.S.F.S. and other government agencies, only one vendor, Great Western Chemical, Nampa, Idaho, is used for all chemical supplies at Stibnite.

An 8 foot high mesh wire fence was constructed around the plant and pads to prevent wildlife and unauthorized personnel from entering the area. To retain any solution spillage and runoff in the plant area, asphalt was laid around all the facilities and insloped toward the storage ponds. Sections of Meadow Creek meandered near the plant area and had to be straightened in order to maintain the required distance of 300 feet from a live body of water. This required permits from both the State of Idaho and the U.S. Corps of Engineers.

Four solution storage ponds are used in the Stibnite leaching process: two 1/3 million gallon ponds, for fresh water and barren solution; and two 3/4 million gallon ponds, for pregnant and clorine solutions. The total capacity of all four ponds is 2,327,000 gallons. The ponds were constructed by first compacting a rock free material along the pond walls and, to provide side slope stabilization and additional protection for the pond liner, a coarse geotextile fabric was installed over the compacted material. The ponds are lined with a 50 mil reinforced hypalon liner. At the start of each operating season, the ponds are tested for leakage.

The area where the pads were constructed was drilled and soil tests run. Results showed that foundation conditions were such that a deflection of 1% could be expected when the pads were loaded. A pad had to be designed that was flexible, yet completely safe from leakage. The design of the consulting soil engineers called for a continuous 30 mil p.v.c. liner protected on the bottom by a 1 inch layer of minus 100 mesh tailings and on the top by a coarse geotextile fabric. A 1 foot layer of washed and open graded crushed gravel was placed above the geotextile fabric. This layer was compacted and topped by a 3 inch layer of sealed asphalt.

There are five leach pads at Stibnite, each approximately 250 feet by 350 feet. The pads are sloped in and down 1% to the drain corner. On the downward side of the pads, a continuous perforated drain pipe was placed on top of the p.v.c. liner to collect any solution weeping through the asphalt layer. Discharge from this pipe flows into the pregnant storage pond. Two feet below the p.v.c. liner, in the same location, is another perforated drain pipe. The purpose of this drain pipe is to collect groundwater flow from beneath the pads and from the adjacent hillside. The flow from this drain pipe is discharged outside the plant area. During the operating season, the outlets of both drain pipes are sampled daily for free cyanide. (Figure 4)

To process the planned tonnage each season, each ore heap is processed in a 50 day cycle, allotting: 10 days for loading; 20 days leaching and draining; 10 days neutralizing/destruction of residual cyanide; and 10 days for unloading. The various functions of the cycle are rotated from pad to pad, giving a continuous operation.

Experience from the first few pads leached showed that a cyanide consumption of .2 pounds sodium cyanide per ton of ore could be expected. It has been the operating practice at Stibnite to add the needed cyanide (6,000 lbs) in the first two days of the leach cycle. This practice lessens the amount of cyanide that has to be neutralized before disposal. The strength of sodium cyanide in the leaching solution will vary from 600 ppm to 1,000 ppm in the first 2 days. Afterwhich it will drop to approximately 200 ppm, remaining at that level throughout the rest of the leach cycle.

The cyanide is added to the leaching solution as it leaves the recovery plant. In one operation, a full 3,000 pound Dupont cyanide flow bin is discharged into the cyanide mixing box. The lid of the mixing box is then closed and the cyanide is allowed to dissolve by the leaching solution passing through the bottom of the box. While adding cyanide, the operator is protected by a rubber rain suit, cyanide approved dust mask, face shield and rubber gloves. There is also a safety shower within 30 feet of the operation.

A 12 foot by 20 foot lunch room equipped with washing facilities is located adjacent to the plant and provides an eating area which is free from cyanide contamination. The lunch room also contains complete first aid supplies, a cyanide antidote kit, a cyanide gas mask, and a self-contained oxygen gas mask. A cyanide gas mask and antidote kit are also kept in the main plant building.

NEUTRALIZATION
(Cyanide Destruction)

The operating permit issued by the U.S.F.S. requires that the free cyanide remaining in the processed heaps must be reduced to an environmentally safe level prior to disposal. The operation has to be accomplished within the 10 day cycle period. The time frame for the neutralization operation is 2 days for draining, 6 days for neutralizing and 2 days for final draining.

During the planning stage, laboratory tests showed that chlorine would be the most effective agent for reducing the free cyanide left in the processed heaps.

For cost saving, alkaline chlorine/calcium hypochlorine is prepared at the site (chlorine gas $.17/lb, lime $.08/lb F.O.B. Stibnite). Pebble lime is stored in a 30 ton hopper. From this hopper, lime is fed into an 8 foot by 8 foot mixing tank where the lime is mixed with water by a 15 hp agitator. The milk of lime produced in this tank is injected into the neutralization spray line by means of a venturi injector. After the milk of lime has been added to the solution, chlorine gas is injected into the same spray line with another venturi injector. The chlorine is regulated with a Pennwalt model

V-8080 chlorinator. To insure an adequate supply of chlorine gas in cold weather, the chlorinator is supplied chlorine gas from 10, one ton chlorine cylinders. To supply the needed energy to operate the venturi injector an additional 25 hp pump is placed in front of the chlorine injector. Chlorine is consumed at the rate of 4,000 pounds per day and lime is added at the rate of 8,000 pounds per day, a 2 to 1 ratio. The resulting solution has a chlorine concentration of approximately 1,000 ppm free chlorine. The solution is sprayed on the heaps using the same sprinkler system used in the leaching cycle. The sprinkler system is composed of #12 Sinninger sprinklers placed at 20 feet by 40 feet centers. After the solution percolates through the heap it is collected in the chlorine pond where it is recycled through the neutralization system. (Figure 5) The effluent from the ponds is sampled at 2 hour intervals until a free cyanide concentration of 0.2 mg/l is achieved. Once the 0.2 mg/l free cyanide concentration is reached, a 24 hour test is initiated with samples taken every hour. Under the company's agreement with the U.S.F.S., in order for the heap to be environmentally suitable for disposal, the 24 hour average free cyanide concentration must not exceed 0.2 mg/l and no single sample can exceed 1.0 mg/l free cyanide. If the 24 hour test fails to meet the average requirement, the entire procedure is repeated.

EPA and U.S. Public Health Service regulations, at the time the Stibnite project was permitted, limited the concentration of cyanide in acceptable drinking water to below 0.2 mg/l free cyanide. Since no process solutions are being discharged to surface or groundwater, the 0.2 mg/l free cyanide was accepted as a safe level for land application of the treated ore.

The first heap that was neutralized in 1982 took 22 days. Since then we have reduced this time to 6 days. The critical parameter in neutralization is to maintain a high pH level. The chlorine feed has been changed from 2,500 lb/day to 4,000 lb/day with no noticeable affect. Even after a full season of operation, no significant accumulation of chloride or heavy metal salts have been noticed. Metal concentrations are given in Table 1 for August 24, 1983.

DISPOSAL OF PROCESSED ORE

Following successful treatment with chlorine, the processed ore is hauled in 10 yard trucks to an old tailing site, spread out in thin layered lifts of 1 to 2 feet and left for a minimum of 10 days to allow further oxidation and volitilization of the remaining cyanide and chlorine.

Disposing of the processed ore at the old tailing site serves an additional purpose. Prior to Superior's activities, fines from these old tailings were eroding into the Salmon River at a rate of approximately 1,000 tons annually and deteriorating the downstream salmon spawning beds. Since the characteristics of the material prevents revegetation, Superior opted in its E.I.S. to stabilize the old tailings and halt the erosion by completely covering them with processed ore and reclaiming the area. At the end of the project, this area will be revegetated according to an approved reclamation plan, resulting in a positive environmental impact for the project.

During the 1983 season, measurements of natural destruction of cyanide in hypochlorite treated waste ore were carried out by James M. Montgomery Consulting Engineers, Inc., (Cryer, 1984). After treated waste ore from each of eight heaps were spread, 10 sampling locations were established with survey stakes. These locations were sampled at 6 to 12 inches below the surface at one, five and ten day intervals. Twenty five grams of the ore were placed in 50 ml of cyanide free caustic soda (NaOH) solution at (20%) strength and allowed to mix until delivery to the laboratory for testing (average 12 to 24 hours). The solution was then analyzed for free cyanide.

The results of the eight, 10 day tests are shown in Figure 6. While no detailed statistical correlation was attempted with this data, the general trend was for the quantity of free cyanide to decrease with time. The average 10 day decrease was approximately 50% of the first day sample, with a range from about 10% for the samples with a very low starting concentration (-0.2 ug/g) to a high of nearly 80% with samples having a higher starting concentration. Only one sample exhibited an increase over time, in this case the free cyanide concentration on the first day sample of that waste ore sample was very low (-0.2 ug/g), and the precision of sampling and analysis is questionable at levels this low.

While no attempt was made to determine the exact mechanism of natural degradation of the residual free cyanide once the treated waste ore was disposed, several pathways are available. Natural degradation is attributable to a combination of physical, chemical and biological mechanisms which include volatilization, oxidation, biodegradation, photodecomposition, conversion to thiocyanates, and formation of stable complexes with available metal cations.

In conclusion, the procedure for treating the waste ore is effective in reducing the free cyanide levels in the ore to a point where it can be disposed of in a safe and environmentally acceptable manner. The exposure to ambient (natural) conditions (oxygen, sunlight, precipitation) appears to further act on the treated waste ore to reduce or degrade the residual free cyanide carried on the ore to even lower levels once it is spread for disposal and left undisturbed for ten days. (Figure 6)

DISPOSAL OF EXCESS WATER

In the Stibnite region, the annual precipitation is in excess of 31 inches. Most of this precipitation comes in the form of snow between the months of December and April. To handle the spring runoff from snow melt, all four ponds at the plant are emptied before the seasonal shutdown. During the off-season, the levels in the ponds are monitored and the ponds are pumped periodically as the snow melts. The criteria set in the permit for the disposal of excess water from the ponds require a 24 hour sampling period prior to discharge during which the average of hourly samples must be less than .2 mg/l free cyanide. While the solution is being discharged from the ponds, samples are taken every hour with none having an excess of .2 mg/l free cyanide. The concentration of free cyanide is reduced by the addition of calcium hypochlorine (HTH) as necessary.

The treated solution is pumped from the ponds at the rate of approximately 200 gpm by using two 25 hp pumps placed in series. The treated solution is pumped through a 4 inch p.v.c. pipeline for a distance of 5,000 feet to the old tailing area where it is discharged as a land application to further oxidize any residual cyanide. The solution is sprayed by a Rain-Bird irrigation sprinkler with a 1 inch orifice.

MONITORING

During the first season of operation a number of methods were tried for testing the low concentration of free cyanide required in environmental sampling. After correlating results of the different methods with outside laboratories, the Hach method became the standard test used at the Stibnite project. The Hach kit has the advantage of being simple to use, and personnel can be trained to use the kit in a few hours and produce reliable results. Samples are regularly analyzed at commercial laboratories for free and total cyanide, providing verification of the Hach method.

Surface water sampling is currently conducted three times each season of operation (last two weeks in May, July, October) at the 15 sites shown in Figure 7. The samples are analyzed for 20 parameters. In addition, there are four sites which are sampled once every seven days for turbidity and free cyanide, and once a month for arsenic and total suspended solids. The surface water monitoring parameters are given in Table 2.

The 10 shallow wells shown in Figure 9 are sampled three times each operating season on the same schedule as the surface water sampling for free cyanide with the analyses conducted by an independent laboratory. In addition, Superior analyzes samples from the same wells for free cyanide (Hach method), pH and residual chlorine on the following schedule during the operating season: Wells #1 - 5, 8 and 9 are sampled twice weekly; Wells #6, 7, 10 and the pad subdrain are sampled daily. During the off season, these wells are sampled and analyzed monthly.

The camp domestic well and the plant utility well are sampled three times each operating season and analyzed for the 11 parameters shown in Table 3, and are monitored for the U.S.E.P.A. drinking water parameters in the spring and early fall of each operating season.

ENVIRONMENTAL PERMITTING

The permitting and operational agreements needed for the Stibnite project have involved dealing with a number of govermental agencies. The national agencies include the U.S. Forest Service, E.P.A. Administration, U.S. Corps of Engineers, and Mine Health and Safety Administration. Among the Idaho State agencies are the Department of Health and Welfare, Department of Lands, Department of Water Resources, Department of Industrial Safety, Department of Fish & Game, and Department of Archaeology. Several local Valley County agencies have also been involved in the project.

Since both the treated ore and solution discharges are disposed of by land application, an NPDES permit has not been required for the project.

To insure the environmental integrity of the project is maintained, a monthly coordination meeting is held between representatives of Superior Mining, the U.S. Forest Service and various other concerned agencies.

ACKNOWLEDGEMENTS

We at the Stibnite project are proud of our record for the safe handling and use of cyanide. To maintain this record, we have relied on the environmental studies and works conducted by E. T. Cryer (principal engineer) and his staff at J. M. Montgomery Engineers, Inc., for the E.I.S., construction permits, and the necessary operating permits.

I am grateful to the Boise staff of Superior Mining Company for their assistance in preparing this paper. I would also like to thank the management of Superior Mining Company for the opportunity to present this paper.

REFERENCES

For additional information regarding the Stibnite project:

Josey, W. L., and others, "Gold Heap Leach Project at Stibnite, Idaho", Preprint No. 84-374 (Presented at SME-AIME Fall Meeting, October, 1984).

Table 1 - Solution Sample of Chlorine Pond

August 24, 1983

Chloride	1,724 mg/l
Arsenic	0.271 mg/l
Antimony	0.021 mg/l
Calcium	560 mg/l
Copper	0.071 mg/l
Iron	0.590 mg/l
Lead	0.034 mg/l
Mercury	0.357 mg/l
Sodium	135 mg/l
Zinc	0.030 mg/l
Cadmium	0.016 mg/l

Table 2 - Surface Water Monitoring Parameters

pH (Lab)	Clorine Residual (Field) sites 12, 24, 11, 6 only
Conductivity	Total Coliform
Temperature (Field)	Turbidity (Lab)
Total Kjeldahal Nitrogen	Total Suspended Solids
Sulfate	Nitrate
Antimony	Total Phosphorus
Sodium	Arsenic
Lead	Hardness ($CaCO_3$)
Zinc	Iron
Free Cyanide sites 4, 12, 24, 11, 6 only	Mercury

All analyses are according to Standard Methods for the Examination of Water and Waste-water, 15th Edition (a.k.a. SMWW) except as otherwise noted.

Table 3 - Camp Domestic Well and Plant Utility Well Monitoring Parameters

Cyanide	Calcium
Aluminum	Magnesium
Arsenic	Sodium
Antimony	Iron
Hardness	Mercury
pH	

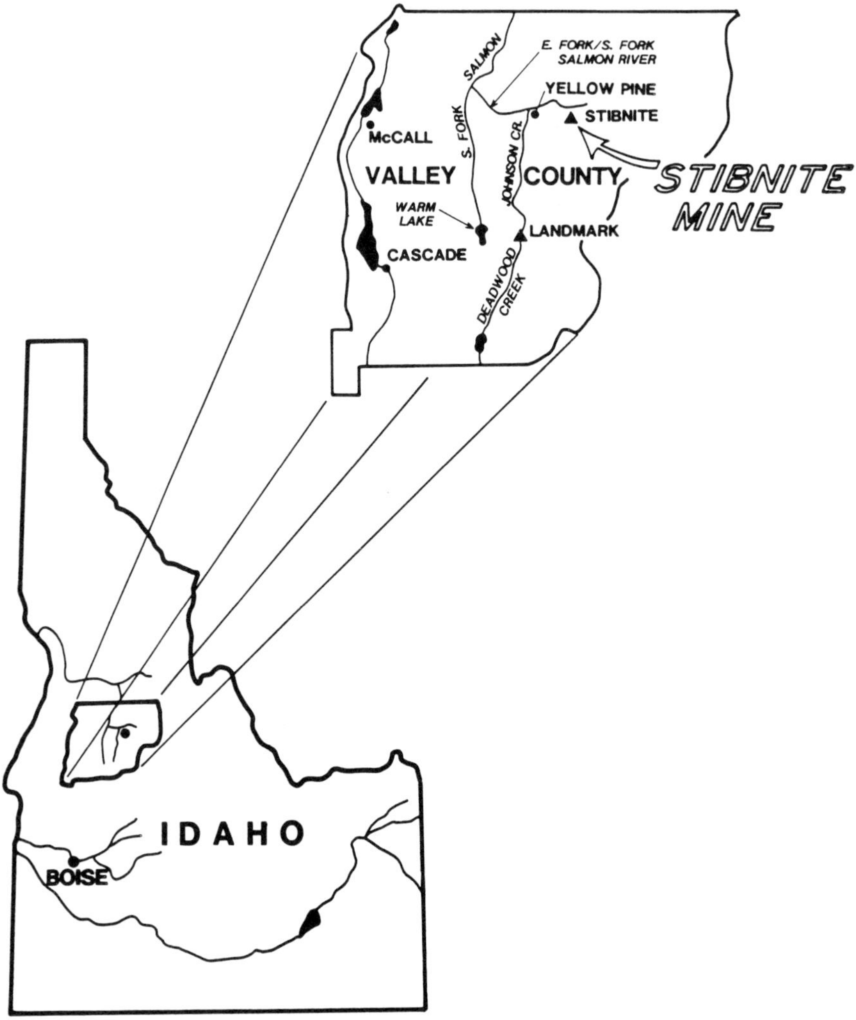

STIBNITE MINE LOCATION
FIGURE 1

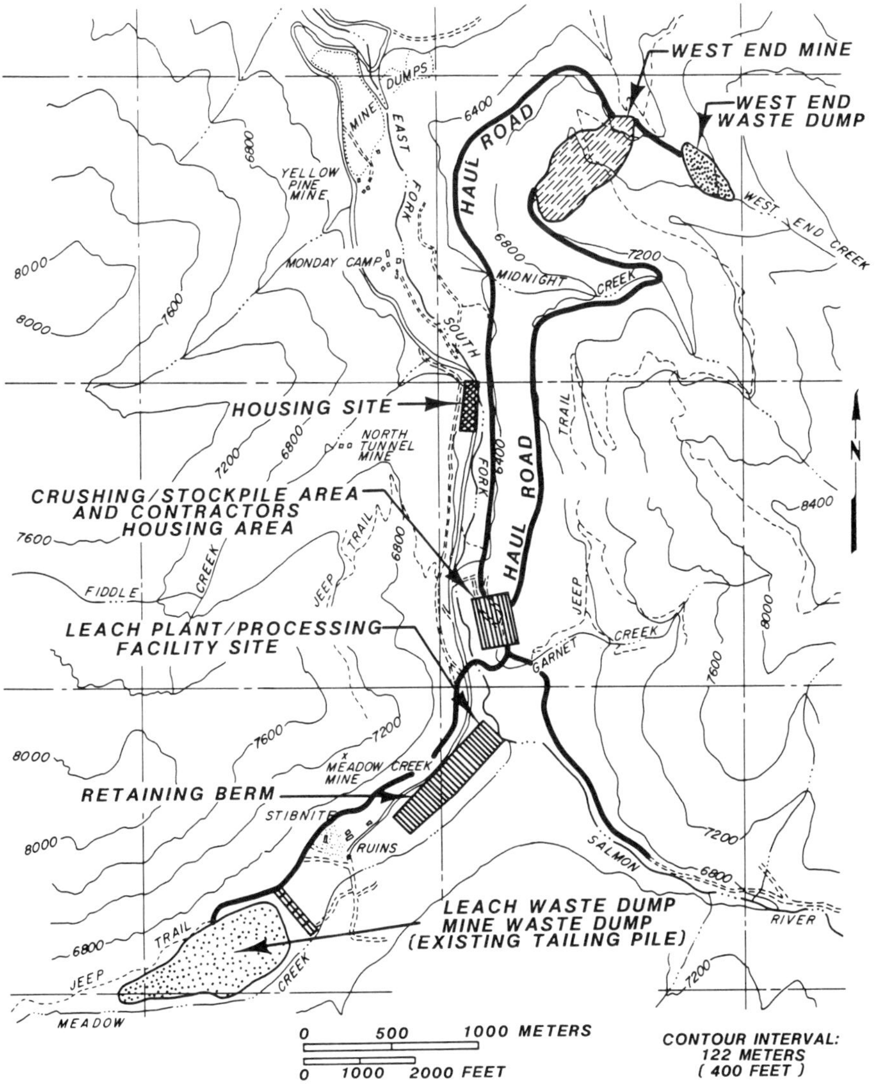

PROJECT SITE FACILITIES

FIGURE 2

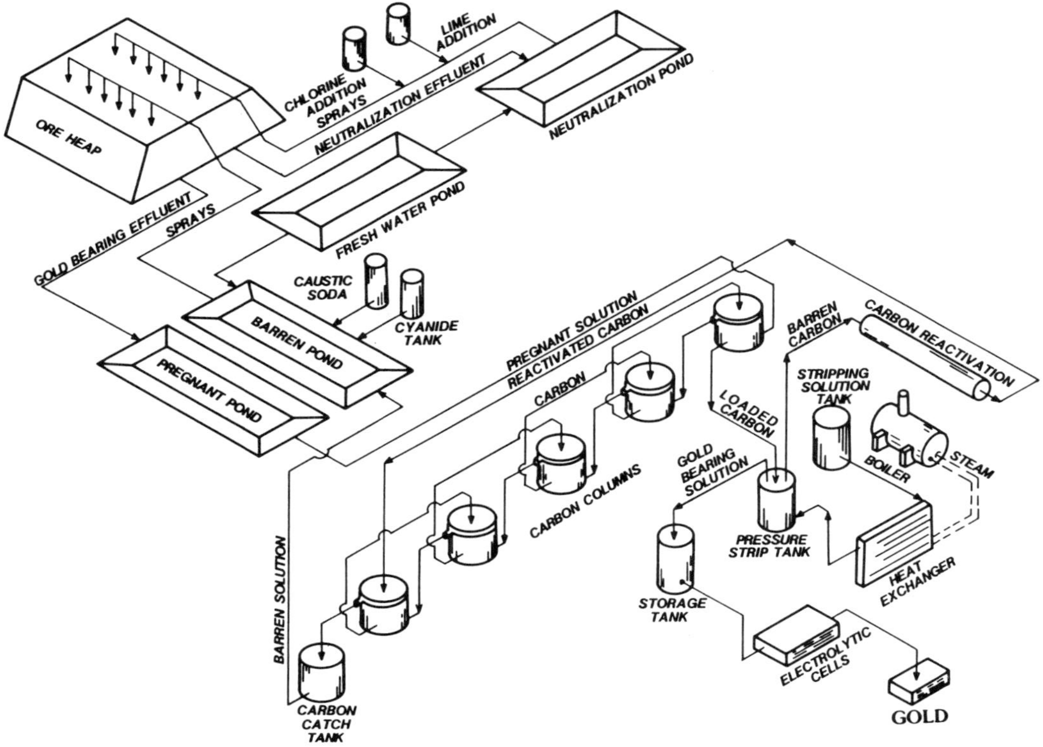

STIBNITE GOLD RECOVERY CIRCUIT

FIGURE 3

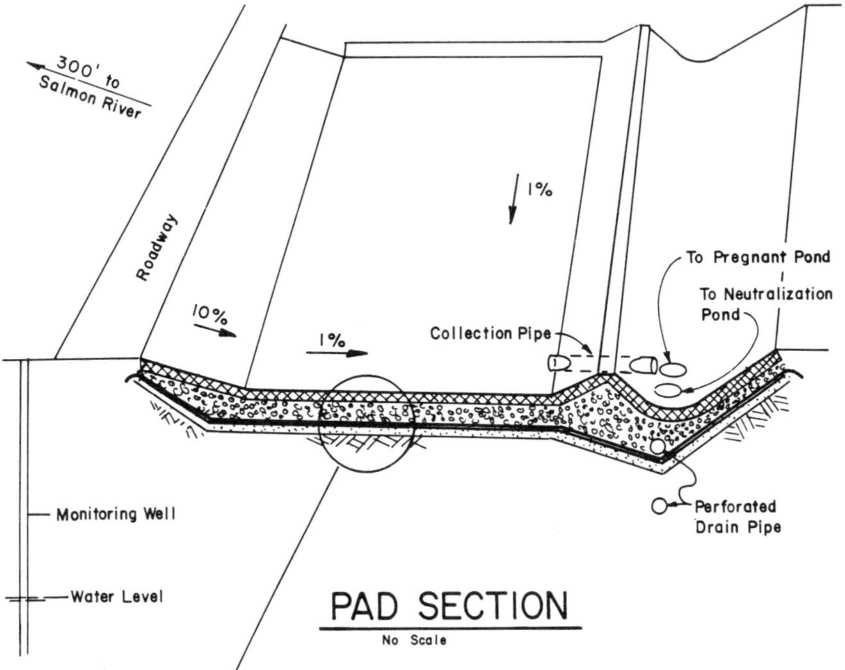

PAD SECTION

No Scale

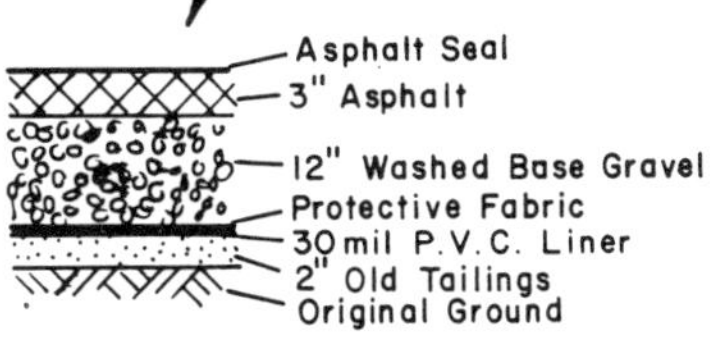

TYPICAL BUILD-UP

No Scale

FIGURE 4

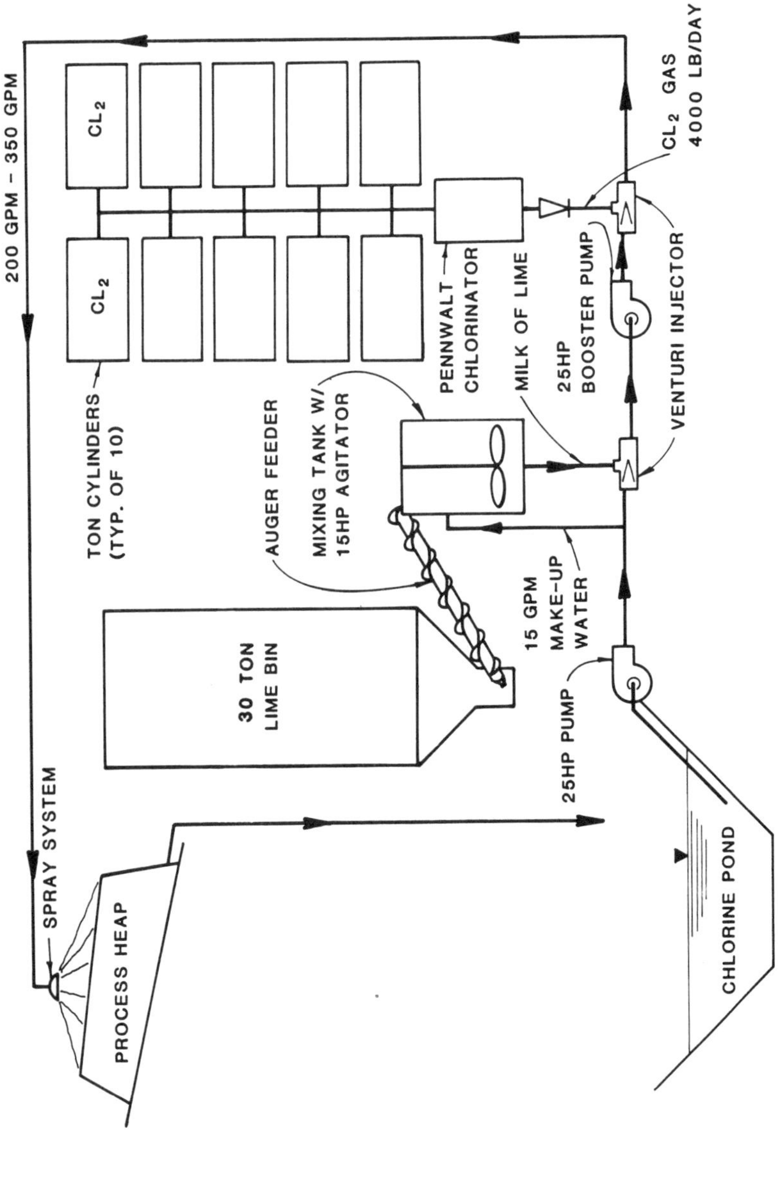

CHLORINATION CIRCUIT
STIBNITE PLANT

FIGURE 5

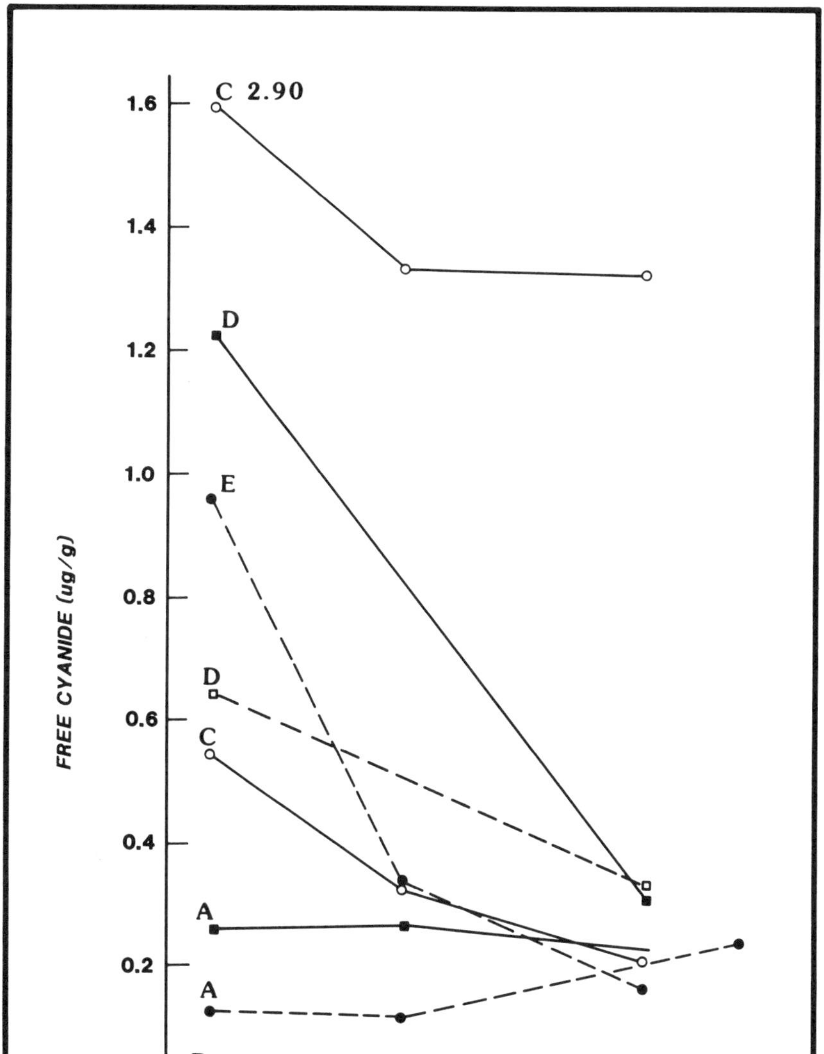

CYANIDE DEGRADATION IN TREATED WASTE ORE
FIGURE 6

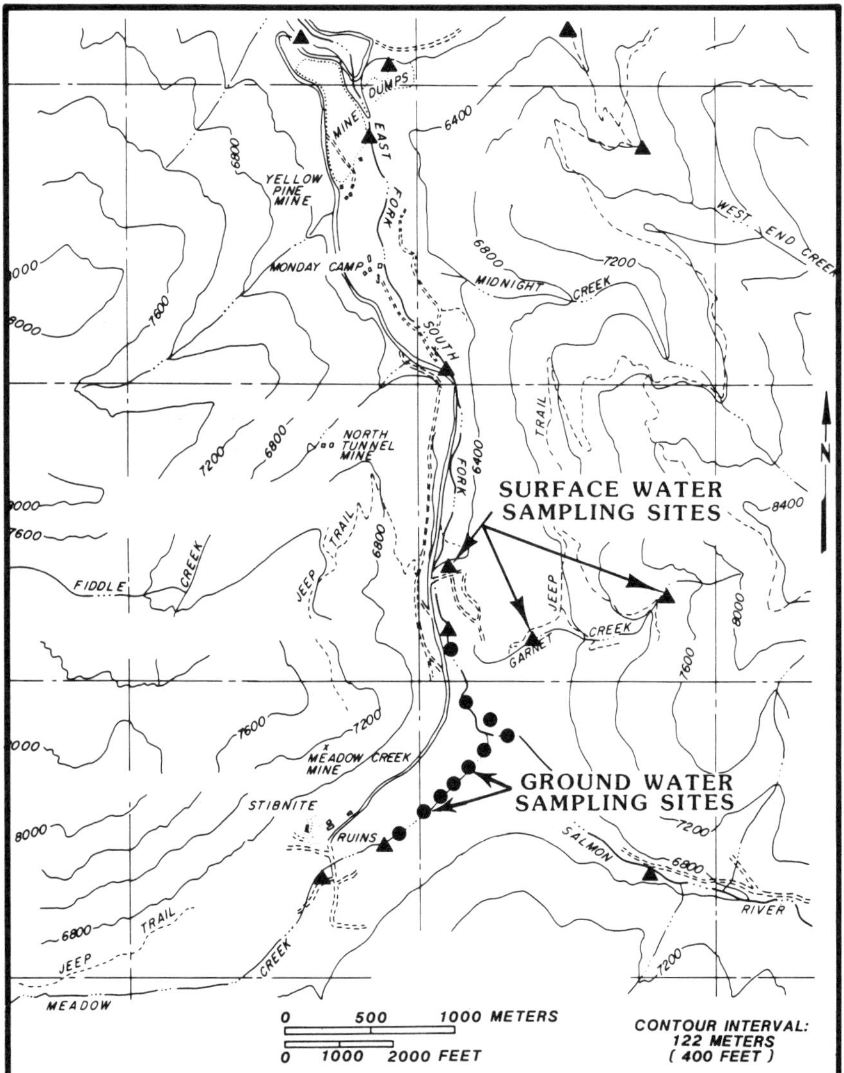

SURFACE AND GROUND WATER SAMPLING SITES FIGURE 7

DISCUSSION

Question (P. Saletta): What about drainage control and topsoiling at the Idaho site? Were there any requirements on this for final reclamation?

Answer (W. Stotts): This is covered in the final reclamation plan. The site is in mountainous terrain and there is no topsoil. We have done vegetation studies to find species that will grow on the material.

Question (P. Saletta): So there was no specific sloping required for your final disposition of the tailings to control drainage?

Answer (W. Stotts): Yes, this is in the plan. Very gentle slopes are provided.

Question (P. Saletta): Also, Mr. Stotts, have you had any problems with the asphalt pad durability at your site, or do you anticipate any during the life of the operation?

Answer (W. Stotts): We've had no problems.

Question (P. Saletta): Do you attribute the fact that you've had no cracking problems to the gravelly subgrade material there?

Answer (W. Stotts): Yes. We put a lot of effort into building it because we were in a very sensitive area. We had engineers watching every bit of fill that went in and all the seams on the PVC. It was very important for us to do it right.

Question: Bill, you have two collection pipes in your system. Would you tell us what becomes of those samples, for instance the artificial aquifer between the liners in the first pipe and the control sample from underneath?

Answer (W. Stotts): We use the samples from pipes on top of the PVC liner for our own assay and we don't make them available to the Forest Service. The results from the pipes underneath the PVC liner are all public and are reported.

CONFERENCE ON CYANIDE AND THE ENVIRONMENT
Tucson, Arizona • December 1984
Published by Geotechnical Engineering Program • Colorado State University • Fort Collins, Colorado 80523

IMPOUNDMENT DESIGN FOR CYANIDED TAILINGS - CASE HISTORY OF THE CANNON MINE PROJECT

by
Jack A. Caldwell[1], Don Moore[2],
and Adrian Smith[1]

INTRODUCTION

One of the reagents used in the recovery of gold from ore is sodium cyanide. The toxicity of free cyanide is such that the disposal of tailings, which may contain cyanide, requires significant engineering effort to avoid possible loss of cyanide to the environment. The design of systems for the economic disposal and environmentally sound containment of the tailings from mines and mills, that employ cyanide in the metal recovery process, involves consideration of possible metallurgical processes, tailings treatment options, suitable disposal sites, and appropriate disposal methods. This paper discusses the options open to the metallurgist and the geotechnical engineer in planning an economic and well engineered disposal facility for tailings that may contain cyanide. The paper illustrates these issues by describing a case history of an impoundment, designed and currently under construction, at a mine where cyanide will be used in the recovery of gold from the ore.

GOLD ORE PROCESSING AT THE CANNON MINE

There are a number of unit processes to recover gold from ore. The process which is selected is usually based upon laboratory or pilot plant tests or both. Selection criteria include recovery, capital and operating costs, cyanide leaching amenability, etc.

[1] Jack A. Caldwell and Adrian Smith, Steffen Robertson and Kirsten, 7510 West Mississippi Ave., Suite 210, Lakewood, Colorado 80226.
[2] Don Moore, Mill Superintendent, Asamera Minerals, 1201 Circle Street, Wenatchee, Washington 98801.

The flowsheet selected for processing Cannon Mine ore is shown in Figure 1. The ore is initially crushed underground with secondary crushing performed on the surface. Crushed ore is ground in a conventional rod mill-ball circuit using reclaim water. Cyclone overflow is sent to rougher flotation. Rougher tailings are thickened and then pumped to the flotation impoundment. Rougher concentrate is cleaned twice with cleaner tailings reporting to the head of rougher flotation. After thickening and filtering, the concentrate is leached with cyanide for eight hours. Pregnant solution is processed in a Merrill-Crowe unit to recover soluble gold and silver. Precipitate is melted in an induction furnace and the cooled slag is returned to the grinding circuit. Bullion is cooled into bars.

Primary cyanide leach tailings are sent to the autoclave plant for oxidation of the sulfides and some carbon. After neutralization with limestone and lime, the slurry is again leached with cyanide in a secondary leach section. After eight hours of agitated leach, the slurry is filtered with the pregnant solution being sent to the Merrill-Crowe plant. Secondary leach solids are sent to chlorine neutralization to destroy any residual free cyanide. This tailings slurry is sent to the flotation tailings sump. The combined flotation-leach tailings are sent to the tailings impoundment.

CYANIDED TAILINGS DESIGN OPTIONS

Prior to the adoption of strict pollution control laws, cyanide had been used in the recovery of gold and the tailings discharged, after little or no treatment, to impoundments. Natural processes on the surface of the impoundment, within the tailings, and in the foundation subsoils and rocks at the impoundment, were usually sufficient to preclude or reduce detrimental environmental impact. Increasing awareness of the potential for the impact of tailings on surface and ground water, has led to the passage of laws and regulations that impose a need for tailings disposal options with a lesser impact than those previously considered reasonable.

For these reasons different options for the proper disposal of tailings that may contain cyanide have been defined. Options considered in this paper include:

- Avoid the use of cyanide by adopting an alternative reagent or metallurgical process.

- Destroy the cyanide before the tailings leaves the plant (oxidation with either chlorine or ozone are two possible options).

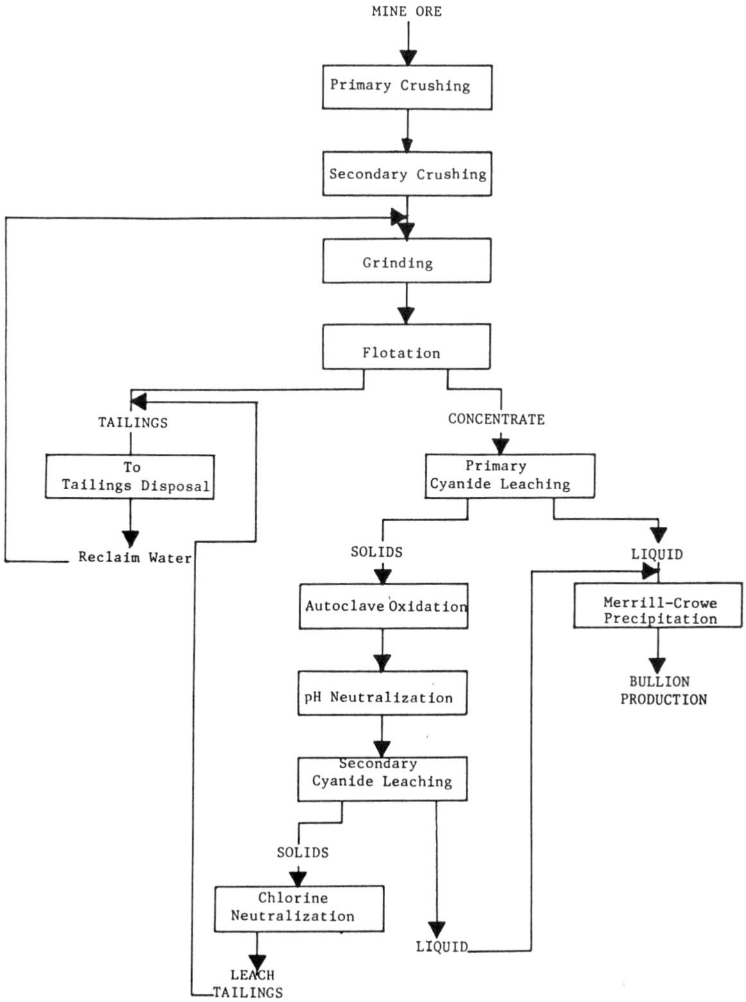

ASMAERA MINERALS (U.S.) INC.
Cannon Mine
Flowsheet

Figure 1

- Deposit the tailings in a "tight" impoundment, i.e. one from which significant seepage is unlikely.

- Deposit the tailings to maximize the natural degradation of cyanide by sunlight and oxidation.

- Remove as much water as possible from the tailings before disposing of them in "dry" tailing disposal facilities, hence minimizing the potential for seepage, and thus solute transport from the impoundment.

- Select and place the tailings at a site where the capacity of the foundation materials to attenuate cyanide in water seeping from the impoundment is sufficient to prevent significant environmental impact.

DISPOSAL OPTIONS

The choice of a disposal option for tailings that may contain cyanide is influenced by economics, laws and regulations, and the availability of suitable sites. Because of attitudes to cyanide, public opinion may play a part in selecting a suitable disposal option.

In many states, tailings may be classified according to their level of chemical constituents. The waste classification may in turn dictate adoption of a particular disposal option.

The most economic disposal option is discharge of untreated tailings to the facility. The hydraulic conductivity of the foundation soils and rocks of a site suitable for such a disposal option must be low.

If available sites have high foundation hydraulic conductivities, the cost of installing cutoffs or liners should be compared with the cost of treatment in the plant to destroy the cyanide prior to tailings discharge. Thus the most economic solution may be identified.

If the cyanide is not destroyed in the mill, consideration must also be given to the transport of the tailings from the mill to the impoundment. If the mill is distant from the impoundment, and the pipeline traverses property where a tailings spill would be unacceptable, it may be necessary to consider relocating the mill to a site close to the impoundment.

Whatever solution is adopted to protect the environment from cyanide contamination, the designer must keep in mind the possibility that the ore or the actual process employed in the mill may involve the use of considerably more cyanide than initially envisaged. The tailings in the impoundment may, as described by Robertson et al (1984) contain very high levels of cyanide. Hence the water seeping from the impoundment may contain elevated levels of cyanide. To deal with such an eventuality, provision should be made in the design to collect and treat the seepage water for release, or to return the seepage water to the impoundment.

The designer of the cyanide tailings impoundment should also consider the following possible problem: seepage through an undetected or ungrouted joint may be more rapid than anticipated. Therefore less attenuation than anticipated may occur, and seepage water quality may be affected. Possible approaches to this problem are a carefully designed and installed grout curtain and an impoundment layout that makes it possible to collect and treat unacceptable seepage.

If the impoundment is to be constructed in a hot, dry climate, and the topography is relatively flat, the impoundment can be designed to rise slowly and have large flat pools. Exposure of supernatant to wind and sun breaks down the cyanide. As discussed by Smith et al (1984), this occurs in South African tailings impoundments and has been adopted at a number of mines in the USA. Such an approach to the control of cyanide is seldom feasible for impoundments in wet, cool climates or where the site is steep and narrow.

On the basis of the discussion above we may conclude that selection of a suitable site for an impoundment to contain tailings from a mill where cyanide is used in the recovery of gold involves detailed consideration of economic, legal, and engineering factors.

CASE HISTORY: CANNON MINE, WENATCHEE, WASHINGTON

The Cannon Mine is just southwest of Wenatchee, Washington, a town about 160 km east of Seattle. The tailings impoundment will contain between five and ten million tons of gold tailings deposited over ten to fifteen years. The site chosen after a detailed site selection study is up Dry Gulch to the west of the mine.

Dry Gulch is part of a valley and ridge system that rises from the flatter, alluvial terrace on which the mine and the town of Wenatchee are situated. The elevation of the Gulch rises from 300 m at the alluvial terrace, to about 480 m at the impoundment site, to about 1,500 m at the upper end of the catchment boundary. The climate of the area is relatively mild and dry. Winters are characterized by light precipitation and cool temperatures, while summers are hot and dry. The mean annual precipitation is 230 mm and the annual evaporation is 760 mm.

The rocks at the site, Tertiary sandstones and siltstones of the Wenatchee Formation, are generally massive and constitute a strong and competent foundation. Bedrock hydraulic conductivity decreases from 10-6 m/sec at the surface to less than 10-10 m/sec at about 50 m depth.

The gold occurs as a hydrothermal deposit in the siltstone of the Swauk Formation. The ore will be ground to ninety percent less than 200 mesh and the gold will be extracted by the process illustrated in Figure 1. As indicated, the cyanide leach slurry will be neutralized with chlorine, then mixed with the flotation tailings before discharge at the impoundment.

Table 1 gives the chemistry of the mixed tailings and the flotation tailings supernatant liquids. The bulk of the cyanide is chemically complexed (compare total cyanide at 284 mg/l with free cyanide at 0.35 mg/l), hence chemically unreactive and not harmful. The free cyanide level of 0.35 mg/l presents no problem at the neutral pH of the tailings solution, although it exceeds the U.S. Public Health Services limit of 0.2 mg/l.

The chemical composition of seepage from the tailings impoundment is not necessarily the same as the slurry liquid composition at the time of tailings deposition. It is subject to modification by a number of processes, the most important of which are: re-leaching of the tailings solids with rainwater and snowmelt and hydrochemical reduction in the tailings mass.

In order to assess the potential for modification of the tailings liquid chemistry that might occur in the pool on top of the impoundment, mixed tailings were equilibrated with simulated rainwater (distilled water with hydrochloric acid to pH 5). The resultant chemistry of the supernatant is given in Table 2. The table indicates an increase in the levels of free cyanide and iron, and shows that overall the leaching by rainfall and snowmelt will improve or not significantly alter the seepage liquid chemistry from the tailings impoundment.

To simulate hydrochemical reduction of interstitial tailings liquid, a sample of the mixed tailings was equilibrated with a 10-percent mass-to-volume sodium bisulphite (Na2S203) solution. Sodium bisulphite was selected as a chemically conservative reducing agent that

TABLE 1

CHEMISTRY OF "MIXED" TAILINGS AND FLOTATION TAILINGS LIQUIDS

Parameter	Mixed Tailings Supernatant	Floatation Tailings Supernatant
pH value (units)	7.17	7.30
Total dissolved solids	4320	440
Sulphate	1660	170
Chloride	1040	15.5
Total cyanide	284	<0.05
Free cyanide	0.35	<0.05
Sodium	480	90
Iron	10	<0.05
Arsenic	0.07	0.01
Cadmium	<0.01	<0.01
Cobalt	0.33	<0.01
Copper	0.03	<0.01
Lead	<0.01	<0.01
Mercury	0.0024	<0.0003
Nickel	<0.05	<0.05
Selenium	<0.01	<0.01
Silver	<0.01	<0.01

Note: All values in mg/l, except pH

TABLE 2

REACTION PRODUCTS CHEMISTRY OF "MIXED" TAILINGS

Parameter	Mixed Tailings Reduced with $Na_2S_2O_3$	Mixed Tailings Leached with Rainwater
pH value (units)	5.17	4.80
Total dissolved solids	N/A	2750
Sulphate	N/A	1587
Chloride	3750	202
Total cyanide	<0.05	57
Free cyanide	<0.05	2.58
Sodium	N/A	87
Iron	1100	18
Arsenic	<0.01	0.08
Cadmium	<0.01	<0.01
Cobalt	0.55	0.08
Copper	<0.01	<0.01
Lead	<0.01	<0.01
Mercury	0.0062	0.0011
Nickel	5.4	<0.05
Selenium	<0.01	<0.01
Silver	<0.01	<0.01

Note: All values in mg/l, except pH

would not interfere with the results. The chemical composition of the resultant equilibrium solution is given in Table 1. The important observation is that both the total and the free cyanide and copper are decreased to below analytical detection limits.

Seepage from the impoundment will occur in the upper fifty feet of the sandstones. Attenuation will occur in this zone. The yellow-brown rocks in the upper zone are oxidized and weathered. The lower rocks are relatively reduced and gray. The attenuation capacity of both zones was tested according to standard EPA procedures (1977). This involved agitation for 24 hours of the sample at a 16:1 liquid to solid ratio with the mixed tailings. Table 3 summarizes the partition coefficients describing the attenuation capacity of the two rock types. The results indicate significant attenuation of total cyanide, but no attenuation of free cyanide.

A one-dimensional solute transport model was used to predict the rate and extent of solute migration in the near-surface groundwater downstream from the impoundment. Seven cases were analyzed using the parameters given in Table 4 and for values of the partition coefficient varying from zero to ten. The chemistry of the seepage from the tailings was assumed to be the worst case that could possibly occur. The results of the simulations are given in Table 5. This table shows that, with no attenuation, dispersion causes a fifty-percent reduction in solute concentrations at the downstream toe of the embankment. For partition coefficient values above three, the downstream solute concentrations are radically reduced to less than 0.0001 percent of the original seepage concentrations. Sulphate, total cyanide, arsenic, cobalt, and copper are reduced to below detection limits before the downstream toe of the impoundment embankment. Non-attenuated free cyanide is reduced to fifty percent of the initial value.

The work described above shows that seepage from the tailings impoundment will have no apparent effect on the downstream groundwater quality, even near the impoundment itself. Attenuation of total cyanide and oxidation of the free cyanide in the impoundment, together with immobilization of the free cyanide in the tailings mass, are important reasons for this result.

Figure 2 is a cross section through the embankment. The zone 1 material is a clayey silt with a low hydraulic conductivity. This will inhibit seepage from the tailings. A grout curtain will be installed beneath the core. The grout curtain will prevent seepage through joints in the rock. The seepage and attenuation studies did not consider the presence of the curtain, which will further tend to reduce flow rates and the possibility of solute transport.

At the Cannon Mine, the decision to deal with cyanided tailings by treatment in the mill prior to discharge to the impoundment was based as

TABLE 3 PARTITION COEFFICIENT VALUES: "MIXED" TAILINGS ATTENUATION TESTS

Parameter	Oxidized		Reduced		Alluvium	Mean (Where Applicable)
	1	2	1	2		
Sulphate	3.95	4.24	4.05	3.57	3.43	4 (3.4 for alluvium)
Total dissolved solids	3.12	1.44	3.07	3.26	2.52	3.2 (2.5 for alluvium)
Total cyanide	8.2	6.66	14.1	11.5	6.3	Variable*
Sodium	3.66	3.66	3.96	3.96	2.97	3.8 (3 for alluvium)
Arsenic	11.4	13.7	13.7	13.7	9.14	>10
Cobalt	0.97	1.45	1.45	0.97	1.45	1.24
Copper	>10.7	>10.7	>10.7	>10.7	>10.7	>10

* 7.4 oxidized, 12.8 reduced, and 6.3 alluvium

Notes: 1) Cadmium, lead, nickel, selenium, and silver are not present.

2) Iron, free cyanide, and mercury show no attenuation.

TABLE 4 INPUT PARAMETERS FOR 1-D SOLUTE TRANSPORT MODEL: METRIC AND IMPERIAL EQUIVALENT UNITS

Parameters	Metric	Imperial
Flow		
Path length 1*	365 m	1200 ft
Path length 2*	548 m	1800 ft
Distance increment	27.5 m	90 ft
Time		
Total simulation	18,250 days	18,250 days
Time increment	1,825 days	1,825 days
Dispersivity		
Longitudinal	5 m	16.5 ft
Velocity	0.0078 m/day	0.0256 ft/day
Attenuation		
Bulk density	2.59 g/cm^3	162 lbs/ft^3
Porosity	0.4	0.4
Partition coefficient	Variable (0- 10)	Variable

Notes: 1* Distance to downstream toe of embankment

2* Distance to seepage control dam

TABLE 5 PREDICTED DOWNSTREAM CONCENTRATIONS BY THE SOLUTE TRANSPORT "MIXED" TAILINGS DISPOSAL

Parameter	Partition Coefficient (Kd)	Initial Concentration (Co)	Concentration (C_1) @ 365 m	Concentration (C_2) @ 548 m
Sulphate	4	1660	<0.2	<0.2
Total dissolved solids	3.2	4320	86	0.4
Total cyanide	>7	284	<0.03	<0.03
Free cyanide	--	0.35	0.18	0.105
Sodium	3.8	480	5	0.05
Iron	--	10	5.1	3
Arsenic	>10	0.07	<0.0001	<0.0001
Cobalt	1.24	0.33	< 0.008	<0.0001
Copper	>10	0.03	<0.0001	<0.0001
Mercury	--	0.0024	0.0012	0.0007

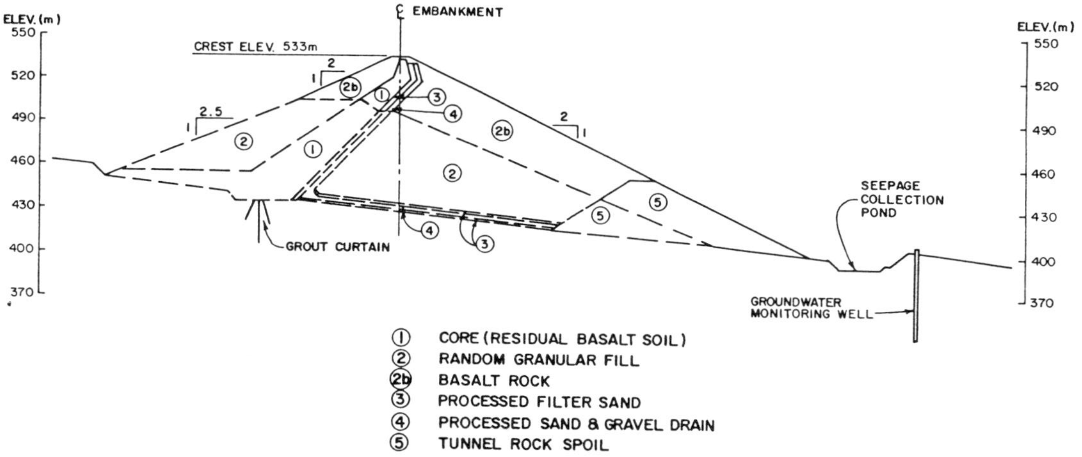

FIGURE 2. CANNON MINE TYPICAL EMBANKMENT CROSS SECTION

much on the proximity of the project to the town, as on the hydraulic conductivity of the impoundment foundation bedrock, and the desire to create a tailings pile with insignificant pollution potential.

DISCUSSION

The approach adopted for discharge of tailings from a mill that uses cyanide in the extraction of gold, as described in the case history, is not the only one that is possible. As described by Smith et al (1984) the standard approach in South Africa, and one that has been adopted at a number of mines in the USA and Canada, is not to treat the tailings to suppress cyanide before discharge.

Instead the tailings are discharged from the perimeter of the impoundment to form thin layers; each layer is, to the maximum extent possible, allowed to sun dry before deposition of another layer. Only a small amount of water is kept on the pool which is maintained in the center of the impoundment. This deposition technique effectively dries the tailings in situ, thus reducing the water available for seepage from the impoundment. Exposure to sunlight serves to degrade the cyanide.

If the impoundment site is far from the mine, environmental considerations may make it undesirable to transport the cyanided tailings in a pipeline to the impoundment--a break of the pipeline and a spill would be difficult to countenance. In such a case the ore may be slurried at the mine and pumped to a process plant at or closer to the impoundment. The cyanide is employed in the plant close to the impoundment and hence the tailings discharge directly to the impoundment. It may even be possible in this case to locate the plant above the impoundment so that any spill from the plant flows directly to the tailings discharge facility. This provides additional environmental protection against accidents involving the use of cyanide in the extraction of gold.

If the approach of discharge of untreated tailings in drying layers can be used at a site where the hydraulic conductivity of the soils and bedrock at the site is low, the designer is double blessed. In this case he can select a site and adopt a tailings discharge system that economically and effectively meets social concerns, complies with State requirements, maximizes the destruction of cyanide by natural processes, and prevents significant environmental alteration.

CONCLUSIONS

This paper has described design options for impoundments for the disposal of tailings that may contain cyanide. The case history illustrates the implementation of certain of the principles.

On the basis of the case history and the options available, we conclude that economic, well engineered, and sound tailings impoundments may be designed and constructed to contain tailings from mills where cyanide is used in the recovery of gold. Such impoundments meet the requirements of the various new laws that regulate the disposal of such tailings, and hence the environment may be protected from significant or unacceptable impact.

REFERENCES

E.P.A., 1977, Methods of evaluations of solid waste materials.

Robertson, A. MacG., Hutchison, I. P. G., Ferguson, K. A., Ash, W., and Fisher, J. W., 1984, Cyanide control options: Lessons from case histories, Conference on Cyanide and the Environment, Tucson, Ariz., Dec. 12-14.

Smith, Adrian, Dehrmann, Alison, and Pullen, Rob, 1984, The effects of cyanide-bearing, gold tailings disposal on water quality in the Witwatersrand, Conference on Cyanide and the Environment, Tucson, Ariz., Dec. 12-14.

CONFERENCE ON CYANIDE AND THE ENVIRONMENT
Tucson, Arizona • December 1984
Published by Geotechnical Engineering Program • Colorado State University • Fort Collins, Colorado 80523

FATE OF CYANIDE TAILINGS - AN UPDATE

by
James L. Hendrix*, John H. Nelson **
and Mojtaba Ahmadiantehrani ***

ABSTRACT

This paper is intended to give the reader an update on the work being done at the Mackay School of Mines about the fate of cyanide in precious metals mill tailings waste. Although the project is at an infancy stage, we believe some of our initial observations (and trials) may be of interest to others. To date, little has been determined about the fate of cyanides within the tailings we have examined, but amounts of cyanides currently present have been evaluated. The most succinct method to explain our current results and our projected methodology is to discuss sample collection, sample preservation, preparation, and sample analyses and characterization.

SAMPLE COLLECTION

So far, two sites have been sampled extensively. Several other sites will be investigated before the completion of the project. The sites sampled represent a contrast in tailings impoundments. The first site has multiple impoundments and the gold cyanide mill has not operated during the past 16 years. It is thought that little or no treatment of cyanide in the mill tails was done. The second site is active and there is currently treatment of the effluent.

Samples were collected by using a hand auger made by Art's Manufacturing Supply. The auger can be equipped with various types of heads able to take samples in the wet or dry regimes. A sample is contained within the head, or bucket, and is generally 10 cm in diameter and 20 to 25 cm in depth. At the first location, the one with many small impoundments, samples were taken along a line starting at the mouth of the former effluent stream to the outermost dike of the tailings. Five separate impoundments were sampled at distances between 50m and 100m, depending on the individual impoundment size. At each sampling point, samples were taken at depth intervals starting at the surface to seven meters or until native earth was reached. At the second site samples were taken along lines perpendicular to each other.

The hand auger was able to be used because of the characteristics of the tailings. First, since the tailings had been previously milled, there was little difficulty in digging the hold. Also, the moisture

* James L. Hendrix, Professor of Chemical Engineering, University of Nevada-Reno, Reno, NV 89557.
** John H. Nelson, Professor of Chemistry, University of Nevada-Reno, Reno, NV 89557
*** Mojtaba Ahmadiantehrani, Research Associate, University of Nevada-Reno, Reno, NV 89557

content and the particle size distribution was such that the hole was stable, with no caveins, and little material falling into the hole if the operators were careful. We estimate less than five percent of the material used as a sample was alien to the depth sampled. It should be noted that when the material was greater than 40 percent moisture, it was difficult to obtain representative samples. Caveins could occur and it was difficult to hold the sample in the auger head as the auger was being withdrawn from the hold.

In summation, we have found the hand auger to be an adequate method for sampling milled tailings. It's inexpensive, introduces little energy to the sampled material, and samples relatively free of mixing can be obtained.

SAMPLE PRESERVATION

From previous studies[1,2] it is known that cyanide can decompose in the presence of oxygen and light. Therefore care was taken to minimize the augered sample's exposure to light and air. Samples were immediately placed in labeled plastic bags and the bags were stored either in sealed plastic pails or ice chests. Some samples were iced down for the trip from the tailings site to the laboratory in Reno. After their arrival in Reno, the samples were frozen until they could be analyzed.

SAMPLE PREPARATION

No part of the procedure is as difficult as the preparation of the samples. We have been specifically interested in the cyanide contained within the solids part of the tailings. The material from the first site, and to a certain extent the second site, is variable even within the 20 cm of core used as a sample. Complete color changes in the material can occur within one centimeter of depth. Therefore, the preparation of a homogeneous sample, without losing cyanide, has been paramount. Variation of the material is not the only problem encountered. The clay-like fineness of the material can cause lumping of the tailings into balls when samples are dried.

During the past three months we have tried different schemes for sample preparation. Some schemes did not produce a homogeneous sample in terms of cyanide present. Other schemes produced homogeneous samples, but with much of the cyanide escaping or decomposing.

The first method attempted was rolling the sample over a plastic sheet to get as homogenized sample as possible. It was unsuccessful because of the high moisture content and the chunks of clay material observed in the samples.

It was decided to evaluate the preparation procedure of using a bottle roll. Approximately 500 g of sample was put into a plastic jar and 500 ml of distilled water and 10 g of lead carbonate ($PbCO_3$) was added. The jar was then rolled for 30 minutes. When the sample was analyzed for total and free cyanides, the results were reproducible, but low. To verify that cyanide is lost during the process of rolling and filtering, 8.45 mg of potassium cyanide (KCN) was mixed with 500 grams of silica sand and then the water was added to the jar. Again the mixture was rolled for 30 minutes. Twenty five percent of the cyanide was lost.

The effect of thermal drying on the cyanide analyses was investigated. A wet sample was confined in a flask. That flask was connected to a second flask by a tube. The second flask contained sodium hydroxide (NaOH) solution so the off gases from the heated wet sample could be absorbed. The material was dried at approximately 80°C. Analyses were made on the absorption solution and the dried sample. It was determined that nearly one half of the cyanide found was in the caustic solution.

From the tests it was determined that solution mixing and heating could not be used to prepare the tailings samples. Finally, it was decided to dry samples using an inert gas stream. About ninety grams of wet sample was dried in a closed tube in the presence of anhydrous calcium chloride by blowing nitrogen gas over the sample while applying a vacuum to the other side of the tube. The sample stayed in the tube for 24 hours, but the N_2 gas was applied for approximately 10 hours. Seven percent of the sample was evaporated. The sample was dried enough to mix uniformly. Five gram samples of the dried solids, and five gram portions of the wet solids were analyzed for total and free cyanide. The results are given in the following Table.

TABLE I.
Wet Mixing vs. Dry Mixing in Terms of Cyanide Analysis

	Sample (site 2, 3 meter depth	
	Total CN , ppm	Free CN , ppm
Wet (mixed)	3.75	1.0
Wet (mixed)	4.63	1.03
Dried with N_2	5.5	1.16
Dried with N_2	5.5	1.16
Dried with N_2	5.6	1.16

Obviously, the reproducibility of the analyses improved by drying the samples at ambient conditions using nitrogen and then well mixing.

SAMPLE CHARACTERIZATION AND ANALYSIS

As mentioned earlier, there was variability from site to site, sample to sample, and even within the sample. For all samples, which now numbers over 100, size distribution and moisture content will be determined. Moisture content will be determined by differences in weight between wet and dried material. Some moisture analyses have been done. Representative of the first site are the data from a hole in the middle of the first tailings impoundment.

TABLE II

Moisture Content of Tailings (Site 1, Hole A-4)

Depth, m	Percentage Moisture
surface	24
1	27
2	26
3	25
4	27
5	36
6	27
7	28

When considering the moisture content it should be noted that the samples were taken in late July from an area that can be described as high altitude, middle latitude desert. The area had received an insignificant amount of precipitation during the past three months.

Particle size distribution for the samples was hard to determine because of the difficulty of the clay forming balls. The problem was solved in the following manner. The sample was weighed and then placed in a mortar and pestle. The sample was lightly broken, breaking only the clay nodules. Then the sample was rotapped for 15 minutes. Any remaining clay nodules were broken up using a rubber stopper. This was rotapped again for 15 minutes. Each size was weighed and recorded.

TABLE III

Results of Size Distribution Analysis (Hole A-4)

Sample Depth:	Surface	1m	2m	3m	4m	5m	6m	7m
Size								
+65 mesh	12.76%	29.40%	17.96%	44.50%	13.83%	5.26%	7.68%	18.42%
-65+100	23.60%	23.80%	38.61%	26.60%	13.96%	8.61%	12.40%	21.55%
-100+150	22.44%	15.40%	8.47%	12.06%	13.16%	8.29%	17.38%	24.86%
-150+200	16.44%	10.8%	4.89%	6.17%	12.63%	8.93%	17.92%	16.39%
-200+325	14.51%	10.40%	6.57%	5.36%	19.41%	16.27%	18.46%	10.13%
-325	10.25%	10.20%	23.22%	8.31%	29.99%	52.63%	26.14%	8.66%

On selected samples inductively coupled plasma analysis (ICP) and x-ray diffraction has been, and will be done. Rather than completely dissolving the sample, we have elected to run ICP's on solutions that were obtained by, first, mixing five grams of sample with 250 ml of distilled water; second, mixing five grams of sample with 20 ml of concentrated sulfuric acid (H_2SO_4) and 230 ml of water at ambient temperature; and third, using the same acid mixture and heating. We were not so much interested in the exact composition of the sample, but rather what might be soluble when the samples were treated analytically to measure the cyanide contained. Some of the elements reported from a sample obtained from the first site are found in Table IV.

TABLE IV

Inductively Coupled Plasma Analysis (reported in ppm in the solutions).

Sample	Al	As	Au	Ca	Co
in H_2O	<3	<2	<5	<3	<0.2
in H_2SO_4 (cold)	<3	49	<5	90	<0.2
in H_2SO_4 (heated)	55	34	<5	87	<0.2

Sample	Fe	Mn	Na	Pb	Zn
in H_2O	<0.2	<0.02	<3	<8	<0.2
in H_2SO_4 (cold)	200	2.6	<3	<8	<0.2
in H_2SO_4 (heated)	200	2.6	<3	<8	<0.2

Little has been reported[3] about the analysis for cyanides contained in solid materials. Obviously much work needs to be done. Although we are interested in new analytical techniques, we decided if a recognized method of cyanide determination could be modified successfully for our purposes we could commence our studies about cyanides in tailings.

The ASTM method[4] for the analysis of total cyanide was selected for the base procedure. This method, which is for determination of cyanide in water, is based on the decomposition of nearly all the metallo-cyanide complexes (cyanide in some cyanocomplexes of some transition metals such as cobalt, gold, and platinum is not completely decomposed) plus the free or simple cyanides from a strongly acidified sample during a one hour reflux distillation. The cyanide gas is absorbed in a basic (NaOH) solution. Then the cyanide content of the absorption solution is determined either by titration, colorimetry, or by using a selective ion electrode. In our procedure, 50 ml of 1:1 H_2SO_4 and 10 ml of 510 g/l magnesium chloride ($MgCl_2$) are being used for acid decomposition and catalyst, respectively. A spectronic 21 is being used for the colorimetric determination.

Solid samples were directly dropped into the distillation flask. Initially, two gram samples were used, but to obtain higher intensity and better absorbance, the amount of samples was increased to five grams. A few results using this method are given in Table V. When a sample number is given in any table, the last digit of the number represents the depth in meters of the sample and the first letters and numbers correspond to the hole location.

TABLE V

Cyanide Reported in Some Samples Using the ASTM Method

Sample No.	Total Cn^-, ppm	Sample Size, g
A4-3	0.23	5
A4-4	0.0	5
A4-5	0.3	5

Even with the five gram samples, the absorbance was low and the reproducibility was very poor. It was thought the samples contain some sulfides which slowly convert the cyanide in the sample to thiocyanate.[4] At high thiocyanate levels, some interference has been observed in measuring very low levels of cyanides. To remove these sulfides, as it is suggested,[3] a small amount of lead carbonate ($PbCO_3$), about 200 mg, was added to the five grams of the sample that was to be analyzed. As can be seen from Table VI, the problem of reproducibility was not solved by the addition of $PbCO_3$.

TABLE VI
Results Using the ASTM Method Plus $PbCO_3$

Sample No.	Total CN^-, ppm	Sample Size, g
A4-surface	0	5
A4-1	0.21	5
A4-3	0.25	2
A4-3	16.13	2
A4-3	1.2	5
A4-4	0.21	5
A4-4	0	5
A4-4	2.72	2
A4-5	0.21	2
A4-6	0.28	5
A4-6	0.25	2
A4-7	0.25	2
A4-7	0.28	5

Next, the samples were analyzed for weak dissociable cyanide complexes and free cyanide according to the ASTM method for water analysis. Samples were distilled directly in the flask by addition of 10 ml each of the acetate buffer and zinc acetate solutions. The results, in general, showed higher free cyanide content than the corresponding total cyanide content of the same sample. We believed this happened because the interferences are lower. Perhaps, by using a weak acid (acetate buffer) in the procedure, the sulfur, sulfide, compounds in the tailings material did not decompose during the acid digestion-distillation. Some sulfur compounds may decompose during the acid digestion-distillation conditions, releasing hydrogen sulfide (H_2S) gas into the absorption solution and later being oxidized by the colorimetric reagent, Chloramine-T. Therefore, the color intensity would be reduced.

To overcome the interference problem, we decided to mix the sample with 20 ml of 1N NaOH and about 200 mg of $PbCO_3$ and filter into the distillation flask. Using the filtrate, the ASTM methods for the analysis of total and free cyanide were followed. We also employed a second catalyst, HgCl2, while doing the filtration method. The results are shown in Table VII.

TABLE VII
Analytical Results Using a Filtration Pretreatment Step
(Sample A4-3 used throughout)

Test	CN^-, ppm	sample wt., g	Distillation time, hr
Filtered, total	10.81	2	1
Filtered, total	10.64	2	1
Filtered, total	10.2	2	2
Filtered, free	0	2	1
Filtered, free	0	2	1
Filtered, $HgCl_2$, total	12.64	2	2
Filtered, $HgCl_2$, total	14.99	2	1
Filtered, $HgCl_2$, total	13.2	2	1

The results from the filtration experiments indicate: one, filtration increases the recovery of the total cyanide because it reduces the sulfur content inside the distillation flask; two, the recovery of free cyanide is reduced, perhaps, because the free cyanide is so little that it's lost during filtration; three, the addition of the second catalyst, $HgCl_2$, slightly increased the total cyanide recovery; and four, increasing the distillation time did not impact the results.

We were curious if ferri- and ferrocyanides were recovered when we employ the filtration technique. As seen in the ICP results, one of the most soluble components found in the first tailings is iron. We hypothesized that some of the cyanide found in the tailings will be in the form of the iron cyanides. Our enthusiasm for our hypothesis has been tempered somewhat by not identifying any iron cyanides by electrochemical or infra-red spectroscopy techniques in the samples tested. Anyway, the recovery of ferri-ferrocyanides, when using the filtration procedure, was tested by introducing 10 mg of potassium ferri and ferro cyanide to five grams of sample. All the cyanide added plus some of the cyanide from the sample were recovered.

The effects of iron sulfide (FeS) on the analytical results were evaluated. Fifty milligrams of FeS was added to five grams of sample and tested three different ways. The first method was to mix the sample plus the FeS with 1N NaOH and then filter into the distillation flask. We believe nearly all the cyanide was recovered. The second method was to mix the FeS plus the sample with distilled water and then filter. There was no cyanide recovery. For the third method the FeS and sample were distilled directly. This method also produced no cyanide recovery. These tests show that the presence of sulfide compounds in the distillation flask interfer in the total cyanide procedure.

For reproducible results the samples must be dried and well mixed to achieve a homogeneous sample. For the total cyanide procedure, the sample should be mixed with NaOH solution and then filtered into the distillation flask. For free cyanide the sample should enter the distillation flask without the caustic-filtration pretreatment.

CONCLUSIONS

Although our techniques for sample collection, preservation, preparation, and analysis are still in the need of refinement, we now are able to obtain reproducible results for total and free cyanides in tailings samples. It should be noted that the samples represent a composite of 20 to 25 cm in length of a nonhomogeneous material. Also, the material tested is not bone dry, but contains probably 10 to 18 percent residual moisture.

Although, by necessity, this update paper is a discussion of our various techniques, one interesting result can be stated at this time. At both sites, to date, we have found no cyanide at the surface of the tailings impounds. What cyanide which is not quickly percolated downward is decomposed at the surface.

ACKNOWLEDGEMENTS

The authors wish to acknowledge the companies which graciously consented to having their tailings impoundments sampled.

Also, the authors wish to acknowledge the financial support of the United States Bureau of Mines under the Mining and Minerals Resources Research Institute Generic Center program (grant number G1125132-Mineral Industry Waste Treatment and Recovery Generic Center).

LITERATURE CITED

1. Ecological Analysts, Inc. 1979. Cyanide, An Overview and Analysis of the Literautre on Chemistry, Fate, Toxicity, and Detection in Surface Waters. Prepared for the Inter-Industry Cyanide Group.

2. Broderius, S. J., 1978, Quarterly Report. Influence of External F-actors on the Toxicity of Iron and Copper Cyanide Forms. Jan. 1-March 31, 1978. EPA Grant # R80529-01-0. Univ. of Minnesota.

3. Pohlandt, C., E. A. Jones, and A. F. Lee, 1983. A Critical Evaluation of Methods Applicable to the Determination of Cyanides, Journal of the South African Institute of Mining and Metallurgy, January pp 11-16.

4. ASTM. 1982. Annual Book of Standards. American Society for Testing and Materials.

CONFERENCE ON CYANIDE AND THE ENVIRONMENT
Tucson, Arizona • December 1984
Published by Geotechnical Engineering Program • Colorado State University • Fort Collins, Colorado 80523

CYANIDE CONTROL OPTIONS - LESSONS FROM CASE HISTORIES

Ian P.G. Hutchison[1], Wayne M. Ash[2], John W. Fisher[3]

INTRODUCTION

Safe, long-term disposal of cyanide gold tailings, particularly in wet climates can be difficult. Because of the regulatory environment in North America and because of the general perception that cyanide is extremely toxic, mines are put under significant pressure to prevent, at all costs, the escape of cyanide to the environment. In some cases, this is achieved by chemically treating the tailings to remove cyanide before disposal. In other cases, disposal occurs in water-tight impoundments formed generally by constructing an earthen embankment across a valley.

The writers have been dealing extensively with the design and operation of such waste disposal systems in the U.S. and Canada. This paper outlines some of the problems that were encountered at three operating facilities and describes how these were dealt with.

The three projects that are discussed are as follows;

- Scottie Gold Project, British Columbia;
- Carolin Mines Project, 100 miles east of Vancouver, British Columbia; and
- Noranda's Grey Eagle Project, Siskiyou County, California.

The following sections describe the occurrences at each of these projects in turn. The Scottie and Carolin projects deal with the disposal of treated tailings and highlight problems that can be encountered with cyanide treatment systems. The Grey Eagle case history deals mainly with the disposal of untreated tailings and highlights problems that can be encountered when operating a zero discharge tailings impoundment. Specific lessons that were learned from each project are discussed. The paper concludes with a summary of the general lessons learned.

1 Steffen Robertson and Kirsten (Colorado) Inc.

2 ADTEK Mining Consultants Inc., Vancouver, B.C., Canada

3 Consultant, Vancouver, B.C., Canada

CASE 1 - SCOTTIE GOLD PROJECT

Background

Scottie Gold's cyanide mill started production September, 1981. the design milling rate of 200 tons/day was not achieved on a continuous basis for any significant length of time during the first year. In an attempt to release free gold retained in the ball mill, the circuit was revised in March, 1982 to operate with cyanide added to the grinding section. It continued this way for the next five months. During this period, alkaline chlorination was used to destroy residual cyanide in mill tailings pulp to achieve discharge standards (0.1 ppm total cyanide) before disposal. The chlorination treatment was, however, unsuccessful. As a result, INCO's SO_2 air cyanide removal process was tested, found to be satisfactory, and implemented. The INCO process has performed well with only isolated instancs of "off-spec" effluent analyses during the past 27 months.

Case History

Scottie's operation is generally not easy. The mill is in an isolated area of northern British Columbia and is situated underground. Mill feed is somewhat variable and contains massive amounts of pyrrhotite with traces of copper minerals. In order to minimize cyanide consumption, this type of ore is usually milled in freshwater and the milled pulp is aerated at high pH with litharge added to oxidize and tie up the cyanicides (notably pyrrhotite and some copper minerals). The original mill process for Scottie was developed on this basis, and apart from the five-month period (March-July, 1982) when cyanide was added to the grinding circuit, it has operated in this way.

Scottie's experience with the alkaline chlorination process is difficult to assess objectively for the following reasons:

1) The mill did not operate under steady conditions.
2) Cyanide addition in the process was not controlled and levels of cyanide concentration were extremely variable.
3) Water input to the process and barren solution bled from the circuit was virtually uncontrolled.
4) Mill tailings were not washed effectively on the disc filters and repulped tailings leaving the second stage of filtration were mixed with barren bleed solution. Pulp density and cyanide content were extremely variable.
5) Vaporization and control of chlorine addition was not always reliable.
6) Sampling and analysis of mill tailings products from the chlorination stages were not established on a regular basis.

In addition to these factors, higher levels of cyanide complexes and free cyanide were brought about by the temporary addition of cyanide to the grinding circuit. In the absence of pre-aeration, the cyanide consumption was increased threefold to approximately 7.5 lbs/ton solids during this period.

Toward the latter part of July, 1982, a combination of high-grade ore and higher grade reactive pyrrhotite resulted in total loss of control of both extraction and the ability to recover gold from the pregnant solution. As a result of this, the mill was shut down and the circuit revised to the original basis of a freshwater grind. During this period, INCO's technical staff implemented the SO_2-air process which had already been tested in the laboratory.

Subsequent experience with the SO_2-air process at Scottie has shown it to be remarkably successful. In the development of this waste treatment system, the barren solution bled from the circuit is processed separately and this treated effluent is subsequently recombined with mill tailings which have been filtered and washed effectively using freshwater. Good control of the mill process has been established and waste management sampling has been given the same priority as the routine mill control samples.

During the past six months, both pH and redox potential in the waste treatment reactors have been monitored and controlled automatically. This has made the operator's tasks much easier. However, optimization of reagent use from the SO_2-air process has not been established. In the writers' opinion, further cost savings may be possible.

Table 1 shows the average daily data pertaining to Scottie's mill operation during the first nine months of 1984.

TABLE 1

ORE (TONS)	NacN (LB)	BARREN (TONS)	SOLN BLEED @(LBS NACN PER TON)	TREATMENT DOSAGE (SOD.SULFITE) (LBS)	(METABISULFITE) (LBS)	(COPPER SULFATE) (LBS)
180	345	130	@ 0.6	1700	550	55

Cost of reagents (Canadian funds) are as follows:

Sodium Sulfite	32¢/lb
Sodium Metabisulfite	32¢/lb
Copper Sulfate	115¢/lb

The approximate reagent costs to treat each lb. of free cyanide and associated weak cyanide complexes is $10.-(Canadian). At Scottie this is equivalent to $4.33 per ton of ore milled. However, the process is successful and problems due to inadequate waste treatment have been minimal. Discharge of final tailings is, with very few and occasional exceptions, within the requirements necessary to comply with environmental regulations.

Lessons Learned

Experience at Scottie has shown that the important lessons learned are:

1. Good steady control of the mill circuit, with minimal use of cyanide, is essential.
2. Effective washing, with freshwater, of the mill tailings produces a a clean filter cake containing minimal amount of dissolved gold (0.5 oz/day) and associated low levels of free cyanide.
3. Effective treatment of barren solution bled from the circuit is best achieved with automatic control of both pH and redox potential.

4. Treated barren solution containing a slight excess of reagents is effective as a means of removing the trace amounts of cyanide remaining in the washed mill tailings when they are remixed and aerated prior to final discharge.

The relatively high cost of reagents at Scottie may, conceivably, be reduced if gaseous SO_2 could be used instead of the sulfite and metabisulfite products. That this technology appears as yet not to be commercially available for small gold milling operations, is surprising.

The simple concept of treating mill effluents to produce a reusable water product would seem to be an easier way to go than to have to treat effluents to the extent required for compliance with tough environmental standards. If developed successfully, it should be more economical than present methods.

CASE 2 - CAROLIN MINES PROJECT

Background

Carolin Mines Ltd., loacted some 100 miles east of Vancouver, British Columbia, operates a 1,300 ton-per-day flotation-cyanidation plant for the recovery of gold. The raw ore, containing approximately 0.10 oz. Au/ton, is made up of 90% quartz, 9% pyrrhotite and 1% graphite, with minor arsenic and copper components.

Case History

A gold-bearing sulphide-carbon concentrate is floated off while the quartz tailings is pumped to the tailings impoundment. The sulphide-carbon concentrate is then cyanided and the gold is recovered using the Merrill-Crowe process. While the process may seem straight-forward, the concentrates are most difficult to process. The pyrrhotite is extremely reactive and iron cyanide is rapidly produced when un-pre-aerated concentrate is subjected to cyanide. The rate of iron cyanide production increased dramatically 12 hours after the first cyanidation. At times, iron cyanide content of up to 4,000 ppm had been measured, but normally varies from several hundred to 2,000 ppm in the barren solution.

Pre-aeration essentially eliminates iron cyanide problem but produces dissolved sulphur compounds which, when subjected to cyanide, are combined to form thiocyanate. At times, the thiocyanate can reach over 2,000 ppm but normally ranges from 700 to 1,800 ppm. In standard-strength cyanide solutions, the gold dissolved from the phyrrhotite is re-precipitated on the carbon (graphite) while high-strength cyanide solutions results in extremely high iron cyanide production.

In summary, the operation of the circuit is extremely delicately balanced. As a result, extreme fluctuations in both gold recovery and quality of the barren solution occur. As is described below, this in turn led to problems in treating and disposing of the tailings.

In order to reduce cyanide levels in the waste stream, the company originally installed an alkaline chlorination system to treat the liquid portion of the tailings. However, this process proved ineffectual due to the high thiocyanate and iron cyanide content of the barren solution. As a result, after the first six months of operation the iron cyanide in the pond climbed to over 100 ppm and when the spring rains and snowmelt made a pond discharge inevitable the mine was shut down by the Provincial Government. During the shutdown, the chlorination system was greatly enlarged and a secondary Alkaline Chlorination system was installed to treat the pond water effluent prior to discharge to the environment. During the eight month shutdown, the total cyanide in the pond was gradually destroyed by nature.

After the next six months of production the total cyanide in the pond once again reached 80 ppm and the mine was once more forced to suspend operations.

The problems with Alkaline Chlorinates stemmed from the following:

1. The chlorine had to destroy the thiocyanate (the substance most susceptible to chlorination) before the chlorine would attack even the free cyanide. The high thiocyanate content resulted in chlorine consumption that peaked at $105,000 per month.

2. Only 1/3 of the iron cyanide in the barren was destroyed by alkaline chlorination. The other 2/3 ended up in the tailings pond. Under winter conditions the iron cyanide was not subjected to ultraviolet light and consequently a build up of iron cyanide in the tailings pond occurred.

3. Chlorine reacted so vigorously with pyrrhotite that the cyanide associated with the solids (estimated at between 5 and 10%) could not be treated. This source thus contributed substantially to the cyanide content in the pond.

The principals of Adtec Mining Consultants Inc. who had been instrumental in the installation and early operation of the INCO Sulphur-dioxide-air process at Scottie Gold Mines Ltd. were then consulted. On-site pilot plant test work with the INCO process showed that an immediate improvement in effluent quality could be achieved. The company was allowed to resume production once more and the new system was installed at a cost of $55,000. The new INCO process went on stream in October 1983 while the cyanide in the tailings pond was still at 12 ppm. After the first 7 months of operation the total cyanide in the pond had risen only 3 ppm, up to 15 ppm. The secondary treatment system still operated by using alkaline chlorination. This performance is considered remarkable in the face of the financial constraints placed upon the project in which a system to treat the solid fraction of the tailings could not be afforded.

The monthly reagent bill for cyanide destruction fell to $30,000 from an average of $85,000 when chlorine was used, and the savings resulted in full payback of the new installation within 2½ months. Because of the mixed treatment mode, continuously increasing amounts of chlorine were required at the secondary treatment system to deal with thiocyanate levels. Further refinements to the treatment system would have been required to keep treatemtn costs to an economic level. However, Carolin Mines has since received such favorable smelter rates that they were able to drop cyanidation in favor of sending their concentrates directly to a smelter.

Lessons Learned

For the specific conditions encountered at Carolin Mines, cyanide destruction by the INCO process had several major advantages over alkaline chlorination:

1. It is less expensive to install.
2. Operating costs are much lower.
3. The cyanide associated with the solids can be effectively treated.
4. The reaction continues in the tailings pond, even under winter conditions. It is, therefore, more forgiving than alkaline chlorination.
5. The final effluent is of much better quality when compared to alkaline chlorination.

The INCO process has two minor disadvantages:

1. It is marginally more complicated than alkaline chlorination and thus more operator training is required.
2. A royalty must be paid to INCO for the use of the process. This however, was not a serious problem since the royalty constituted only about 1/3 of the savings that were achieved, when compared to alkaline chlorination.

CASE 3 - GREY EAGLE MINE

Background

The Grey Eagle Mine is located in Siskiyou County, Northern California. Operated by Noranda, it processes 500 tons/day of gold ore using a conventional CIP process. The tailings are disposed of behind a fill dam constructed of clay and granular material obtained from the open pit.

With annual precipitation of 66 inches, control of excess water in the tailings impoundment is a critical item. To reduce the inflow of runoff water, a diversion ditch is located around portions of the impoundment. The steep topography made a complete peripheral ditch unpractical. Makeup water use in the mill circuit was minimized. In spite of these measures, an alkaline chlorination treatment plant had to be constructed to deal with the anticipated buildup of water containing cyanide in the impoundment. This treatment plant reduces the residual cyanide and metal concentrations down to regulatory standards and then discharges the excess water to a land application site. Provision was made for the installation of a dam seepage collection and pump-back system to prevent the escape of any contaminated fluids from the impoundment.

Unforeseen problems started arising when the plant went into operation in October, 1982. Because of higher than expected copper values and due to shakedown problems in the mill, the cyanide consumption was considerably higher than the pilot scale test results had indicated. This in turn led to high levels of both free and total cyanide in the tailings pond; 100 ppm, and 400 ppm, respectively. Mechanical problems were also experienced with the chemical feed systems in the water treatment plant which was called on to deliver very high rates of liquid chlorine. Further problems were encountered with scale development on the intake pump impellors and volutes, and clogging of the clarifiers. As a result, the treatment plant did not operate at design capacity for the first six months.

To compound the mine's problems, the first two years of operation were among the wettest in Northern California's history. Water accumulated in the impoundment and construction of the final stages of the tailings impoundment were advanced to the summer of 1983 to eliminate the risk of overtopping. A final problem developed which further aggravated the operating conditions. Three months after starting deposition in the tailings impoundment, dam seepage rates of the order of 25 gpm developed. Before exiting at the toe of the dam, this seepage was diluted by precipitation infiltrating through the downstream shell of the dam resulting in flow rates of up to 400 gpm that had to be pumped back into the impoundment. This seepage contained residual values of cyanide, both free and total. Levels within the dam's internal drainage system were approximately 20 ppm free and 100 ppm total. At the toe of the dam, these were considerably diluted by the shell infiltration. This seepage, which demonstrated unattenuated cyanide, was not expected. The additional volume of water that was pumped back added to the disturbance of the water balance in the impoundment.

In order to respond to these problems, Noranda acted quickly. A working group of consultants and in-house experts was assembled to evaluate all possible remedial actions and to assist Noranda on selecting schemes which could be implemented. A wide range of options were studied. These included removing the tailings to alternative sites, treating the tailings stream using chlorine or the SO_2 air process, constructing an additional water treatment plant, methods of sealing the dam, and treating the deposited tailings.

It was found to be impractical and prohibitively expensive to construct an alternative site. Because of the extremely steep terrain and the very wet climate, it was difficult to envisage an alternative site working without an excessive amount of engineering effort to prevent contamination of ground and surface waters. Furthermore, additional disposal sites would have in turn generated their own environmental impact. Treating the tailings stream was also rejected. It would not have solved the problem associated with the 150,000 tons already in the impoundment. For similar reasons, various combinations of treatment and removal of portions of the tailings were rejected. Sealing of the dam was not considered to be practical. Because it has an upstream sloping clay core and because of the nature of the jointing in the foundation, it was not feasible to consider installing a further grout curtain or a slurry trench. Construction of an upstream impermeable blanket was also ruled out because of the retrofitting difficulties and the presence of fairly permeable colluvium and alluvium which would act to convey seepage under any partial liner. Fully lining the impoundment was impractical because of the presence of tailings and the very steep impoundment walls. Finally, detailed studies of tailings consolidation and infiltration through the impounded tailings revealed that the contaminated dam toe seepage could occur for many years after reclamation of the impoundment. Any proposed remedial program would also have to deal with this.

The final program adopted involved an eight point program as follows:

1. Early completion of the tailings dam to its ultimate height.
2. Construction of diversion channels and drains on and around the downstream shell to reduce infiltration.
3. Enlargement of the dam toe seepage pumpback system.
4. Construction of a new water treatment plant to treat the dam toe seepage.
5. Improvements to the existing treatment plant.
6. Sealing of an old adit which was discharging into the tailings pond.
7. Reduction of cyanide consumption in the mill.
8. Committing to a long term operations plan which would deal with any seepage problems after closure.

This program was started during mid 1983 and immediately had an effect. As stated above, the raising of the dam eliminated any possibility of overtopping. The downstream shell engineering measures reduced the amount of water being pumped back to the impoundment. The metallurgical work in the mill reduced the cyanide consumption considerably and lowered cyanide levels in the pond. This, coupled with improvements made to enlarge the hydraulic capacity of the treatment plant, dramatically increased the rate of water removal from the pond. A start was made with the design and construction of the proposed lower treatment plant.

The situation today is much improved. Because of the relatively dry 1983/84 winter and the good performance of the existing water treatment plant, completion of the dam toe seepage plant has been postponed. It may even be possible to postpone it until closure. The dam seepage has stabilized and the situation is well under control.

Lessons Learned

The lessons to be learned from this case history are as follows:

Generally, a cyanide waste disposal system in a mining operation is fairly complex and is influenced by the ore metallurgy, mill process, water treatment facilities, climate and the condition of the ultimate containment structure. All of these are variable to some degree. Assessment of the possible range in variation must be made during the initial design stage and flexibility built into the waste disposal system. The design should take into account both operating and post decommissioning requirements.

More specifically, it may be appropriate to incorporate some redundancies or overdesigns in a project. These could include capability to easily increase treatment capacity and the chemical addition in treatment plants, as well as some backup measures to the reliance only on attenuation to deal with cyanide seepage loss. The degree of redundancy would obviously depend on the environment in which the waste is disposed of, as well as the amount of study and engineering effort put into refining the disposal concepts. Extremely wet climate and steep terrain are inheritly difficult conditions for waste disposal and certainly appear to warrant inclusion of some of these redundant features.

SUMMARY

The Scottie Mine's example demonstrated that cyanide destruct or treatment systems require very carful monitoring and control of both the process and the treatment systems. In this case, it is believed that either alkaline chlorination or the INCO process may have worked successfully. The Carolin Mines' case history also indicated that cyanide treatment systems require very careful control. The INCO process proved to be superior. It also demonstrated that mixed mode treatment systems (i.e. both INCO and alkaline chlorination) can create problems. Grey Eagle proved that disposal of cyanide waste in a wet climate behind an earthen embankment can be difficult and may involve some long-term commitment by the mining company to maintain environmental protection measures after mine closure.

In all cases, it can be said that the problems encountered are not unsurmountable. Having learned these lessons, it will be possible to more carefully plan and design the safe cyanide waste disposal facilities in the future and avoid many of the past pitfalls.

ACKNOWLEDGEMENTS

The writers are grateful to the management of Scottie Gold Mine for permission to publish this paper, in particular to Mr. M. F. Lindsay, (General Manager of Mine) who provided specific information on the waste management aspects of the operation. The cooperation and input from Carolin Mines and Noranda Mining (Inc.) are also gratefully acknowledged.

DISCUSSION

Question (P. Saletta): Mr. Hutchison, concerning Grey Eagle, at the time seepage was discovered at the dam, what were the water quality requirements on that water?

Answer (I. Hutchison): The requirement was a zero discharge system. There could be seepage, but it had to be returned to the pond.

Question (P. Saletta): So they just recirculated it?

Answer (I. Hutchison): Yes.

Question (H. Van Drielin): What do you consider the most effective way of depositing tailings in the tailings pond?

Answer (I. Hutchison): Gray Eagle was a difficult site at which to do any tailings management. We had very steep reservoir sides and high precipitation so there was very little you could control, other than discharge the tailings in the pond and try to form a beach and get some oxidation going on the surface. A large percentage of the time the tailings are covered by water. In other new impoundments, like some of them in California in drier climates where we can get a flatter tailings impoundment basin, we would try some sort of sub-aerial deposition. We would try to create as large a beach as possible either from a point discharge or using a spreader bar, keeping the pool away from the tailings as far as possible, and discharging uphill to get the tailings to spread out, dry, and allow oxidation. That is what we generally would try to do in a water-impoundment-type disposal system. Adrian Smith can probably describe practices in South Africa where this technique is used far more extensively.

Comment (A. Smith): The mode of tailings deposition is often dictated by the grind of the ore and therefore how the tailings must be handled to facilitate dewatering. If the coarse fraction is reasonably large, the tailings can be separated by cycloning; if not, some form of beaching must be used. In South Africa we use a self-build principle of tailings deposition. Rather than an impoundment we use a ring-dike construction where the coarse fraction is deposited on the outside and the finer fraction gravitates to the middle on a very shallow beach angle with a very small depth but a wide wall area around the decant tower. During day operations, the wall is usually built up higher on the outside by digging it out. During the night there is a night wall that is located closer to the centre of the impoundment and tailings are deposited straight into that. We try to maintain a very shallow angle beach to maximize the surface area and the evaporative losses and the potential for the breakdown of things like cyanide.

Question: What about the dust potential on those big, relatively dry beaches?

Answer (A. Smith): This is a serious problem. There is a semi-cementing effect from residual pyrite: the sides of these impoundments are actually solid enough to climb. The problem we do see is dusting on the drier parts of the beaches, so operations management becomes a balancing act between maximizing evaporation and trying to keep the beach wet. Discharge is regulated from one of the points on the ring dike to try to optimize that situation.

Question: Could you amplify on your comment that the Inco SO_2/air process is difficult to control?

Answer (B. Conard): It is important to understand the context in which Mr. Hutchison is discussing process control at the Scottie Gold and Carolin's Ladner Creek operations. Inco installed the SO_2-air process at both sites in a retro-fit mode using available equipment. To limit capital costs, no automatic process control was installed, except for pH control. At both sites operator interaction in a manual mode was imperative for control. The Inco process does not require sophisticated control methods. Indeed, we believe our control is simpler than the ORP used in alkaline chlorination or than that reported for the Degussa H_2O_2 control reported elsewhere at this conference. However, in the absence of automatic control and without proper operator attention, any process, no matter how simple, can fail.

The control methodology, whether automatic or manual, of the Inco process consists of providing a set amount of well-dispersed air, and either bleeding into that air a set amount of SO_2(g) or feeding sulfite solutions at a set rate into the reactor. The SO_2 delivery rate can be set daily, for example, based on ratioing it to the flow of feed and the feed CN content. Any time the CN load to the reactor is known to change, then the SO_2 delivery must be adjusted correspondingly. The only other variable is the Cu^{++} addition (if any is required) and this can be set in ratio to the Fe in the feed. A pH set-point is easily maintained provided electrodes are properly maintained, but this remark is the same for any number of CN removal processes requiring set pH.

At Inco/Queenston's McBean mill the success of CN removal is judged by the color of the effluent. This judgement is easily made by the operator in a 10-second stop. If the color is different than nominal, then a troubleshooting guide is referred to and he follows steps depending on the color he observes. ORP may be helpful also in recovering the system to good operation. Efficient operator interaction with the circuit does require a certain amount of training and exerience, but this is the case for any industrial operation.

Comment (J. Scott): I'd like to say a little bit about control of the Inco process, particularly at the McBean property. At the McBean property, I've been told that it takes the operator about one hour a day to apply control to the Inco process as utilized there. The pH is automatically controlled, but the metabisulfate is controlled manually. Control is based mainly on analyses of the solution going to the reactor, using a few simple calculations to determine the demand for metabisulfate. In the applications I'm aware of, the Inco process has not appeared difficult to control.

Safe Handling of Cyanide

CONFERENCE ON CYANIDE AND THE ENVIRONMENT
Tucson, Arizona • December 1984
Published by Geotechnical Engineering Program • Colorado State University • Fort Collins, Colorado 80523

SAFE HANDLING OF CYANIDE
Panel Discussion

The conference on Cyanide and the Environment was opened with an afternoon session on the safe handling of cyanide. During the first part of the session, a slide series on safe handling used by the Dupont Company as a training program was shown by F.W. DeVries. Subsequent comments by three speakers formed the basis for further discussions. They described recent experience in the states of Arizona and Nevada with cyanide problems and solutions. The three speakers were Dr. Theodore Tong of the Arizona Poison Control System, Mr. Bill Fellows of the Arizona State Mine Inspector's Office, and Mr. Norton Pickett from the Nevada State Division of Mine Inspection. Their comments were recorded and transcribed, and are briefly summarized below. A summary of the discussion session is also presented.

Theodore Tong, Arizona Poison Control System

In his opening remarks, Dr. Tong profiled the Arizona Poison Control System with which he is associated. This program, as he indicated, is state-supported and serves as a poison information and treatment referral service for the citizens of Arizona. In 1983 the Arizona Poison Control System received nearly 65,000 calls from consumers and health professionals primarily in the state of Arizona. Of those 65,000 calls, nearly 80% dealt with cases of actual exposure or contact with something that was potentially hazardous, poisonous or toxic, and nearly two dozen during that period were cyanide-related questions. Fortunately, none of those involved exposure of individuals, but rather were questions about how to obtain the so-called cyanide antidote kit.

In toxicology - the science of poisons and other substances that injure biological systems - there are very few antidotes, drugs or medications that act specifically when given to reverse the toxic effect of a particular poison. However, in the case of cyanide, there is an antidote, actually a series of medications, available to reverse the toxic effects. From a scientific point of view, it is fascinating to have something so specific as amyl nitrite and sodium nitrite work to reverse the effects of cyanide at the cellular level. Cyanide is a respiratory or cellular asphyxiant that poisons by making tissues unable to utilize oxygen. Despite the fact that the oxygen may be in the blood, the tissues are unable to pick it up, and become hypoxic. Cyanide acts by converting the iron on the hemoglobin and in the cytochrome oxidase system in the cellular mitochondria to the ferric form which complexes specifically with cyanide. The antidote for cyanide poisoning produces a condition known in medicine as methemoglobinemia, characterized by a chocolate brown-colored appearance of the blood.

The addition of thiosulfate then permits the cyanmethemoglobin complex to be carried away and eliminated in a soluble and less toxic thiocyanate form through the kidneys.

The antidote kit contains amyl nitrite, 3% sodium nitrite and 25% sodium thiosulfate. Before administering these drugs, it is vital to know exactly what the problem is, that is, to be sure that the case is one of cyanide poisoning. It is also important to ascertain how poisoning or exposure occurred. Treatment of cyanide poisoning from inhalation of vapors differs from that due to ingestion, both with respect to when the antidote is used, and how it is given, whether orally or by injection. Oxygen should be administered as soon as treatment is begun and should be continued throughout.

Checking up on your antidote kit frequently is important, to make certain that the supply of any of the components has not been depleted and that the materials are fresh and still usable. The color and physical characteristics of the solutions can indicate whether the materials are stable or otherwise. It is strongly suggested that people who may have occasion to use the antidote kit take a course in cardiopulmonary resuscitation (CPR) techniques and remain updated on these procedures. Another important point to keep in mind is that hazardous materials, particularly such materials as cyanide, may adhere to the clothing of individuals who have been exposed to them. Because of this, the clothing of those who handle victims must be protected. Prolonged contact with the skin may allow enough systemic absorption to produce toxicity. Toxic materials can adhere to clothing or medical equipment which may be used by many people in an emergency setting, and there have been cases in which the rescuers developed symptoms of exposure to the poison they were attempting to control, due to this type of contamination.

Bill Fellows, Arizona Mine Inspector's Office

Bill Fellows, head of the Education and Training Division in the Arizona State Mine Inspector's Office, spoke on Arizona's experience with cyanide handling problems. In 1980 the Office became quite concerned about the increasing use of cyanide for gold and silver extraction in Arizona. Problems were foreseen not only for the miners themselves, but also for the general public in communities near operations where cyanide is utilized. The office was able to obtain the cooperation of the one cyanide supplier in the United States, the Dupont Company, which produced an excellent educational assistance package for Arizona and other concerned states, dealing with the safe handling of cyanide. Arizona has 'personalized' the multi-media presentation to fit the state's specific needs and has also produced versions geared to the non-technical public. These training programs have been very successful and are credited directly with the saving of two miners' lives.

The number of mining operations in Arizona which make use of cyanide has increased from 30 to 50 between the years 1980 and 1983, and the number of miners has grown proportionately. Arizona will soon become the first state to enact regulations governing the use of cyanide. A set of regulations formulated by Jim McCutcheon, State Mine Inspector, with help from others, has undergone a public hearing and comments on it are under consideration at the present time (December 1984). These regulations will be published soon, and will assist the growing mining industry to maintain safe operations as well as establish a basis for enforcement and control of some of the abuses.

It is worth emphasizing the necessity for us, as professional engineers who are usually in positions of deciding on the lay-out of an operation, to concern ourselves with the safety of the workers. This is an area often neglected. Likewise, public opinion can become an extremely important factor in the success or failure of an operation. Public education should accompany the start of an operation to avoid later misunderstandings which may occur if the general public and the media are not informed about it and about safety measures in a timely fashion.

Norton Pickett, Nevada State Division of Mine Inspection

Nevada has 386 mining operations, of which 83 are either cyanide leaching operations, or utilize cyanide in some fashion. The mining population is approximately 6000, with some 2800 people working with cyanide. About 30% of the state's mining activity is associated in some way with cyanide. The new, or revised, technology for gold recovery by cyanide heap leaching has made it possible for people without large sources of revenue to establish gold operations. Nevada was the major gold producer in the United States last year (1983), and this probably accounts for the high percentage of mining operations which use cyanide in the state.

Nevada has developed its own slide program as an educational tool on cyanide use and safety, following guidelines set out by the Dupont Company and incorporating information from doctors, individuals who have handled cyanide for many years, and other sources. The slide show, which was shown at the meeting, includes examples of typical operations, both well- and poorly-managed with respect to cyanide safety.

The State Mine Inspector's records date back to 1908, and since that date the state has never had a mining-related cyanide fatality. However, there have been some very close calls, which prompted the current effort to familiarize miners with cyanide, its effects, and what to do if exposed to it. One example of the sort of problem which can occur because of lack of knowledge is an actual incident which involved a new worker in a small operation in the central part of Nevada. She was a mill helper, and the mill had just installed some new PVC line for their solution handline system. They were in such a hurry to get operations going that they didn't give the epoxy on the PVC adequate time to set, so that when the pump was turned on and the line was subjected to pressure, the connections blew apart. The mill helper was drenched with cyanide solution. Not knowing what she was experiencing, she panicked and ran from the mill screaming: 'I'm dying, I'm dying'. What she was actually suffering from was physical shock.

She had been so scared that she had been exposed to a large dose of cyanide that she went into a state of shock and had to be hospitalized for several days for that reason. This was due to a lack of education, a lack of training.

Another incident, which took place not far from Carson City, demonstrates the fact that, in many cases, the general public and even officials responsible for public protection are not very knowledgeable about cyanide and how it should be handled. Two young men had been out roaming the hills on their dirt bikes and had wandered into one of the old mining sites where some cyanide had been left, abandoned. They helped themselves to it, not knowing what it was, but out of curiosity, and took several pounds of it home with them. Fortunately, one of the young men's fathers recognized it, or at least suspected what it was, and turned it over to the sheriff's department. The sheriff then called the State Mine Inspector's office, asking how to dispose of it. He was advised to give it to a working operation which could put it to use. This is considered the best way to deal with cyanide, both not to waste it and to avoid the problem of how to otherwise dispose of it safely. In Carson City itself, a young man 15 years old burglarized a laboratory and took what he thought was cocaine. He gave it to a friend, a 14-year old boy, who took it and died: the substance was actually cyanide. This incident raised interest in the issue of toxic chemicals hazard control, both in the general public and in the agencies concerned with this problem.

Not too long ago, in the central part of Nevada, one of the larger mining operations experienced three closely connected cyanide incidents. Again, they involved people actually working with cyanide, but unfamiliar with it or its effects. A pump failed, allowing a sump to overflow and flooding the mill floor wth cyanide solution. There were three people involved in the clean-up: a supervisor and two maintenance workers. Shortly after they began the cleaning, the supervisor said that he felt very nauseous, attributing this to a case of the flu; he vomited and went home. The others continued to work, and by the end of seven hours one of them was experiencing nausea, severe headache, and difficulty in breathing. At this point it was suspected that they were being over-exposed to cyanide. The cyanide antidote, amyl nitrite, was administered to them and they were rushed to the local hospital, about 40 miles away. By the time they arrived at the hospital the one worker was in a semi-conscious condition, although the other did not appear to be much affected. They were both kept in the hospital overnight: the more seriously-affected man continued to receive doses of the antidote, while the other, who was experiencing headache and nausea, was given only oxygen. In many cases, oxygen is all that is necessary if it can be administered soon enough. Both men suffered severe caustic burns on their feet after working for seven hours in the high-pH cyanide slurry wearing only leather boots. However, the strange thing was that although one of them experienced cyanide poisoning by absorption through the skin, the other came out with nothing but caustic burns on his feet. The doctors were unable to explain why the effects were so different between the two men, but different individual response to exposure to cyanide is an observed fact. The supervisor suffered no lasting effects at all and was back at work the following day.

In all areas where cyanide is used, warning signs should of course be posted, as well as no smoking and no eating signs. After handling cyanide in solution or solid form, there is a possibility that some residue may remain on the hands or clothes, so slight that it cannot be seen. If a person should eat or smoke without washing his hands, cyanide poisoning is possible. Good personal hygiene is important for this reason, and to avoid contaminating street clothes and the family at home. The potential which exists for poisoning others in the family was demonstrated by a case involving a worker in one of the larger operations in central Nevada who lived about 60 miles from the mine and travelled to and from his job on weekends, living at the mine during the week. Each weekend he would take his laundry home for his wife to wash. Suddenly, his two-year old daughter became inexplicably ill, and they took her to a doctor thinking it was a case of the flu. By the time they got her to the doctor, though, she had recovered on her own. This happened a second time, and after a more thorough investigation of what was causing her reaction, they found she was suffering from mild cyanide poisoning. The little girl had been helping her mother with the washing and playing in the laundry room, transferring the minute residue of cyanide from the father's clothes to her mouth. Very little was necessary to make the small child quite ill. Again, this occurred because of a lack of knowledge and recognition of the symptoms of cyanide poisoning. Therefore, all operations should be posted with the appropriate, and legible, signs. Like many other states, Nevada requires that leaching operations be fenced and secured against free access, and that the ponds be monitored for leakage.

Remember that a particle the size of a grain of rice is enough cyanide to prove fatal to the average person. Although it is true that cyanide does not accumulate in the system, continuous exposure over a period of days may result in a build-up of cyanide in the body because it does not have the opportunity to discharge it. For instance, a case came up in a cyanide leaching operation where the people working in the counter-current decantation system were experiencing true cyanide-poisoning symptoms. Even though the exposure was less than the 10 ppm mandated by the federal government, nevertheless by the end of the week, these workers had raspy throats, upset stomachs, especially if they had eaten lunch on the job, and their wives attested to their irritability. The symptoms became worse as the week went on, but after the weekend off they had disappeared. This is attributed to the body's inability to cleanse itself each day of the daily dosage, so that a build-up occurs throughout the working week until the weekend when the body has the chance to catch up. The logical way of dealing with this is to educate the workers themselves and encourage them to practice the proper procedures in handling cyanide.

A Draeger monitor for detecting HCN should be available at all cyanide operations, and is required by regulations. The gas detector should be used to monitor all areas of the plant where anyone is working, especially enclosed areas where minor quantities of HCN can be trapped. If cyanide is detected, the area should be posted or ventilated adequately. Personal protective equipment is mandatory for all operations, including helmets with face shields and respirators. It is recommended that the respirator be a positive type, even though regulations require only a dust type. This is because there is no definite proof that a dust type respirator is working adequately unless it can be tested for a tight seal.

When over-exposure occurs to the point that breathing becomes difficult or even stops, artificial respiration is the single most important thing to do to restore or at least sustain breathing. The use of oxygen is vital and every operation dealing with cyanide should have an oxygen unit available. In fact, few operations work without some type of oxygen, even if only an oxygen acetylene tank. Early administration of oxygen can sometimes be all that is necessary if the symptoms are recognized in time. The pre-major oxygen unit is the most appropriate and beneficial as long as the individual is still breathing. If breathing stops altogether, either some form of artificial respiration, or a resucitator, must be utilized. Because an average of only about 3% of the population is familiar with the use of a resucitator, hands-on practice in its use is part of Nevada's first aid training program.

The cyanide antidote kit, of course, must be readily available. The two workers involved in the incident related earlier, who suffered cyanide poisoning symptoms after cleaning up an overflow of cyanide slurry, were lucky that the kit was available at the mine so that they could receive the amyl nitrite pearl on the way to the hospital. At the same mine, a week later, a lab technician was overcome by HCN and collapsed. He was treated with amyl nitrite as the two other workers had been. However, the hospital had reported the previous incident to the state emergency service, claiming that the men had been overdosed with amyl nitrite, so that the ambulance called in the second case was reluctant to transport the patient or the antidote kit. Amyl nitrite is classified as a dangerous drug and is prohibited in ambulances in the state of Nevada. This case helped prompt the State Inspector's office to begin its program of miner education, soliciting the cooperation of state emergency medical services and the State Board of Pharmacy. A program was developed for presentation to the mine workers to enable them to respond immediately in case of an incident. Mr. Elliot King, executive secretary of the State Board of Pharmacy, sat in on one of the first presentations given to miners, and gave it his complete support. To date, more than half of the 2800 people working with cyanide in Nevada have received the training. The program is currently in wide use and is very successful.

In Nevada, the anidote kit is one of the first aid materials required at all cyanide-using operations by law. To provide any first aid that may be necessary the mines must have a trained person who can administer the antidote, and the program responds to this need. The potential for abuse of amyl nitrite, or misuse of it as an antidote, presents a problem to having the cyanide kits available at the mines. For this reason, the Nevada training program issues a certificate of completion of training and a wallet card. As long as the person uses amyl nitrite properly according to the recommended procedures, he is protected in a manner similar to protection under the good samaritan law in the event of adverse effects due to the administration of amyl nitrite. This program has now been sanctioned by both the state emergency medical service and the State Board of Pharmacy. There is no guarantee that a person carrying such a certificate cannot be sued, but he would have the backing of the State Mine Inspector's Office, as well as that of the state emergency medical services and the Board of Pharmacy, which would be good in a court of law. To be certified, a person must complete the approximately 3-hour course, which gives hands-on training in the use of the cyanide kit and other techniques, with a score of 70% or better.

The State Board of Pharmacy has also accepted a new method, devised by the State Mine Inspector's office, which makes it more feasible to administer sodium thiosulfate in cases of ingestion of cyanide dust or solution. Although amyl nitrite can be used in these situations, sodium thiosulfate works more directly in the stomach to provoke elimination of the cyanide. Ordinarily, sodium thiosulfate is included in the antidote kit, but the amount required for the prescribed 1% solution must be measured out and mixed up during the actual emergency. Several administrations of the antidote may be necessary if vomiting is induced. They are continued until the next dose is retained in the stomach. In order to facilitate the use of thiosulfate, individual doses are premeasured into small vials and included in the antidote kit, along with a dark-colored pint bottle which protects the solution from sunlight after the thiosulfate is mixed with tap water. This idea has been well received by the mining companies and enhances their capability to deal with cyanide poisoning.

Another problem with the antidote kit is that the component amyl nitrite, and the kit itself, are expensive. The kits cost about 65 and last only a year or two, after which they must be replaced. In Nevada the State Board of Pharmacy has responded to these problems by offering the amyl nitrite at a rate reduced to about 50% of the over-the-counter cost, through the Office of the State Mine Inspector.

DISCUSSION

Comment: There is an excellent cyanide antidote that has been used in France, a cobalt complex that reacts with cyanide to make vitamin B-12. It is my understanding that, at the moment, a change-over to this new antidote appears to present problems of such scope that there is no real movement to implement such a change.

Comment (C. Chase): This is a little story that I think the people in this group should know about. I have a friend who personally saved 6 men in 2 minutes in a cyanide accident. He came from a family in Mexico that was used to mining and cyanide plants. One day he was alone in the Sierra Madre of Mexico when he walked into a cyanide mill and saw the operators keeling over eveywhere. Being very quick of mind, he held his breath, rushed in and dragged them out into the fresh air, saving all six. He knew what the problem was, he recognized it and figured out a quick way to cope with it. What had happened at the mill was that one of the operators had dumped a bottle of concentrated sulfuric acid into the mill circuit.

Question (G. Potter): For a hypothetical case of a 1500-ton-per-day operation, would one of the panel please sketch what would be a very safe way to dissolve the cyanide solution and distribute it to the leach liquor?

Answer (F. DeVries): If they're using our Flo-Bins, there are about 3000 pounds in the bin. Most people make up a 10% solution, which for 3000 pounds would take about 3000 gallons of water. 50 pounds of caustic per 1000 gallons should be added in an agitated tank. There are really very minor dusting problems from briquetted cyanide. A very modest hood might be placed over the area - certainly the tank area will have toxic fumes over it, so that if it is indoors some kind of exhaust must be provided. If the tank is outdoors, just be sure to stay well removed from it.

The Flo-Bins are usually readily emptied. The design of the gates underneath the Flo-Bins made by Dupont was changed about 4 years ago. The new style of bins has a much longer rectangular opening on the bottom and different slopes on the two sides so that there is less of a tendency to bridge. Occasionally, some effort is required to break a bridge at the bottom, but generally, since cyanide is so readily soluble, it will fall out quickly once it gets started. The tank has to be agitated, of course, so that briquettes do not just accumulate at the bottom. Generally this 10% solution is then metered into the recycling barrens to make up whatever solution concentration is desired. My understanding is that this is usually on the order of a tenth of one percent, which is 1000 ppm. Some operations use even lower concentrations in the actual leach.

Operations which use large amounts of cyanide would use the Wet-Flo tank car, 65,000 pounds of cyanide at once, and make up about 30,000 gallons for a 22 or 23% solution. Those large-scale operations require much more engineering.

Question (G. Potter): As you discharge the Flo-Bins into the stirred agitator, do you catch those eggs in a sort of basket with a steel grille and prevent the agitated solution circulating through the basket, or do you just let them fall loose into the tank?

Answer (F. DeVries): If the eggs are put into a basket, less agitation will be required because you won't have to resuspend the ones that fell out.

Question (M. El Tawil): In a couple of the presentations, the figure pH 12 was mentioned. I wonder if that is realistic, both metallurgically and in terms of just maintaining that high pH. It's fine for a stock solution, but for process solutions that is not practical.

Answer (F. DeVries): We're talking about solutions of 1% or higher. Nobody leaches at pH 12, but nobody leaches at a 1% concentration, either. For safety, the pH should be as high as possible, but there are many ores that the metallurgists would like to leach at as low a pH as possible. This is a matter of balancing safety precautions against yield of metal. The lower the pH, the more HCN you will lose out the flue, so to some extent cyanide economics enter into this. There are very few operations where the pH is maintained at even 11.0, with concentrations no higher than 0.1% cyanide. Certainly pH 11 and 0.1% is pretty comfortable. Where pH is allowed to fall to 10 or 9.9, the surrounding atmosphere will be pretty thick. This creates somewhat of a hazard and does not produce good yields, but it may be the only way to recover the metals.

Comment (N. Pickett): We recommend a pH of 12 in the mixing tank, and not less than 10.5 in the leaching cycle which gives a margin of safety there. The important thing is to maintain a concentration of less than 10 ppm in the atmosphere, regardless of the pH. 10.5 is realistic and in most cases appears to work well.

Question: This has to do with the survival of cyanide in solutions and of hydrogen cyanide in the atmosphere: what is the rate of degradation under idealized conditions?

Answer (F. DeVries): Hydrogen cyanide, with a molecular weight of 27, is slightly lighter than air, and therefore rises and enters the stratosphere where cyanide occurs naturally. A study made by the National Oceanic and Atmospheric Administration in Boulder about a year and a half ago showed that HCN that reaches the stratosphere from man-made sources equilibrates with the naturally occurring cyanide and has no effect whatsoever on the earth's atmosphere, the ultraviolet rays coming through or the ozone. By the way, cyanide is a galactic material and one of the building blocks of life.

Comment (F. DeVries): I don't believe in describing the sensation of what cyanide tastes or smells like so that people can depend on experiencing those sensations to tell whether cyanide is present or not. Everybody is different and everyone who works with cyanide should be directly exposed to it once so that he can learn his own way of distinguishing it. Some people taste it, others smell it or feel it tingling on the lips. I happen to taste it; sometimes I even taste it when it's not there because I am so aware of it. One of our men was walking down Fifth Avenue in New York with his wife one day, and as they were fond of the candies put out by a place called Baracini, they bought a box full of these lovely chocolate-covered candies. He bit into one of them as they were walking, and to his wife's horror, instictively spat the whole candy on the sidewalk. It was a reflex action on his part: the taste reminded him of cyanide.

I don't think we should talk about cyanide having the odor of almonds or the taste of burnt meat, which is what it tastes like to me. Everybody should be exposed to learn to detect cyanide and find out what his own reaction to it is. When Dupont began producing hydrogen cyanide at our Memphis plant in 1951, the cyanide sniff test was standard procedure. If you could not detect cyanide in the sniff test, you were not allowed to work in that area. But the number of people who cannot be trained to detect cyanide is very small.

Comment (B. Fellows): In Arizona, everyone who takes our training course is exposed to this sniff test which we have picked up from Dupont. After that they know for sure if and how they can detect it, and few people find that they cannot smell or detect it in any way.

Comment (N. Pickett): One of the first questions we pose to the people in our groups is whether they have experienced the odor of cyanide around their operations. Those who haven't smelled it are certainly in the minority; almost everyone has experienced the sensation of it, and again, it is different to everyone. If you ask ten different people what cyanide smells like, you may get ten different answers. The guideline should be to make sure they do recognize cyanide and know what steps to take if they detect it.

Question: Is a solution of sodium thiosulfate taken orally effective as an antidote if poisoning has been caused by breathing HCN?

Answer (N. Pickett): We do not advocate the use of sodium thiosulfate for poisoning by HCN, but only in cases of ingestion of cyanide solutions or in solid form. If HCN is involved, it would have to be administered by intravenous injection, similar to sodium nitrite.

Question (P. Saletta): How effective are the air-test tube samplers, and what do you know about the presence of H_2S making them more difficult to read?

Answer (F. DeVries): That's a good issue. Probably the Draeger air tester is the most common and most accurate on the market, but it is not 100% accurate. The margin of error is probably plus or minus 10. One thing you should keep in mind is to keep the tubes updated. If you have outdated tubes the reading might vary more than that.

Comment: One thing to remember is that, although H_2S may read as HCN, the error is in the right direction in that it is better to read too high than too low. The acid gases may give you an erroneously high reading but never a low one. Most of the mining operations don't generate much H_2S so it is not usually around, but if it is, it will present a problem since there is a potential for interference by the acid gases.

Question (R. Soniassy): Do you have further information on the availability of CN detectors in air (tubes)? If they are available off the shelf, please give the name and address of the supplier. Can they can be prepared in a laboratory with standard reagents?

Answer (F. DeVries): Two suppliers/manufacturers are:

Draeger Multi-Gas Detector: National Mine Service Co.
300 Koppers Bldg.
Pittsburgh, PA 15219

and: Mine Safety Appliance Co.
301 N. Braddock Ave.
Pittsburgh, PA 15235

It is not reasonable to make up tubes from a recipe in a laboratory.

The following material is from Quality Criteria for Water, compiled by the Office of Water Planning and Standards of the U.S. Environmental Protection Agency and published July 1976.

CYANIDE

CRITERION

5.0 ug/l for freshwater and marine aquatic life and wildlife.

INTRODUCTION

Cyanide is one of the simplest and most readily formed organic moieties. Cyanide and compounds of cyanide are almost universally present where life and industry are found. Besides being very important in a number of manufacturing processes, they are found in many plants and animals as metabolic intermediates which generally are not stored for long periods of time.

In addition to the simple hydrocyanic acid (HCN), the alkali metal salts such as potassium cyanide (KCN) and sodium cyanide (NaCN), are commonly occurring forms and sources of cyanide. The latter compounds are readily dissolved in water; the extent of HCN formation is pH-dependent. A significant fraction of the cyanide exists as HCN molecules up to pH of approximately 8, and the fraction increases rapidly as the pH of the solution decreases. When these simple salts dissociate in aqueous solution, the cyanide ion combines with the hydrogen ion to form hydrocyanic acid, which is toxic to aquatic life. Chemically, the cyanide ion behaves similarly to the halide ions–chloride, fluoride, bromide, and iodide.

The cyanide ion combines with numerous heavy metal ions to form metallocyanide complexes. The stability of these anions is highly variable. Those formed with zinc and cadmium are not stable; dissociation and production of hydrocyanic acid in near neutral or acidic environments is rapid. In turn, some of the metallocyanide anions are extremely stable. Cobaltocyanide is difficult to destroy with highly destructive acid distillation in a laboratory. The iron cyanides are also very stable but exhibit the phenomenon of photodecomposition. In the presence of sunlight they dissociate to release the cyanide ion, thus affecting toxicity; at night the reaction may reverse to produce a less toxic form or state.

A wide variety of organic compounds may contain cyanide functional groups. These compounds belong to a class of organic chemicals called nitriles, few of which dissociate to liberate cyanide ions or molecular HCN. In addition, there are also complex organic acids, alcohols, esters, and amides that contain the cyanide radical. These organic compounds are used for numerous products or may be waste byproducts. Their toxicity, persistence, and chemistry in the aquatic environment are not well known except for a few specific compounds.

Cyanide toxicity is essentially an inhibition of oxygen metabolism, i.e., rendering the tissues incapable of exchanging oxygen. The cyanogen compounds are true, noncumulative, protoplasmic poisons (can be detoxified readily) since they arrest the activity of all forms of animal life. Cyanide shows a very specific type of toxic action. It inhibits the cytochrome oxidase system which functions in the electron transfer from reduced metabolites to molecular oxygen. The ferric iron-porphyrin molecule responsible for the catalytic action of cytochrome oxidase is the reactive site where cyanide combines with ferric (+ + +) iron atoms to form a reversible complex. Other enzymes containing a metal porphyrin molecule, e.g., peroxidases and xanthine oxidase, are also strongly inhibited by cyanide. Only undissociated HCN inhibits the consumption of oxygen in the tissues, causing cellular asphyxia (histotoxic anoxia) by attaching itself to the iron of the prosthetic group of the enzyme cytochrome oxidase.

Hydrocyanic acid can be absorbed readily and carried in the plasma but does not combine with hemoglobin because its iron atom is divalent (ferrous). Instead, cyanide combines with methemoglobin, a mildly oxidized form of hemoglobin in which the iron atom is trivalent (ferric). Methemoglobin, which cannot carry oxygen, normally represents only a small fraction of the total hemoglobin. Since it forms an irreversible and innocuous complex with cyanide, it is an active cyanide detoxifying agent. Amyl nitrite and other agents can be used to increase the level of methemoglobin to counteract cyanide toxicity. A few of the ways in which cyanide can be metabolized within a pattern of normal physiology are by the production of thiocyanate, reaction with hydroxocobalamin to form the harmless cyanocobalamin, combination with amino acids, oxidation to carbon dioxide and formate, et cetera. The conversion of only free cyanide and not organically bound cyano groups to thiocyanate (SCN^-) by action of the enzyme rhodanese is considered to be the primary method of detoxification of cyanide. Rhodanese is absent from blood and skeletal muscle but is abundant in the liver. Thiocyanate is eliminated irregularly and slowly in the urine.

The action of cyanide on the respiration of the cell and the primary methods of detoxification of cyanide have been noted above. However, it should be pointed out that cyanide does not completely abolish cellular respiration. It is possible that a small amount of residual respiratory activity is made possible by cytochrome b activity, since this substance does not require the cyanide-susceptible cytochrome oxidase. An alternative explanation of residual respiratory activity of the cyanide-poisoned system is found in the action of the flavin aerobic dehydrogenases, which can transfer hydrogen to molecular oxygen without the cytochrome system.

The persistence of cyanide in water is highly variable. This variability is dependent upon the chemical form of cyanide in the water, the concentration of cyanide, and the nature of other constituents. Cyanide may be destroyed by strong oxidizing agents such as permanganates and chlorine. Chlorine is commonly used to oxidize strong cyanide solutions to produce carbon dioxide and ammonia; if the reaction is not carried through to completion, cyanogen chloride may remain as a residual and this material is also toxic. If the pH of the receiving waterway is acid and the stream is well aerated, gaseous hydrogen cyanide may evolve from the waterway to the atmosphere. At low concentrations or toxicity and with acclimated microflora, cyanide may be decomposed by microorganisms in both anaerobic and aerobic environments or waste treatment systems.

Hydrocyanic acid probably is the most toxic form of cyanide in water. The ratio of hydrocyanic acid to total cyanide is quite variable. Under natural conditions the variation is due to fluctuations in pH. Photochemical action can also affect this ratio. Fluctuation in pH is caused by acid wastewater discharges, and photosynthetic and respiration cycles of aquatic plant life affect the formation, stability, and toxicity of HCN. Since such chemical and physical conditions will dictate the form of cyanide, the cyanide criterion must be based on the concentration of total cyanide present in the water.

RATIONALE

Cyanide ingested by humans at quantities of 10 mg or less per day is not toxic and is biotransformed to the less toxic thiocyanate. Lethal toxic effects from the ingestion of water containing cyanide occur only when cyanide concentrations are high and overwhelm the detoxifying mechanisms of the human body. Continuous long term consumption of up to nearly 5 mg per day has shown no injurious effects (Bodansky and Levy, 1923).

A review of the available pertinent data on the acute toxicity of simple cyanides to fish reveals the following minimum lethal (threshold) concentrations of free cyanide in ug/l from data obtained from experiments ranging from 12 minutes to 10 days: brook trout, *Salvelinus fontinalis*, 50, (Karsten, 1934); rainbow trout, *Salmo gairdneri*, 70 (60 determined concentration), (Herbert and Merkens, 1952); brown trout, *Salmo trutta*, 70, (Burdick, et al. 1958); smallmouth bass, *Micropterus dolomieui*, 104, (Burdick, et al. 1958); bluegills, *Lepomis macrochirus*, 150, (Doudoroff, et al. 1966); and fathead minnows, *Pimephales promelas*, 180, (Doudoroff, 1956).

Research at the University of Minnesota has revealed that the minimum lethal (threshold) concentrations, as determined from continuous flow bioassays in which routine analyses for cyanide were performed, are generally lower than the above reported values. The threshold concentrations, expressed as mg/l cyanide, were: for the brook trout, *Salvelinus fontinalis*, 0.057 at 10°C; bluegill, *Lepomis macrochirus*, 0.104 at 25°C; and fathead minnow, *Pimephales promelas*, 0.120 at 25°C (Broderius, 1974).

In review it can be concluded that free cyanide concentrations in the range from 50 to 100 ug/l as cyanide have proven eventually fatal to many sensitive fishes and levels much above 200 ug/l probably are rapidly fatal to most fish species.

Downing (1954), Cairns and Scheier (1958), and Burdick, et al. (1958) have shown that the toxicity of free cyanides increases with any reduction in dissolved oxygen below the 100 percent saturation level.

Cairns and Scheier (1958) observed that even periodic lowering of dissolved oxygen decreased the tolerance of bluegills to cyanide.

The tolerance of fish to cyanide solutions that are rapidly lethal has been reported to decrease with a rise in temperature. This increased toxicity may be explained in part by the increased metabolism of fish at higher temperatures.

Contradictory information from the literature indicates the uncertainty between the relationship of toxicity of simple cyanides to fish and the pH of the test solution. However, since undissociated hydrogen cyanide has been demonstrated to be the toxic cyanide species in simple cyanide solutions, changes in the pH of natural waters below a value of about 8.3 should have no measurable effect on the acute toxicity of simple cyanides to fish. There is no apparent relationship among toxicity to fish, the alkalinity, and the hardness of the dilution water.

Cyanide is acutely toxic to most fishes at concentrations ranging from 50 to 200 ug/l (Herbert and Merkens, 1952; Burdick, et al. 1958; Cairns and Scheier, 1958; Doudoroff, 1956; Turnbull, et al. 1954; Lipschuetz and Cooper, 1955; Washburn, 1948).

Some information on chronic or sublethal effects of cyanide is also available. Leduc (1966) found increased intestinal secretions in the fish, *Cichlasoma bimaculatum*, at concentrations as low as 20 ug/l and reduced swimming capability at concentrations of 40 ug/l. Costa (1965) reported that three common species of fish detected and avoided cyanide concentrations of 26 ug/l in approximately an hour or less. Exposure to cyanide concentrations as low as 10 ug/l reduced the swimming ability or endurance of brook trout, *Salvelinus fontinalis* (Neil, 1957). Growth, or food conversion efficiency of coho salmon, *Oncorhynchus kisutch*, was reduced at hydrogen cyanide concentrations of 20 ug/l. Small freshwater fish of the family *Cichlidae* exposed to a cyanide concentration of 15 ug/l lost weight more rapidly than the control fish in water free from cyanide (Leduc, 1966).

The effects of cyanide on marine life have not been investigated adequately to determine separate water quality criteria, but based on the physiological mechanisms of cyanide, toxicity to marine life probably is similar to that of freshwater life. Since marine waters generally are alkaline, the toxicity of cyanide should be less than in fresh waters where pH fluctuations occur more readily and frequently. Thus, an additional factor exists to provide a margin of safety and compensation for a lack of specific data on which to base the criterion for marine aquatic life.

Cyanide has not been reported to have any direct effect on recreational uses of water other than its effects on aquatic life. No information is available on adverse effects of cyanide in agricultural practices nor in industrial uses of water containing cyanide.

Since cyanide concentrations as low as 10 ug/l have been reported to cause adverse effects on fish, an ambient concentration of 5 ug/l is believed to provide protection with a reasonable margin of safety.

REFERENCES CITED

Bodansky, M., and M.D. Levy. 1923. I: Some factors influencing the detoxication of cyanides in health and disease. Arch. Int. Med. 31: 373.

Broderius, S.J. 1974. Testimony in the matter of proposed toxic pollutant effluent standards for Aldrin-Dieldrin, et al. Federal Water Pollution Control Act Amendments (307) Docket No. 1.

Burdick, G.E., et al. 1958. Toxicity of cyanide to brown trout and smallmouth bass. New York Fish and Game Jour. 5: 133.

Cairns, J., Jr., and A. Scheier. 1958. The effect of periodic low oxygen upon toxicity of various chemicals to aquatic organisms. Proc. 12th Industr. Waste Conf., Purdue University Eng. Bull. 42: 165.

Costa, H.H. 1965. Responses of freshwater animals to sodium cyanide solutions. Ceylon Jour. Sci., Biol. Sci. 5: 41.

Doudoroff, P. 1956. Some experiments on the toxicity of complex cyanides to fish. Sew. and Ind. Wastes, 28: 1020.

Doudoroff, P., et al. 1966. Acute toxicity to fish of solutions containing complex metal cyanides, in relation to concentrations of molecular hydrocyanic acid. Trans. Amer. Fish. Soc. 95: 6.

Downing, K.M. 1954. The influence of dissolved oxygen on the toxicity of potassium cyanide to rainbow trout. Jour. Exp. Biol. 31: 161.

Herbert, D.W.M., and J.C. Merkens. 1952. The toxicity of potassium cyanide to trout. Jour. Exp. Biol. 29:632.

Karsten, A. 1934. Investigation of the effect of cyanide on Black Hills trout. South Dakota School of Mines Black Hills Engineer, 22: 145.

Leduc, H. 1966. Some physiological and biochemical responses of fish to chronic poisoning by cyanide. Ph.D. Thesis, Oregon State University, Corvallis.

Lipschuetz, M., and A.L. Cooper. 1955. Comparative toxicities of potassium cyanide and potassium cuprocyanide to the western black-nosed dace (*Rhinichthys atratulus meleagris*). New York Fish and Game Jour. 2: 194.

Neil, J.H. 1957. Some effects of potassium cyanide on speckled trout, *Salvelinus fontinalis*. 4th Ontario Industrial Wastes Conference, Water Poll. Advisory Committee, Ontario Water Resources Commission, p. 74–96.

Turnbull, H., et al. 1954. Toxicity of various refinery materials to freshwater fish. Ind. and Eng. Chem. 46: 24.

Washburn, G.H. 1948. The toxicity to warm water fishes of certain cyanide plating and carburizing salts before and after treatment by the alkali-chlorination method. Sew. Works Jour. 20: 1074.

AUTHOR INDEX